Applied Longitudinal Data Analysis for Medical Science

Applied Longitudinal Data Analysis for Medical Science

A Practical Guide

Jos W. R. Twisk
Amsterdam University Medical Centers

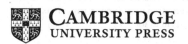

CAMBRIDGE
UNIVERSITY PRESS

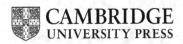
CAMBRIDGE
UNIVERSITY PRESS

Shaftesbury Road, Cambridge CB2 8EA, United Kingdom

One Liberty Plaza, 20th Floor, New York, NY 10006, USA

477 Williamstown Road, Port Melbourne, VIC 3207, Australia

314–321, 3rd Floor, Plot 3, Splendor Forum, Jasola District Centre, New Delhi – 110025, India

103 Penang Road, #05-06/07, Visioncrest Commercial, Singapore 238467

Cambridge University Press is part of Cambridge University Press & Assessment, a department of the University of Cambridge.

We share the University's mission to contribute to society through the pursuit of education, learning and research at the highest international levels of excellence.

www.cambridge.org
Information on this title: www.cambridge.org/9781009288040

DOI: 10.1017/9781009288002

© Jos W. R. Twisk 2023

First published 2023
A catalogue record for this publication is available from the British Library.

Library of Congress Cataloging-in-Publication Data
Names: Twisk, Jos W. R., 1962- author.
Title: Applied longitudinal data analysis for medical science : a practical guide / Jos W.R. Twisk.
Other titles: Applied longitudinal data analysis for epidemiology
Description: 3. | Cambridge, United Kingdom ; New York, NY : Cambridge University Press, 2023. | Preceded by Applied longitudinal data analysis for epidemiology / Jos W.R. Twisk. Second edition. 2013. | Includes bibliographical references and index.
Identifiers: LCCN 2022053460 (print) | LCCN 2022053461 (ebook) | ISBN 9781009288040 (hardback) | ISBN 9781009288033 (paperback) | ISBN 9781009288002 (epub)
Subjects: MESH: Longitudinal Studies | Data Analysis | Data Interpretation, Statistical | Models, Statistical
Classification: LCC RA652.2.M3 (print) | LCC RA652.2.M3 (ebook) | NLM WA 950 | DDC 614.4072/7–dc23/eng/20230125
LC record available at https://lccn.loc.gov/2022053460
LC ebook record available at https://lccn.loc.gov/2022053461

ISBN 978-1-009-28804-0 Hardback
ISBN 978-1-009-28803-3 Paperback

[Medical disclaimer:]
....

Every effort has been made in preparing this book to provide accurate and up-to-date information that is in accord with accepted standards and practice at the time of publication. Although case histories are drawn from actual cases, every effort has been made to disguise the identities of the individuals involved. Nevertheless, the authors, editors, and publishers can make no warranties that the information contained herein is totally free from error, not least because clinical standards are constantly changing through research and regulation. The authors, editors, and publishers therefore disclaim all liability for direct or consequential damages resulting from the use of material contained in this book. Readers are strongly advised to pay careful attention to information provided by the manufacturer of any drugs or equipment that they plan to use.

To Marjon, Mike and Nick

Content

Preface

The most important feature of this book is the word applied in the title. This implies that the emphasis of this book lies more on the application of statistical methods for longitudinal data analysis and not so much on the mathematical background. In most other books on longitudinal data analysis, the mathematical background is the major issue, which may not be surprising since (nearly) all the books on this topic have been written by statisticians. Although statisticians fully understand the difficult mathematical material underlying longitudinal data analysis, they often have difficulty in explaining this complex material in a way that is understandable for the researchers who have to use the method or interpret the results. Therefore, this book is not written by a statistician, but by an applied medical researcher. In fact, an applied researcher is not primarily interested in the basic (difficult) mathematical background of the statistical methods, but in finding the answer to a specific research question; the applied researcher wants to know how to apply a statistical method and how to interpret the results. Owing to their different basic interests and different level of thinking, communication problems between statisticians and applied researchers are quite common. This, in addition to the growing interest in longitudinal studies, initiated the writing of this book: a book on longitudinal data analysis, which is especially suitable for non-statistical applied researchers. The aim of this book is to provide a practical guide on how to handle data from a longitudinal study. The purpose of this book is to build a bridge over the communication gap that exists between statisticians and applied researchers regarding the (complicated) topic of longitudinal data analysis.

Acknowledgements

I am very grateful to all my colleagues and students who came to me with (mostly) practical questions on longitudinal data analysis. This book is based on all those questions.

Introduction

1.1 Introduction

Longitudinal studies are defined as studies in which the outcome variable is repeatedly measured; i.e. the outcome variable is measured in the same subject on several occasions. In longitudinal studies, the observations of a subject over time are not independent of each other, and therefore it is necessary to apply special statistical methods, which take into account the fact that the repeated observations within a subject are correlated. The definition of longitudinal studies (used in this book) implicates that statistical methods like survival analyses are beyond the scope of this book. Those methods basically are not longitudinal data analysing methods because (in general) the outcome variable is an irreversible endpoint and therefore strictly speaking only measured at one occasion. After the occurrence of an event no more observations are carried out on that particular subject.

Why are longitudinal studies so popular these days? One of the reasons for this popularity is that there is a general belief that with longitudinal studies the problem of causality can be solved. This is, however, a typical misunderstanding and is only partly true. Table 1.1 shows the most important criteria for causality, which can be found in every epidemiological textbook. Only one of them is specific for a longitudinal study:

Table 1.1 Criteria for causality

Strength of the relationship

Consistency in different populations and under different circumstances

Specificity (cause leads to a single effect)

Temporality (cause precedes effect in time)

Biological gradient (dose–response relationship)

Biological plausibility

Experimental evidence

the rule of temporality. There has to be a time-lag between the outcome variable (effect) and the covariate (cause); in time the cause has to precede the effect. The question of whether or not causality exists can only be (partly) answered in specific longitudinal studies (e.g. randomized controlled trials) and certainly not in all longitudinal studies. In Chapter 6 the problem of causality in observational longitudinal studies will be discussed, while Chapter 10 deals with the analysis of data from randomised controlled trials.

What then is the advantage of performing a longitudinal study? A longitudinal study is expensive, time consuming, and the data are difficult to analyse. If there are no advantages over cross-sectional studies why bother? The main advantage of a longitudinal study compared to a cross-sectional study is that the individual development of a certain outcome variable over time can be studied. In addition to this, the individual development of an outcome variable can be related to the individual development of particular covariates.

1.2 Study Design

Medical studies can be roughly divided into observational and intervention studies (see Figure 1.1). Observational studies can be further divided into case-control studies and cohort studies. Case-control studies are never longitudinal, in the way that longitudinal studies were defined in Section 1.1. The outcome variable (a dichotomous outcome variable distinguishing case from control) is measured only once. Furthermore, case-control studies are always retrospective in design. The outcome variable is observed at a certain time-point, and the covariates are measured retrospectively.

In general, observational cohort studies can be divided into prospective, retrospective and cross-sectional cohort studies. A prospective cohort study is the only cohort study that can be characterized as a longitudinal study. Prospective cohort

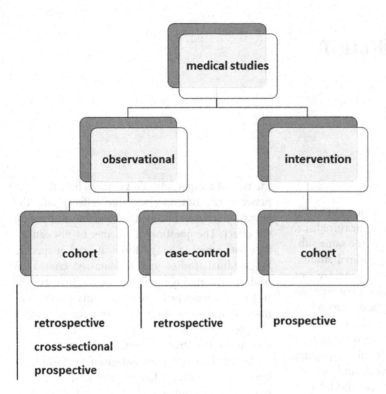

Figure 1.1 Schematic illustration of different medical study designs.

studies are usually designed to analyse the longitudinal development of a certain outcome over time. It is argued that this longitudinal development concerns growth processes. However, in studies investigating the elderly, the process of deterioration is the focus of the study, whereas in other developmental processes, growth and deterioration can alternately follow each other. Moreover, in many studies one is interested not only in the actual growth or deterioration over time, but also in the longitudinal relationship between an outcome and several covariates. Intervention studies, e.g. randomised controlled trials, are by definition prospective, i.e. longitudinal. The outcome variable is measured at least twice (the classical pre-test, post-test design), and other intermediate measures are usually also added to the research design in order to evaluate short-term and long-term effects of the particular intervention.

1.2.1 Observational Longitudinal Studies

In observational longitudinal studies investigating individual development, each measurement taken on a subject at a particular time-point is influenced by three factors: (1) age (time from date of birth to date of measurement), (2) period (time or moment at which the measurement is taken), and (3) birth cohort (group of subjects born in the same year). When studying individual development, one is mainly interested in the age effect. One of the problems of most of the designs used in longitudinal studies of development is that the main age effect cannot be distinguished from the period and cohort effects.

There is an extensive amount of literature describing age, period and cohort effects (e.g. Lebowitz, 1996; Robertson et al., 1999; Holford et al., 2005). However, most of the literature deals with classical age–period–cohort models, which are used to describe and analyse trends in (disease-specific) morbidity and mortality (e.g. Kupper et al., 1985; Mayer and Huinink, 1990; Holford, 1992; McNally et al., 1997; Robertson and Boyle, 1998; Rosenberg and Anderson, 2010). In this book, the main interests are the individual development over time, and the longitudinal relationship between an outcome and several covariates. In this respect, period effects or time of measurement effects are often related to a change in measurement method over time, or to specific environmental conditions at a particular time of measurement. A hypothetical example is given in Figure 1.2. This figure shows the

physical activity (arbitrary units)

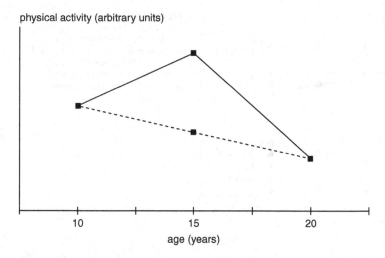

age (years)

Figure 1.2 Illustration of a possible time of measurement effect (dotted line: real age trend, solid line: observed age trend).

body height (arbitrary units)

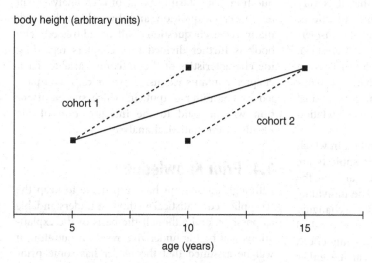

age (years)

Figure 1.3 Illustration of a possible cohort effect (dotted line: cohort specific, solid line: observed).

longitudinal development of physical activity with age. Physical activity patterns were measured with a five-year interval, and were measured during the summer in order to minimise seasonal influences. The first measurement was taken during a summer with normal weather conditions. During the summer when the second measurement was taken, the weather conditions were extremely good, resulting in activity levels that were very high. At the time of the third measurement, the weather conditions were comparable to the weather conditions at the first measurement, and therefore the physical activity levels were much lower than those recorded at the second measurement. When all the results are presented in a graph, it is obvious that the observed age trend is highly biased by the period effect at the second measurement.

One of the most striking examples of a cohort effect is the development of body height with age.

There is an increase in body height with age, but this increase is highly influenced by the increase in height of the birth cohort. This phenomenon is illustrated in Figure 1.3. In this hypothetical study, two repeated measurements were carried out in two different cohorts. The purpose of the study was to detect the age trend in body height. The first cohort had an initial age of five years; the second cohort had an initial age of 10 years. At the age of five, only the first cohort was measured, at the age of 10, both cohorts were measured, and at the age of 15 only the second cohort was measured. The body height obtained at the age of 10 is the average value of the two cohorts. Combining all measurements in order to detect an age trend will lead to a much flatter age trend than the age trends observed in both cohorts separately.

Both cohort and period effects can have an influence on the interpretation of results of longitudinal

performance (arbitrary units)

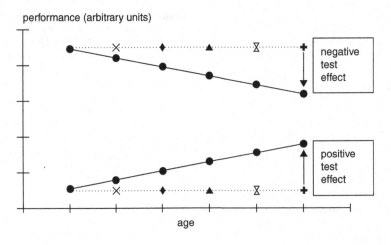

Figure 1.4 Test or learning effects; comparison of repeated measurements of the same subjects with non-repeated measurements in comparable subjects (different symbols indicate different subjects, dotted line: cross-sectional, solid line: longitudinal).

negative test effect

positive test effect

age

studies. An additional problem is that it is very difficult to disentangle the two types of effects. They can easily occur together. Logical considerations regarding the type of variable of interest can give some insight into the plausibility of either a cohort or a period effect. When there are (confounding) cohort or period effects in a longitudinal study, one should be careful with the interpretation of age-related results.

In studies investigating development, in which repeated measurements of the same subjects are performed, cohort and period effects are not the only possible confounding effects. The individual measurements can also be influenced by a changing attitude towards the measurement itself, a so-called test or learning effect. This test or learning effect, which is illustrated in Figure 1.4, can be either positive or negative.

One of the most striking examples of a positive test effect is the measurement of memory in older subjects. It is assumed that with increasing age, memory decreases. However, even when the time interval between subsequent measurements is as long as three years, an increase in memory performance with increasing age can be observed: an increase which is totally due to a learning effect (Dik et al., 2001).

1.3 General Approach

The general approach to explain the statistical methods covered in this book will be: the research question as basis for analysis. Although it may seem quite obvious, it is important to realise that a statistical analysis has to be carried out in order to obtain an answer to a particular research question. The starting point of each analysis will be a research question, and throughout the book many research questions will be addressed. The book is further divided into chapters regarding the characteristics of the outcome variable. Each chapter contains extensive examples, accompanied by computer output, in which special attention will be paid to the interpretation of the results of the statistical analyses.

1.4 Prior Knowledge

Although an attempt has been made to keep the (complicated) statistical methods as understandable as possible, and although the basis of the explanations will be the underlying research question, it will be assumed that the reader has some prior knowledge about (simple) cross-sectional statistical methods such as linear regression analysis, logistic regression analysis, and analysis of variance.

1.5 Example

In general, the examples used throughout this book are taken from the same longitudinal dataset. The dataset is taken from the Amsterdam Growth and Health Longitudinal Study, an observational longitudinal study investigating the longitudinal relation between lifestyle and health in adolescence and young adulthood (Kemper, 1995).

This dataset consists of a continuous outcome variable (serum cholesterol in mmol/liter) which is measured six times on the same subjects. In the examples, in general, two covariates are used. Body fatness, which is operationalised by the sum of the thickness of four skinfolds, is continuous

Table 1.2 Descriptive information[1] for the data used in most of the examples

Time-point	Cholesterol (mmol/liter)	Sum of skinfolds (cm)	Sex
1	4.43 (0.67)	3.26 (1.24)	69/78
2	4.32 (0.67)	3.36 (1.34)	69/78
3	4.27 (0.71)	3.57 (1.46)	69/78
4	4.17 (0.70)	3.76 (1.50)	69/78
5	4.67 (0.78)	4.35 (1.68)	69/78
6	5.12 (0.92)	4.16 (1.61)	69/78

[1] For cholesterol and sum of skinfolds, mean and between brackets standard deviation are given, while for sex the numbers (males/females) are given.

Table 1.3 Illustration of two different data structures

			Broad data structure			
Id	Y_{t1}	Y_{t2}	Y_{t3}	$X1_{t1}$	$X1_{t2}$	$X1_{t3}$	X2
1	3	5	8	10	14	16	1
2	2	4	9	13	15	15	1
3	4	6	7	12	13	16	0

		Long data structure		
Id	Y	X1	X2	Time
1	3	10	1	1
1	5	14	1	2
1	8	16	1	3
2	2	13	1	1
2	4	15	1	2
2	9	15	1	3
3	4	12	0	1
3	6	13	0	2
3	7	16	0	3

and also measured six times on the same subjects and sex, which is dichotomous and which is measured only once and has the same value at all six repeated measurements.

In the chapter dealing with dichotomous outcome variables (i.e. Chapter 7), the continuous outcome variable cholesterol is dichotomised (i.e. the highest tertile versus the other two tertiles) and in the chapter dealing with categorical outcome variables (i.e. Chapter 8), the continuous outcome variable cholesterol is divided into three equal groups based on tertiles. Table 1.2 shows descriptive information for the variables used in the example.

All the example datasets used throughout the book are available on request by jwr.twisk@amsterdamumc.nl.

1.6 Software

Most of the example analyses performed in this book are performed in STATA (version 17).

However, SPSS (version 26) is also used for some of the example analyses. STATA is chosen as the main software package for the longitudinal data analyses, because almost all statistical analyses can be performed in STATA and because of the simplicity of the syntax and the output. In Chapter 13, an overview (and comparison) will be given of other software packages such as R (version 4.0.3) and SAS (version 8). In all these packages, algorithms to perform longitudinal data analysis are implemented in the main software. Both syntax and output will accompany the overview of the different software packages.

1.7 Data Structure

It is important to realise that different statistical software packages need different data structures in order to perform longitudinal data analyses. In this respect a distinction must be made between a long data structure and a broad data structure. In a long data structure, each subject has as many data records as there are measurements over time, while in a broad data structure each subject has one data record, irrespective of the number of measurements over time (see Table 1.3).

1.8 What is New in the Third Edition?

In addition to changes made throughout the book to update the material and to make some of the explanations clearer, some new chapters have been added. In the new Chapter 5, hybrid models are introduced. Hybrid models are used to disentangle the between- and within-subjects interpretation of the regression coefficient obtained from a longitudinal data analysis. The new Chapter 6 contains a discussion regarding causality in observational longitudinal studies, while in the new Chapter 9, the analysis of outcome variables with floor or ceiling effects is discussed. In Chapter 10, 'Analysis of Longitudinal Intervention Studies', three new sections have been added: one section about an alternative repeated measures analysis to take into account regression to the mean; one section about the analysis of data from a stepped wedge trial design; and one section about the difference in difference method.

2

Continuous Outcome Variables

2.1 Two Measurements

The simplest form of longitudinal study is that in which a continuous outcome variable is measured twice in time. With this simple longitudinal design, the following question can be answered: Does the outcome variable change over time? Or, in other words: Is there a difference in the outcome variable between two time-points?

To obtain an answer to this question, a paired t-test can be used. Consider the hypothetical dataset presented in Table 2.1. The dataset consists of 10 subjects, who were measured on two occasions. The paired t-test is used to test the hypothesis that the mean difference between Y_{t1} and Y_{t2} equals zero. Because the individual differences are used in this statistical test, the longitudinal problem of the dependency of the repeated observations within the subjects is reduced to a cross-sectional problem. The test statistic of the paired t-test is the average of the differences divided by the standard deviation of the differences divided by the square root of the number of subjects (Equation 2.1).

$$t = \overline{d} \Big/ \left(\frac{s_d}{\sqrt{N}} \right) \qquad (2.1)$$

where t is the test statistic, $\overline{d}$ is the average of the differences, s_d is the standard deviation of the differences, and N is the number of subjects.

This test statistic follows a t-distribution with $(N - 1)$ degrees of freedom. The assumptions for using the paired t-test are twofold, namely (1) that the observations of different subjects are independent and (2) that the differences between the two measurements are approximately normally distributed. In research situations in which the number of subjects is quite large (say above 25), the paired t-test can be used without any problems. With smaller datasets, however, the assumption of normality becomes important. When the assumption is violated, the non-parametric equivalent of the paired t-test can be used (see Section 2.2). In contrast to its non-parametric equivalent, the paired t-test is not only a testing method. With the paired t-test the average of the paired differences with the corresponding 95% confidence interval can also be estimated.

It should be noted that when the differences are not normally distributed and the sample size is rather large, the paired t-test provides a valid result regarding the p-value, but interpretation of the average differences can be complicated, because the average is not a good indicator of the mid-point of the distribution even when the sample size is large.

2.1.1 Example

One of the limitations of the paired t-test is that the method is only suitable for two measurements over time. It has already been mentioned that the example dataset used throughout this book consists of six repeated measurements. To illustrate the paired t-test in the example dataset, only the first and last measurement of this dataset are used. The question to be answered is: Is there a difference in cholesterol between $t = 1$ and $t = 6$?

Table 2.1 Hypothetical dataset for a longitudinal study with two measurements

Id	Y_{t1}	Y_{t2}	Difference (d)
1	3.5	3.7	−0.2
2	4.1	4.0	0.1
3	3.8	3.5	0.3
4	3.8	3.9	−0.1
5	4.0	4.4	−0.4
6	4.1	4.9	−0.8
7	4.0	3.4	0.6
8	5.1	6.8	−1.7
9	3.7	6.3	−2.6
10	4.1	5.2	−1.1

cholesterol

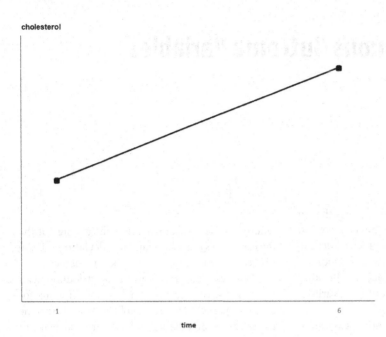

time

1   6

Figure 2.1 Longitudinal development of cholesterol between $t = 1$ and $t = 6$.

Figure 2.1 shows the graphical representation of the data, while Output 2.1 shows the result of the paired t-test.

The first lines of the output show descriptive information (i.e. mean values, standard deviation (SD), number of pairs, etc.), which is not really important in light of the research question. The second part of the output provides the more important information. First of all, the mean of the paired differences is given (i.e. -0.68687), and also the 95% confidence interval around this mean (-0.81072 to -0.56302). A negative value indicates that there is an increase in cholesterol between $t = 1$ and $t = 6$. Furthermore, the result of the actual paired t-test is given: the value of the test statistic ($t = -10.961$), with $(N - 1)$ degrees of freedom (146), and the corresponding p–value (0.000). The result indicates that the increase in cholesterol is statistically significant ($p < 0.001$). The fact that the increase over time is statistically significant was already clear in the 95% confidence interval confidence interval of the mean difference, which did not include zero.

2.2 Non-parametric Equivalent of the Paired t-test

When the assumptions of the paired t-test are violated, it is possible to perform the non-parametric equivalent of the paired t-test, the (Wilcoxon) signed rank sum test. This signed rank sum test is based on the ranking of the individual difference scores, and does not make any assumptions about the distribution of the outcome variable. Consider the hypothetical dataset presented in Table 2.2. Again, the dataset consists of 10 subjects, who were measured on two occasions.

The signed rank sum test evaluates whether the sum of the rank numbers with a positive difference is equal to the sum of the rank numbers with a negative difference. When those two are equal, it suggests that there is no change over time. In the hypothetical dataset, the sum of the rank numbers with a positive difference is 11.5 (i.e. $1.5 + 4 + 6$), while the sum of the rank numbers with a negative difference is 43.5. The exact calculation of the level of significance is complicated, and goes beyond the scope of this book. All statistical handbooks contain tables in which the level of significance can be found (see for instance Altman, 1991), and with all statistical software packages the level of significance can be calculated. For the hypothetical example, the p-value is between 0.2 and 0.1, indicating no significant change over time.

The (Wilcoxon) signed rank sum test can be used in all longitudinal studies with two measurements. It is a testing method which only provides p-values,

Output 2.1 Results of a paired t-test performed to analyse the difference in cholesterol between $t = 1$ and $t = 6$

Paired samples statistics

	Mean	N	Std. deviation	Std. error mean
cholesterol at $t = 1$	4.435	147	.6737	.0556
cholesterol at $t = 6$	5.1216	147	.92353	.07617

Paired samples test

	Paired differences					t	df	Sig. (2-tailed)
	Mean	Std. deviation	Std. error mean	95% confidence interval of the difference				
				Lower	Upper			
cholesterol at $t = 1$ − cholesterol at $t = 6$	−.68687	.75977	.06266	−.81072	−.56302	−10.961	146	.000

Table 2.2 Hypothetical dataset for a longitudinal study with two measurements

Id	Y_{t1}	Y_{t2}	Difference (d)	Rank number
1	3.5	3.7	−0.2	3
2	4.1	4.0	0.1	1.5[1]
3	3.8	3.5	0.3	4
4	3.8	3.9	−0.1	1.5[1]
5	4.0	4.4	−0.4	5
6	4.1	4.9	−0.8	7
7	4.0	3.4	0.6	6
8	5.1	6.8	−1.7	9
9	3.7	6.3	−2.6	10
10	4.1	5.2	−1.1	8

[1] The average rank is used for tied values.

without effect estimation. In real life situations, it will only be used when the sample size is very small (i.e. less than 25).

2.2.1 Example

Although the sample size in the example dataset is large enough to perform a paired t-test, in order to illustrate the method, the (Wilcoxon) signed rank sum test will be used to test whether or not the difference between cholesterol at $t = 1$ and at $t = 6$ is significant. Output 2.2 shows the result of this analysis.

The first part of the output provides the mean rank of the rank numbers with a negative difference and the mean rank of the rank numbers with a positive difference. It also gives the number of cases with a negative and a positive difference. A negative difference corresponds with the situation that cholesterol at $t = 6$ is less than cholesterol at $t = 1$. This corresponds with a decrease in cholesterol over time. A positive difference corresponds with the situation that cholesterol at $t = 6$ is greater than cholesterol at $t = 1$, i.e. corresponds with an increase in cholesterol over time. The last line of the output shows the z-value. Although the (Wilcoxon) signed rank sum test is a non-parametric equivalent of the paired t-test, in many software packages a normal approximation is used to calculate the p-value. This z-value corresponds with a highly significant p-value (0.0000), which indicates that there is a significant change (increase) over time in cholesterol. Because there is a highly significant change over time, the p-value obtained from the paired t-test is the same as the p-value obtained from the signed rank sum test. In general, however, the non-parametric tests are less powerful than the parametric equivalents and will therefore give slightly higher p-values.

2.3 More than Two Measurements

In a longitudinal study with more than two measurements performed on the same subjects (Figure 2.2),

Output 2.2 Results of a (Wilcoxon) matched pairs signed rank sum test to analyse the difference in cholesterol between $t = 1$ and $t = 6$

Wilcoxon matched-pairs signed-ranks test			
cholt1	**cholesterol at t1**		
with cholt6	**cholesterol at t6**		
Mean rank	Cases		
34.84	29	− Ranks	(cholt6 Lt cholt1)
83.62	118	+ Ranks	(cholt6 Gt cholt1)
	0	Ties	(cholt6 Eq cholt1)
	147	Total	
Z = −8.5637	Two-tailed p = 0.0000		

the situation becomes somewhat more complex. A design with only an outcome variable, which is measured several times on the same subjects, is known as a one-within design. This refers to the fact that there is only one factor of interest (i.e. time) and that this factor varies only within-subjects. In a situation with more than two repeated measurements, a paired t-test cannot be carried out. Consider the hypothetical dataset, which is presented in Table 2.3.

The question: Does the outcome variable change over time? can be answered with a generalised linear model (GLM) for repeated measures. The basic idea behind this statistical method, which is also known as multivariate analysis of variance (MANOVA) for repeated measures is the same as for the paired t-test. The statistical test is carried out for the $T - 1$ differences between subsequent measurements. In fact, GLM for repeated measures is a multivariate analysis of these $T - 1$ differences between subsequent time-points. Multivariate refers to the fact that $T - 1$ differences are used simultaneously as outcome variables. The $T - 1$ differences and corresponding variances and covariances form the test statistic for the GLM for repeated measures (Equation 2.2).

$$F = \left(\frac{N - T + 1}{(N - 1)(T - 1)} \right) H^2 \tag{2.2a}$$

$$H^2 = N \times Y_d^t \times \left(S_d^2 \right)^{-1} \times Y_d \tag{2.2b}$$

where F is the test statistic, N is the number of subjects, T is the number of repeated measurements,

Y_d^t is the row vector of differences between subsequent measurements, Y_d is the column vector of differences between subsequent measurements, and S_d^2 is the variance/covariance matrix of the differences between subsequent measurements.

The F-statistic follows an F-distribution with $(T - 1), (N - T + 1)$ degrees of freedom. For a detailed description of how to calculate H^2 using Equation 2.2b, reference should be made to other textbooks (Crowder and Hand, 1990; Hand and Crowder, 1996; Stevens, 1996).[1] As with all statistical methods, GLM for repeated measures is based on several assumptions. These assumptions are more or less comparable to the assumptions of a paired t-test: (1) observations of different subjects at each of the repeated measurements need to be independent, and (2) the observations need to be multivariate normally distributed, which is comparable but slightly more restrictive than the requirement that the differences between subsequent measurements are normally distributed. The calculation described above is called the multivariate approach because several differences are analysed together. However, to answer the same research question, a univariate approach can also be used. This univariate approach is comparable to a simple analysis of variance (ANOVA) and is

---

[1] H^2 is also known as Hotelling's T^2, and is often referred to as T^2. Because throughout this book T is used to denote the number of repeated measurements, H^2 is the preferred notation for this statistic.

Table 2.3 Hypothetical dataset for a longitudinal study with more than two measurements

Id	Y_{t1}	Y_{t2}	d_1	Y_{t3}	d_2	....	Y_{t6}	d_5
1	3.5	3.7	−0.2	3.9	−0.2		3.0	0.2
2	4.1	4.1	0.0	4.2	−0.1		4.6	0.0
3	3.8	3.5	0.3	3.5	0.0		3.4	−0.4
4	3.8	3.9	−0.1	3.8	0.1		3.8	0.3
5	4.0	4.4	−0.4	4.7	−0.3		4.3	−0.3

arbitrary value

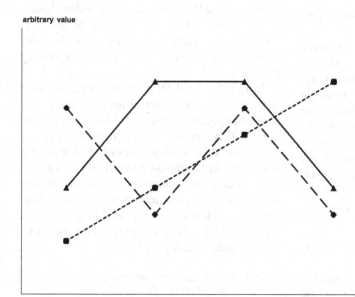

Figure 2.2 A few possible shapes of relationship between a continuous outcome variable and time (- - - linear, • —— quadratic, * – – – cubic).

based on the sum of squares, i.e. the squared differences between observed values and an average value. The univariate approach is only valid when, in addition to the earlier mentioned assumptions, another assumption is met: the assumption of sphericity. This assumption is also known as the compound symmetry assumption. It implies, firstly, that all correlations in the outcome variable between repeated measurements are equal, irrespective of the time interval between the measurements. Secondly, it implies that the variances of the outcome variable are the same at each of the repeated measurements.

Whether or not the assumption of sphericity is met can be expressed by the sphericity coefficient epsilon (noted as ε). In an ideal situation the sphericity coefficient will equal one, and when the assumption is not entirely met, the coefficient will be less than one. When the assumption is not met, the degrees of freedom of the F-test used in the univariate approach can be changed: instead of $(T-1)$, $(N-1)(T-1)$ the degrees of freedom will be $\varepsilon(T-1), \varepsilon(N-1)(T-1)$. It should be noted that the degrees of freedom for the univariate approach are different from the degrees of freedom for the multivariate approach. In many software packages, when GLM for repeated measures is carried out, the sphericity coefficient is automatically estimated and the degrees of freedom are automatically adapted. The sphericity coefficient can also be tested for significance (with the null hypotheses tested: sphericity coefficient $\varepsilon = 1$). However, one must be very careful with the use of this test. If the sample size is large, the test for sphericity will (almost) always give a significant result, whereas in a study with a small sample size the test for sphericity will (almost) never give a significant result. In the first situation, the test is over-powered, which means that even very small violations of the assumption of

11

sphericity will be detected. In studies with small sample sizes, the test will be under-powered, i.e. the power to detect a violation of the assumption of sphericity is too low.

In the next section a numerical example will be given to explain the univariate approach within a GLM for repeated measures.

2.3.1 The Univariate Approach: A Numerical Example

Consider the simple longitudinal dataset presented in Table 2.4.

When the fact that each subject is measured four times is ignored, the question of whether there is a difference between the various time-points can be answered by applying a simple ANOVA, considering the measurements at the four time-points as four independent groups. The ANOVA is then based on a comparison between the between-group (in this case between-time) sum of squares (SS_b) and the within-group (i.e. within-time) sum of squares (SS_w). The latter is also known as the error sum of squares. The sums of squares are calculated as follows:

$$SS_b = \sum_{t=1}^{T} N_t \left(\overline{Y_t} - \overline{Y}\right)^2 \qquad (2.3)$$

where N_t is the number of subjects per group, T is the number of repeated measurements, $\overline{Y_t}$ is the average value of the outcome at time-point t, and $\overline{Y}$ is the overall average of the outcome.

$$SS_w = \sum_{t=1}^{T} \sum_{n=1}^{N} \left(Y_{it} - \overline{Y_t}\right)^2 \qquad (2.4)$$

where T is the number of repeated measurements, N is the number of subjects, Y_{it} are observations of the outcome for subject i at time t, and $\overline{Y_t}$ is the average value of the outcome at time-point t.

Applied to the dataset presented in Table 2.4, $SS_b = 6[(27 - 27)^2 + (28 - 27)^2 + (22.33 - 27)^2 +$

$(30.83 - 27)^2] = 224.79$, and $SS_w = (31 - 27)^2 + (24 - 27)^2 + \cdots + (29 - 30.83)^2 + (34 - 30.83)^2 = 676.17$. These sums of squares are used in the ANOVA's F-test. In this test it is not the total sums of squares that are used, but the mean squares. The mean square (MS) is defined as the sum of squares divided by the degrees of freedom. For SS_b, the degrees of freedom are $(T - 1)$, and for SS_w, the degrees of freedom are $(T) \times (N - 1)$. In the numerical example, $MS_b = 224.79/3 = 74.93$ and $MS_w = 676.17/20 = 33.81$. The F-statistic is equal to MS_b/MS_w and follows an F-distribution with $((T - 1), (T(N - 1))$ degrees of freedom. Applied to the example, the F-statistic is 2.216 with 3 and 20 degrees of freedom. The corresponding p-value (which can be found in a table of the F-distribution, available in all statistical textbooks) is 0.12, i.e. no significant difference between the four time-points. Output 2.3 shows the result of the ANOVA, applied to this numerical example.

It has already been mentioned that in the above calculation the dependency of the observations within the subjects was ignored. It was ignored that the same subject was measured four times. In a design with repeated measurements, the individual sum of squares (SS_i) can be calculated (Equation 2.5)

Table 2.4 Simple longitudinal dataset with four measurements in six subjects

Id	Y_{t1}	Y_{t2}	Y_{t3}	Y_{t4}	Mean
1	31	29	15	26	25.25
2	24	28	20	32	26.00
3	14	20	28	30	23.00
4	38	34	30	34	34.00
5	25	29	25	29	27.00
6	30	28	16	34	27.00
Mean	27.00	28.00	22.33	30.83	27.00

Output 2.3 Results of an ANOVA with a simple longitudinal dataset (see Table 2.4), ignoring the dependency of observations

Source	Sum of squares	df	Mean square	F	Sig.
Between groups	224.792	3	74.931	2.216	0.118
Within groups	676.167	20	33.808		
Total	900.958	23			

$$SS_i = T\sum_{i=1}^{N}\left(\overline{Y_i} - \overline{Y}\right)^2 \tag{2.5}$$

where T is the number of repeated measurements, N is the number of subjects, $\overline{Y_i}$ is the average value of the outcome at all time-points for individual i, and $\overline{Y}$ is the overall average of the outcome.

Applied to the example dataset presented in Table 2.4, $SS_i = 4[(25.25 - 27)^2 + (26 - 27)^2 + \cdots + (27 - 27)^2] = 276.21$. It can be seen that a certain proportion $(276.21/676.17)$ of the error sum of squares (i.e. the within-time sum of squares) can be explained by individual differences. So, in this design with repeated measurements, the total error sum of squares of 676.17 is split into two components. The part which is due to individual differences (276.21) is now removed from the error sum of squares for the time effect. The latter is reduced to 399.96 (i.e. $676.17 - 276.21$). The SS_b is still the same, because this sum of squares reflects the differences between the four time-points. Output 2.4 shows the output of the analysis of this example.

As mentioned before for the ANOVA, to carry out the F-test, the total sum of squares is divided by the degrees of freedom to create the mean square. To obtain the appropriate F-statistic, the mean square of a certain effect is divided by the mean square of the error of that effect. The F-statistic is used in the testing of that particular effect. As can be seen from Output 2.4, the SS_b is divided by $(T - 1)$ degrees of freedom, while the corresponding error term is divided by $(T - 1) \times (N - 1)$ degrees of freedom. The p-value is 0.075, which indicates no significant change over time. Note, however, that this p-value is somewhat lower than the p-value obtained from the ANOVA, in which the dependency of the observations within the subjects was ignored.

The intercept sum of squares, which is also provided in the output, is the sum of squares obtained when an overall average of zero is assumed. In this situation, the intercept sum of squares is useless, but it will be used in the analysis to investigate the shape of the relationship between the outcome and time (see Section 2.3.2)

2.3.2 The Shape of the Relationship between an Outcome Variable and Time

In the preceding sections of this chapter, the question of whether or not there is a change over time in the outcome variable was answered. When such a change over time is found, this implies that there is some kind of relationship between the outcome variable and time. In this section, the shape of the relationship between outcome variable and time will be investigated. In Figure 2.2 a few possible shapes are illustrated.

It is obvious that this question is only of interest when there are more than two measurements. When there are only two measurements, the only possible relationship with time is a linear one. The question about the shape of the relationship can also be answered by applying a GLM for repeated measures. Within GLM for repeated measures, the relationship between the outcome variable and time is compared to a hypothetical linear relationship, a hypothetical quadratic relationship, and so on. When there are T repeated measurements, $T - 1$ possible functions with time can be tested. Although every possible relationship with time can be tested, it is important to have a certain idea or hypothesis of the shape of the relationship between the outcome variable and time. It is highly recommended only to test that

Output 2.4 Results of a GLM for repeated measures with a simple longitudinal dataset (see Table 2.4)

Within-subjects effects					
Source	Sum of squares	df	Mean square	F	Sig.
Time	224.792	3	74.931	2.810	0.075
Error(time)	399.958	15	26.664		
Between-subjects effects					
Source	Sum of squares	df	Mean square	F	Sig
Intercept	17550.042	1	17550.042	317.696	0.000
Error	276.208	5	55.242		

particular hypothesis and not to test all possible relationships routinely.

For each possible relationship, an *F*-statistic is calculated which follows an *F*-distribution with (1), $(N-1)$ degrees of freedom. The shape of the relationship between the outcome variable and time can only be analysed with the univariate approach. In the following section this will be illustrated with a numerical example.

2.3.2.1 A Numerical Example

Consider the same simple longitudinal dataset that was used in Section 2.3.1 and presented in Table 2.4. To answer the question regarding the shape of the relationship between the outcome variable and time, the outcome variable must be transformed. When there are four repeated measurements, the outcome variable is transformed into a linear component, a quadratic component and a cubic component. This transformation is made according to the transformation factors presented in Table 2.5.

Each value of the original dataset is multiplied by the corresponding transformation factor to create a transformed dataset. Table 2.6 presents the linear transformed dataset. The asterisk above the name of a variable indicates that the variable is transformed.

These transformed variables are used to test the different relationships with time. Assume that one is interested in the possible linear relationship with time. Therefore, the individual sum of

squares for the linear transformed variables is related to the individual sum of squares calculated when the overall mean value of the transformed variables is assumed to be zero (i.e. the intercept).

The first step is to calculate the individual sum of squares for the transformed variables according to Equation 2.5. For the transformed dataset $SS_i^* = 4[(-1.62 - 0.33)^2 + (0.89 - 0.33)^2 + \cdots + (0.00 - 0.33)^2] = 54.43$. The next step is to calculate the individual sum of squares when the overall mean value is assumed to be zero. When this calculation is performed for the transformed dataset $SS_i^0 = 4[(-1.62 - 0.00)^2 + (0.89 - 0.00)^2 + \cdots + (0.00 - 0.00)^2] = 56.96$.

The difference between these two individual sums of squares is called the intercept and is shown in the computer output (see Output 2.5). In the example, this intercept is equal to 2.546, and this value is used to test for the linear development over time. The closer this difference comes to zero, the less likely it is that there is a linear relationship with time. In the example, the *p*-value of the intercept is 0.65, which is far from significance, i.e. there is no significant linear relationship between the outcome variable and time.

When a GLM for repeated measures is performed on the original dataset used in Section

Table 2.5 Transformation factors used to test different shapes of the relationship between an outcome variable and time

	Linear	Quadratic	Cubic
Y_{t1}	−0.671	0.500	−0.224
Y_{t2}	−0.224	−0.500	0.671
Y_{t3}	0.224	−0.500	−0.671
Y_{t4}	0.671	0.500	0.224

Table 2.6 Original dataset transformed by linear transformation factors

Id	Y_{t1}^*	Y_{t2}^*	Y_{t3}^*	Y_{t4}^*	Mean
1	−20.8	−6.5	3.4	17.5	−1.62
2	−16.1	−6.3	4.5	21.5	0.89
3	−9.4	−4.5	6.3	20.1	3.13
4	−25.5	−7.6	6.7	22.8	−0.90
5	−16.8	−6.5	5.6	19.5	0.45
6	−20.1	−6.3	3.6	22.8	0.00
Mean					0.33

Output 2.5 Results of a GLM for repeated measures, applied to the linear transformed dataset

Between-subjects effects

Source	Sum of squares	df	Mean square	F	Sig.
Intercept	2.546	1	2.546	0.234	0.649
Error	54.425	5	10.885		

Output 2.6 Results of a GLM for repeated measures with a simple longitudinal dataset (see Table 2.4)

Within-subjects contrasts

Source	Sum of squares	df	Mean square	F	Sig.
Time(linear)	10.208	1	10.208	0.235	0.649
Error(linear)	217.442	5	43.488		

2.3.1, these transformations are automatically carried out and the related test values are shown in the output (see Output 2.6). Because the estimation is slightly different to that explained here, the sum of squares given in this output are the sum of squares given in Output 2.5 multiplied by T. Because it is basically the same method, the p-values are exactly the same.

Exactly the same procedure can be carried out to test for a possible second-order (quadratic) relationship with time and for a possible third-order (cubic) relationship with time.

2.3.3 Example

Output 2.7 shows the result of the GLM for repeated measures performed on the example dataset with six repeated measurements on 147 subjects, while Figure 2.3 shows the graphical representation of the data.

The analysis was performed to answer the question of whether there is a change over time in cholesterol (using the information of all six repeated measurements).

The first part of the output (multivariate tests) shows directly the answer to the question of whether there is a change over time for cholesterol, somewhere between $t = 1$ and $t = 6$. The F-values and the significance levels are based on the multivariate test. In the output there are several multivariate tests available to test the overall time effect. The various tests are named after the statisticians who developed the tests, and they all use slightly different estimation methods. However, the final conclusions of the various tests are almost always the same.

The second part of Output 2.7 provides information on whether or not the assumption of sphericity is met. In this example, the sphericity coefficient (epsilon) calculated by the Greenhouse-Geisser method is 0.741. The output also gives other values for epsilon (Huynh-Feldt and lower-bound), but these values are seldom used. The value

of epsilon can be tested for significance by Mauchly's test of sphericity. The result of this test indicates that epsilon is significantly different from the ideal value of one. This indicates that the degrees of freedom of the F-test should be adjusted. In the computer output presented, this adjustment is automatically carried out and is shown in the next part of the output (tests of within-subjects effects), which shows the result of the univariate approach. The output of the univariate approach gives four different estimates of the overall time effect. The first estimate is the one which assumes sphericity. The other three estimates (Greenhouse-Geisser, Huynh-Feldt and lower-bound) adjust for violations of the assumption of sphericity, by changing the degrees of freedom. The three estimates are slightly different, but it is recommended that the Greenhouse-Geisser adjustment is used, although this adjustment is slightly conservative. From the output it can be seen that the F-values and significance levels are equal for all estimation methods. They are all highly significant, which indicates that there is a significant change over time in cholesterol. From the output, however, there is no indication of whether there is an increase, a decrease or whatever; it only shows a significant difference over time.

The last part of the output (tests of within-subjects contrasts) provides an answer to the second question (what is the shape of the relationship with time?). The first line (linear) indicates the test for a linear development. The F-value (obtained from the mean square (40.322) divided by the error mean square (0.319)) is very high (126.240), and is highly significant (0.000). This result indicates that there is a significant linear development over time. The following lines show the same values belonging to the other functions with time. The second line shows the second-order function (i.e. quadratic), the third line shows the third-order function (i.e. cubic), and so on. All F-values are significant, indicating that all developments over time (second-order, third-

Output 2.7 Results of a GLM for repeated measures to analyse the development over time in cholesterol

		Multivariate tests[a]				
Effect		Value	F	Hypothesis df	Error df	Sig.
Time	Pillai's Trace	.666	56.615[b]	5.000	142.000	.000
	Wilks' Lambda	.334	56.615[b]	5.000	142.000	.000
	Hotelling's Trace	1.993	56.615[b]	5.000	142.000	.000
	Roy's Largest Root	1.993	56.615[b]	5.000	142.000	.000

a. Design: intercept
  Within-subjects design: time

b. Exact statistic

Mauchly's test of sphericity[a]							
Measure: MEASURE_1							
Within-subjects Effect	Mauchly's W	Approx. Chi-Square	df	Sig.	Epsilon[b]		
					Greenhouse-Geisser	Huynh-Feldt	Lower-bound
Time	.435	119.961	14	.000	.741	.763	.200

Tests the null hypothesis that the error covariance matrix of the orthonormalised transformed dependent variables is proportional to an identity matrix.

a. Design: intercept
  Within-subjects design: time

b. May be used to adjust the degrees of freedom for the averaged tests of significance. Corrected tests are displayed in the 'Tests of within-subjects effects' table.

Tests of within-subjects effects						
Measure: MEASURE_1						
Source		Type III sum of squares	Df	Mean Square	F	Sig.
Time	Sphericity assumed	89.987	5	17.997	99.987	.000
	Greenhouse-Geisser	89.987	3.707	24.273	99.987	.000
	Huynh-Feldt	89.987	3.816	23.582	99.987	.000
	Lower-bound	89.987	1.000	89.987	99.987	.000
Error (time)	Sphericity assumed	131.398	730	.180		
	Greenhouse-Geisser	131.398	541.272	.243		
	Huynh-Feldt	131.398	557.126	.236		
	Lower-bound	131.398	146.000	.900		

Tests of within-subjects contrasts

Measure: MEASURE_1

Source	time	Type III sum of squares	df	Mean square	F	Sig.
Time	Linear	40.332	1	40.332	126.240	.000
	Quadratic	44.283	1	44.283	191.356	.000
	Cubic	1.547	1	1.547	11.424	.001
	Order 4	1.555	1	1.555	12.537	.001
	Order 5	2.270	1	2.270	25.322	.000
Error (time)	Linear	46.646	146	.319		
	Quadratic	33.787	146	.231		
	Cubic	19.770	146	.135		
	Order 4	18.108	146	.124		
	Order 5	13.088	146	.090		

Tests of between-subjects effects

Measure: MEASURE_1
Transformed variable: average

Source	Type III sum of squares	df	Mean square	F	Sig.
Intercept	17845.743	1	17845.743	7273.162	.000
Error	358.232	146	2.454		

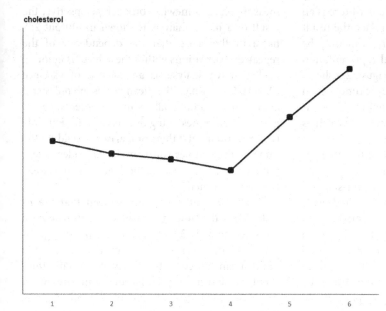

Figure 2.3 Longitudinal development of cholesterol between $t = 1$ and $t = 6$, including the in-between measurements.

Output 2.8 Results of a GLM for repeated measures to analyse the development over time in cholesterol including the explained variance

	Tests of within-subjects effects						
	Measure: MEASURE_1						
Source		Type III sum of squares	df	Mean square	F	Sig.	Partial eta squared
Time	Sphericity assumed	89.987	5	17.997	99.987	.000	.406
	Greenhouse-Geisser	89.987	3.707	24.273	99.987	.000	.406
	Huynh-Feldt	89.987	3.816	23.582	99.987	.000	.406
	Lower-bound	89.987	1.000	89.987	99.987	.000	.406
Error (time)	Sphericity assumed	131.398	730	.180			
	Greenhouse-Geisser	131.398	541.272	.243			
	Huynh-Feldt	131.398	557.126	.236			
	Lower-bound	131.398	146.000	.900			

order, etc.) are statistically significant. The magnitudes of the F-values indicate further that the best way to describe the development over time is a quadratic function, but the simpler linear function with time is also quite good. Again, from the result there is no indication of whether there is an increase or a decrease over time. In fact, the result of the GLM for repeated measures can only be interpreted correctly if a graphical representation of the change over time is made. Figure 2.3 shows that the significant development over time, which was found with a GLM for repeated measures, is first characterised by a small decrease, which is followed by an increase over time.

Within GLM for repeated measures, there is also the possibility to obtain a magnitude of the strength of the effect (i.e. the within-subjects time effect). This magnitude is reflected in a measure called eta squared, which can be seen as an indicator for the explained variance in cholesterol due to a particular effect. Eta squared is calculated as the ratio between the sum of squares of the particular effect and the total sum of squares. Output 2.8 shows part of the output of a GLM for repeated measures including eta squared.

From Output 2.8 it can be seen that eta squared is 0.406 (i.e. 89.99/(131.40 + 89.99)), which indicates that 41% of the variance in cholesterol is explained by the time effect.

To put the result of the GLM for repeated measures in a somewhat broader perspective, the result of a naive analysis is shown in Output 2.9, naive in the sense that the dependency of the repeated observations within the subject is ignored. Such a naive analysis is an analysis of variance (ANOVA), in which the mean values of cholesterol are compared among all six measurements, i.e. six groups, each representing one time-point. For only two measurements, this comparison would be the same as the comparison between an independent sample t-test (the naive method) and a paired t-test (the adjusted method).

From Output 2.9 it can be seen that the F-statistic for the time effect (the effect in which we are interested) is 32.199, which is highly significant (0.000). This result indicates that at least one of the mean values of cholesterol at a certain time-point is significantly different from the mean value of cholesterol at one of the other time-points. However, as has been mentioned before, this method ignores the fact that a longitudinal

Output 2.9 Results of a (naive) analysis of variance (ANOVA) to analyse the development over time in cholesterol, ignoring the dependency of observations

Source	Sum of squares	df	Mean square	F	Sig.
Between groups	89.987	5	17.997	32.199	.000
Within groups	489.630	876	.559		
Total	579.617	881			

study is performed, i.e. that the same subjects are measured on several occasions. The most important difference between the GLM for repeated measures and the naive ANOVA is that the error sum of squares in the ANOVA is much higher than the error sum of squares in the GLM for repeated measures. In the ANOVA, the residual mean square is 0.559 (see Output 2.9), while for the GLM for repeated measures the residual mean square (indicated by Error (TIME) Sphericity Assumed) was more than three times lower, i.e. 0.180 (see Output 2.7). This has to do with the fact that in the GLM for repeated measures, the individual sum of squares is calculated to adjust for the dependency of the observations within the subject. This individual sum of squares is subtracted from the error sum of squares.

2.4 The Univariate or the Multivariate Approach?

Within GLM for repeated measures, a distinction can be made between the multivariate approach (the multivariate extension of a paired *t*-test) and the univariate approach (an extension of ANOVA). The problem is that the two approaches do not produce the same results. So, the question is: Which approach should be used?

One of the differences between the two approaches is the assumption of sphericity. For the multivariate approach this assumption is not necessary, while for the univariate approach it is an important assumption. The restriction of the assumption of sphericity (i.e. equal correlations and equal variances over time) leads to an increase in degrees of freedom, i.e. an increase in power for the univariate approach. This increase

in power becomes more important when the sample size becomes smaller. Historically, the multivariate approach was developed later than the univariate approach, especially for situations when the assumption of sphericity does not hold. So, one could argue that when the assumption of sphericity is violated, the multivariate approach should be used. However, in the univariate approach, adjustments can be made when the assumption of sphericity is not met. So, in principle, both approaches can deal with a situation in which the assumption of sphericity does not hold. It is sometimes argued that when the number of subjects N is less than the number of repeated measurements plus 10, the multivariate approach should not be used. In every other situation, however, it is recommended that the results of both the multivariate and the univariate approach are used to obtain the most valid answer to the research question addressed. Only when both approaches lead to the same conclusion, it is fairly certain that there is either a significant or a non-significant change over time. When both approaches lead to different conclusions, the conclusions must be drawn with many restrictions and considerable caution. In such a situation, it is highly recommended not to use the approach with the lowest (i.e. significant) *p*-value!

2.5 Comparing Groups

In the first sections of this chapter, longitudinal studies were discussed in which a continuous outcome variable is repeatedly measured over time (i.e. the one-within design). In this section, the research situation will be discussed in which the development of a particular continuous outcome variable is compared between different groups. This design is known as the one-within, one-between design. Time is the within-subjects factor and the group variable is the between-subjects factor. This group variable can be either dichotomous or categorical. The question to be addressed is: Is there a difference in change over time for the outcome variable between two or more groups? This question can also be answered with a GLM for repeated measures. The same assumptions as have been mentioned earlier (Section 2.3) apply for this design, but it is also assumed that the covariance matrices of the different groups that are compared to each other are homogeneous. This assumption is comparable with the assumption of equal variances in two groups that are cross-sectionally compared to each other using the independent sample t-test. Although this is an important assumption, in reasonably large samples a violation of this assumption is generally not problematic.

From a one-within, one-between design the following effects can be obtained: (1) an overall time effect, i.e. is there a change over time in the outcome variable for the total population?, (2) a general group effect, i.e. is there on average over time a difference in outcome variable between the compared groups?, and (3) a group by time interaction effect, i.e. is the change over time in the outcome variable different for the compared groups? The within-subjects effects can be calculated in two ways: the multivariate approach, which is based on the multivariate analysis of the differences between subsequent points of measurements, and the univariate approach, which is based on the comparison of several sums of squares (see Section 2.5.1). In most longitudinal studies the group by time interaction effect is probably the most interesting, because it gives an answer to the question of whether there is a difference in change over time between groups.

With respect to the shape of the relationship with time (linear, quadratic, etc.) specific questions can also be answered for the one-within, one-between design, such as is there a difference in the linear development over time between the groups?, is there a difference in the quadratic development over time between the groups?, etc. However, especially for interaction terms, the answers to those questions can be quite complicated; i.e. the result of the GLM for repeated measures can be difficult to interpret.

It should be noted that an important limitation of the GLM for repeated measures is that the between-subjects factor can only be a time-independent dichotomous or categorical variable, such as treatment group, gender, etc.

2.5.1 The Univariate Approach: A Numerical Example

The simple longitudinal dataset used to illustrate the univariate approach in a one-within design will also be used to illustrate the univariate approach in a one-within, one-between design. Therefore, the dataset used in the earlier example, and presented in Table 2.4, is extended to include a group indicator. The new dataset is presented in Table 2.7.

To estimate the different effects, it should first be noted that part of the remaining error sum of squares is related to the difference between the two groups. To calculate this part, the individual sum of squares (SS_i) must be calculated for each of the groups (see Equation 2.5). For group 1, $SS_i = 4$ $[(25.25 - 24.75)^2 + (26 - 24.75)^2 + (23 - 24.75)^2]$ $= 19.5$, and for group 2, $SS_i = 4[(34 - 29.33)^2 + (27 - 29.33)^2 + (27 - 29.33)^2] = 130.7$.

These two parts can be added together to give a sum of squares of 150.2. If the group indication is ignored, the error sum of squares was 276.2 (see Section 2.3.1). This means that the between-subjects sum of squares caused by group differences is 126.0 (i.e. $276.2 - 150.2$). The next step is to calculate the SS_w and the SS_b for each group. This can be done in the same way as has been described for the whole population (see Equations 2.3 and 2.4). The result is summarised in Table 2.8.

The two within-subjects error sums of squares can be added together to form the total within-subjects error sum of squares (adjusted for group). This total within-subjects error sum of

Table 2.7 Simple longitudinal dataset with four measurements in six subjects divided into two groups

Id	Group	Y_{t1}	Y_{t2}	Y_{t3}	Y_{t4}	Mean
1	1	31	29	15	26	25.25
2	1	24	28	20	32	26.00
3	1	14	20	28	30	23.00
Mean		23.00	25.67	21.00	29.33	24.75
4	2	38	34	30	34	34.00
5	2	25	29	25	29	27.00
6	2	30	28	16	34	27.00
Mean		31.00	30.33	23.67	32.33	29.33

squares is 373.17. Without taking the group into account, a within-subjects error sum of squares of 399.96 was found. The difference between the two is the sum of squares belonging to the interaction between the within-subjects factor time and the between-subjects factor group. This sum of squares is 26.79. Output 2.10 shows the computerized result of the GLM for repeated measures for this numerical example.

2.5.2 Example

In the example dataset with six repeated measurements performed on 147 subjects, sex is a dichotomous time-independent covariate, so this variable will be used as a between-subjects factor in this example. The result of the GLM for repeated measures from a one-within, one-between design is shown in Output 2.11.

Part of Output 2.11 is comparable to the output of the one-within design, shown in Output 2.7. One

Table 2.8 Summary of the different sums of squares calculated for each group separately

	Group 1	Group 2
SS_b	116.9	134.7
SS_w	299.3	224.0
SS_i	19.5	130.7
Within-subjects error sum of squares	299.3 − 19.5 = 279.83	224.0 − 130.7 = 93.33

of the differences is found in the first part of the output, in which the result of the tests of between-subjects effects is given. The F-value belonging to this test is 6.382 and the significance level is 0.013, which indicates that there is an overall (i.e. averaged over time) significant difference between the two groups indicated by sex. The other difference between the two outputs is the addition of a time by sex interaction term. This interaction is interesting, because it answers the question of whether there is a difference in development over time between the two groups indicated by sex (i.e. the difference in development of cholesterol between males and females). The answer to that question can either be obtained with the multivariate approach (Pillai, Wilks, Hotelling, and Roy) or with the univariate approach. For the multivariate approach (multivariate tests), firstly the overall time effect is given and secondly the time by sex interaction. For the univariate approach, again the assumption of sphericity has to hold and from the output it can be seen that this is not the case (Greenhouse-Geisser epsilon = 0.722, and the significance of the sphericity test is 0.000). For this reason, in the univariate approach it is recommended that the Greenhouse-Geisser adjustment is used. From the output of the univariate analysis, firstly the overall time effect (F = 104.344, significance 0.000) and secondly the time by sex interaction effect (F = 8.113, significance 0.000) can be obtained. This result indicates that there is a significant difference in development over time in cholesterol between males and females.

Output 2.10 Results of a GLM for repeated measures with a simple longitudinal dataset with a group indicator (see Table 2.7)

Within-subjects effects

Source	Sum of squares	df	Mean square	F	Sig.
Time	224.792	3	74.931	2.810	0.075
Time × group	26.792	3	8.931	0.287	0.834
Error (TIME)	373.167	12	31.097		

Between-subjects effects

Source	Sum of squares	df	Mean square	F	Sig.
Intercept	17550.042	1	17550.042	317.696	0.000
Group	126.042	1	126.042	3.357	0.141
Error	150.167	4	37.542		

Output 2.11 Results of a GLM for repeated measures to analyse the difference in development over time in cholesterol between males and females

Tests of between-subjects effects

Measure: MEASURE_1
Transformed variable: average

Source	Type III sum of squares	Df	Mean square	F	Sig.
Intercept	17715.454	1	17715.454	7486.233	.000
Sex	15.103	1	15.103	6.382	.013
Error	343.129	145	2.366		

Multivariate tests[a]

Effect		Value	F	Hypothesis df	Error df	Sig.
Time	Pillai's Trace	.669	56.881[b]	5.000	141.000	.000
	Wilks' Lambda	.331	56.881[b]	5.000	141.000	.000
	Hotelling's Trace	2.017	56.881[b]	5.000	141.000	.000
	Roy's Largest Root	2.017	56.881[b]	5.000	141.000	.000
Time * sex	Pillai's Trace	.242	8.980[b]	5.000	141.000	.000
	Wilks' Lambda	.758	8.980[b]	5.000	141.000	.000
	Hotelling's Trace	.318	8.980[b]	5.000	141.000	.000
	Roy's Largest Root	.318	8.980[b]	5.000	141.000	.000

a. Design: intercept + sex
Within-subjects design: time

b. Exact statistic

Mauchly's test of sphericity[a]

Measure: MEASURE_1

Within-subjects Effect	Mauchly's W	Approx. Chi-Square	df	Sig.	Epsilon[b]		
					Greenhouse-Geisser	Huynh-Feldt	Lower-bound
Time	.433	119.736	14	.000	.722	.748	.200

Tests the null hypothesis that the error covariance matrix of the orthonormalised transformed dependent variables is proportional to an identity matrix.

a. Design: intercept + sex
Within-subjects sesign: time

b. May be used to adjust the degrees of freedom for the averaged tests of significance. Corrected tests are displayed in the 'Tests of within-subjects effects' table.

(cont.)

Tests of within-subjects effects						
Measure: MEASURE_1						
Source		Type III sum of squares	Df	Mean square	F	Sig.
Time	Sphericity assumed	89.546	5	17.909	104.344	.000
	Greenhouse-Geisser	89.546	3.612	24.793	104.344	.000
	Huynh-Feldt	89.546	3.741	23.937	104.344	.000
	Lower-bound	89.546	1.000	89.546	104.344	.000
Time * sex	Sphericity assumed	6.962	5	1.392	8.113	.000
	Greenhouse-Geisser	6.962	3.612	1.928	8.113	.000
	Huynh-Feldt	6.962	3.741	1.861	8.113	.000
	Lower-bound	6.962	1.000	6.962	8.113	.005
Error (time)	Sphericity assumed	124.436	725	.172		
	Greenhouse-Geisser	124.436	523.707	.238		
	Huynh-Feldt	124.436	542.443	.229		
	Lower-bound	124.436	145.000	.858		

Tests of within-subjects contrasts						
Measure: MEASURE_1						
Source	Time	Type III sum of squares	df	Mean square	F	Sig.
Time	Linear	38.668	1	38.668	131.084	.000
	Quadratic	45.502	1	45.502	213.307	.000
	Cubic	1.602	1	1.602	11.838	.001
	Order 4	1.562	1	1.562	12.516	.001
	Order 5	2.212	1	2.212	24.645	.000
Time * sex	Linear	3.872	1	3.872	13.127	.000
	Quadratic	2.856	1	2.856	13.388	.000
	Cubic	.154	1	.154	1.142	.287
	Order 4	.008	1	.008	.060	.806
	Order 5	.072	1	.072	.804	.371
Error(time)	Linear	42.773	145	.295		
	Quadratic	30.931	145	.213		
	Cubic	19.616	145	.135		
	Order 4	18.100	145	.125		
	Order 5	13.016	145	.090		

Output 2.12 Results of a GLM for repeated measures to analyse the difference in development over time in cholesterol between males and females, including the explained variance

Tests of within-subjects effects

Measure: MEASURE_1

Source		Type III sum of squares	df	Mean square	F	Sig.	Partial eta squared
Time	Sphericity assumed	89.546	5	17.909	104.344	.000	.418
	Greenhouse-Geisser	89.546	3.612	24.793	104.344	.000	.418
	Huynh-Feldt	89.546	3.741	23.937	104.344	.000	.418
	Lower-bound	89.546	1.000	89.546	104.344	.000	.418
Time * sex	Sphericity assumed	6.962	5	1.392	8.113	.000	.053
	Greenhouse-Geisser	6.962	3.612	1.928	8.113	.000	.053
	Huynh-Feldt	6.962	3.741	1.861	8.113	.000	.053
	Lower-bound	6.962	1.000	6.962	8.113	.005	.053
Error (time)	Sphericity assumed	124.436	725	.172			
	Greenhouse-Geisser	124.436	523.707	.238			
	Huynh-Feldt	124.436	542.443	.229			
	Lower-bound	124.436	145.000	.858			

Tests of between-subjects effects

Measure: MEASURE_1
Transformed variable: average

Source	Type III sum of squares	df	Mean square	F	Sig.	Partial eta squared
Intercept	17715.454	1	17715.454	7486.233	.000	.981
Sex	15.103	1	15.103	6.382	.013	.042
Error	343.129	145	2.366			

From the next part of Output 2.11 (tests of within-subjects contrasts) it can be seen that this difference is significant for both the linear development over time and the quadratic development over time.

For all three effects, the explained variance (which is an indicator of the magnitude of the effect) can also be calculated (see Output 2.12).

From Output 2.12 it can be seen that 42% of the variance in cholesterol is explained by the time effect, that 5% is explained by the time by sex interaction, and that 4% of the variance in cholesterol is explained by the overall group effect. Care must be taken in the interpretation of these explained variances, because they cannot be interpreted together in a straightforward way.

cholesterol

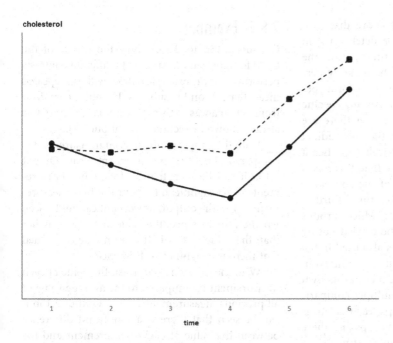

time

Figure 2.4 Difference in development over time in cholesterol between males (solid line) and females (dotted line).

The explained variances for the time effect and the time by group interaction effect are only related to the within-subjects error sum of squares, and not to the total error sum of squares.

As in the case for the one-within design, the result of the GLM for repeated measures for a one-within, one-between design can only be interpreted correctly when a graphical representation is added to the result (see Figure 2.4).

2.6 Comments

One of the problems with GLM for repeated measures is that the time periods under consideration are weighted equally. A non-significant change over a short time period can be relatively greater than a significant change over a long time period. So, when the time periods are unequally spaced, the result of a GLM for repeated measures cannot be interpreted in a straightforward way. The length of the different time intervals must be taken into account.

Another major problem with GLM for repeated measures is that it only takes into account the subjects with complete data, i.e. the subjects who are measured at all time-points. When a subject has no data available for a certain time-point, all other data for that subject is deleted from the analysis. In Chapter 11, the problems and consequences of missing data in longitudinal studies and in the result

obtained from a GLM for repeated measures analysis will be discussed.

Generalised linear model for repeated measures can also be used for more complex study designs, i.e. with more between-subjects and/or more within-subjects factors. Because the ideas and the potential questions to be answered are the same as in the relatively simple designs discussed before, the more complex designs will not be discussed further. It should be kept in mind that the more groups that are compared to each other (given a certain number of subjects), or the more within-subjects factors that are included in the design, the less power there will be to detect significant effects. This is important to realise, because a GLM for repeated measures is basically a testing method, so p-values are used to evaluate the development over time. In principle, no interesting effect estimations are provided by a GLM for repeated measures. As has been mentioned before, the explained variance can be calculated, but the importance of this indicator is rather limited.

2.7 Post-hoc Procedures

With GLM for repeated measures an overall time effect and an overall group effect can be obtained. As in cross-sectional ANOVA, post-hoc procedures can be performed to investigate further the observed overall relationships. In longitudinal analysis there are two types of these post-hoc procedures. (1) When there are more than two repeated measurements, it can be determined in which part of the longitudinal time period the observed effects occur. This can be done by performing a GLM for repeated measures for a specific (shorter) time period or by analysing specific contrasts (see Section 2.7). (2) When there are more than two groups for which the longitudinal development is analysed, a statistically significant between-subjects effect indicates that there is a difference between at least two of the compared groups in the average value over time. Further analysis can determine between which groups the differences occur. This can be carried out by applying the post-hoc procedures also used in the cross-sectional ANOVA (e.g. Tukey, Bonferroni or Scheffe). Each post-hoc procedure has its own particularities, but in essence multiple comparisons are made between all groups; each group is pairwise compared to the other groups and there is a certain adjustment for multiple testing.

2.8 Different Contrasts

In an earlier part of this chapter, attention was paid to answering the question: What is the shape of the relationship between the outcome variable and time? In the example it was mentioned that the answer to that question can be found in the output section: test of within-subjects contrasts. In the example a so-called polynomial contrast was used in order to investigate whether one is dealing with a linear development over time, a quadratic development over time, and so on. In longitudinal research this is an important contrast, but there are many other possible contrasts (depending on the software package used). With a simple contrast, for instance, the value at each measurement is related to the first measurement. With a difference contrast, the value of each measurement is compared to the average of all previous measurements. A Helmert contrast is comparable to the difference contrast, however, the value at a particular measurement is compared to the average of all subsequent measurements. With the repeated contrast, the value of each measurement is compared to the value of the first subsequent measurement. In Section 2.3 it was mentioned that the testing of a polynomial contrast was based on transformed variables. In fact, the testing of all contrasts is based on transformed variables. However, for each contrast, different transformation coefficients are used.

2.8.1 Example

Outputs 2.13a to 2.13d show the results of the GLM for repeated measures with different contrasts performed on the example dataset with six repeated measurements on 147 subjects. The output obtained from the analysis with a polynomial contrast was already shown in Section 2.4 (Output 2.7).

With the simple contrast, each measurement is compared to the first measurement. From Output 2.13a it can be seen that all follow-up measurements differ significantly from the first measurement. From the output, however, it cannot be seen whether, for instance, the value at $t = 2$ is higher than the value at $t = 1$. It can only be concluded that there is a significant difference.

With the difference contrast, the value at each measurement is compared to the average value of all previous measurements. From Output 2.13b it can be seen that there is a significant difference between the value at each measurement and the average value of all previous measurements.

The Helmert contrast (Output 2.13c) is comparable to the difference contrast, but the other way around. The value at each measurement is compared to the average value of all subsequent measurements. All these differences are also highly significant. Only if we compare the first measurement with the average value of the other five measurements, is the p-value of borderline significance (0.047).

With the repeated contrast, the value of each measurement is compared to the value of the first subsequent measurement. From Output 2.13d it can be seen that the cholesterol value at $t = 2$ is not significantly different from the cholesterol value at $t = 3$ ($p = 0.136$). All the other differences investigated were statistically significant. Again, it must be stressed that there is no information about whether the value at a particular time-point is higher or lower than the value at the first subsequent time-point. Like all other results obtained from the GLM for repeated measures, the results of the analysis with different contrasts can only be interpreted correctly if they are combined with a graphical representation of the development of the outcome variable, i.e. cholesterol.

When there are more than two groups to be compared with a GLM for repeated measures, contrasts can also be used to perform post-hoc procedures for the overall group effect. With the traditional post-hoc procedures discussed in Section 2.7 all groups are pairwise compared, while with contrasts

Output 2.13a Results of a GLM for repeated measures to analyse the development over time in cholesterol with a simple contrast

Within-subject contrasts

Source	Sum of squares	df	Mean square	F	Sig.
Level 2 vs Level1	1.830	1	1.830	8.345	0.004
Level 3 vs Level 1	4.184	1	4.184	14.792	0.000
Level 4 vs Level 1	10.031	1	10.031	32.096	0.000
Level 5 vs Level 1	8.139	1	8.139	20.629	0.000
Level 6 vs Level 1	69.353	1	69.353	120.144	0.000
Error					
Level 2 vs Level 1	32.010	146	0.219		
Level 3 vs Level 1	41.296	146	0.283		
Level 4 vs Level 1	45.629	146	0.313		
Level 5 vs Level 1	57.606	146	0.395		
Level 6 vs Level 1	84.279	146	0.577		

Output 2.13b Results of a GLM for repeated measures to analyse the development over time in cholesterol with a difference contrast

Within-subject contrasts

Source	Sum of squares	Df	Mean square	F	Sig.
Level 1 vs Level 2	1.830	1	1.830	8.345	0.004
Level 2 vs Previous	1.875	1	1.875	9.679	0.002
Level 3 vs Previous	4.139	1	4.139	28.639	0.000
Level 4 vs Previous	20.198	1	20.198	79.380	0.000
Level 5 vs Previous	82.271	1	82.271	196.280	0.000
Error					
Level 1 vs Level 2	32.010	146	0.219		
Level 2 vs Previous	28.260	146	0.194		
Level 3 vs Previous	21.101	146	0.145		
Level 4 vs Previous	37.150	146	0.254		
Level 5 vs Previous	61.196	146	0.419		

Output 2.13c Results of a GLM for repeated measures to analyse the development over time in cholesterol with a Helmert contrast

Within-subject contrasts

Source	Sum of squares	df	Mean square	F	Sig.
Level 1 vs Later	0.852	1	0.852	4.005	0.047
Level 2 vs Later	8.092	1	8.092	41.189	0.000
Level 3 vs Later	22.247	1	22.247	113.533	0.000
Level 4 vs Later	76.695	1	76.695	277.405	0.000
Level 5 vs Level 6	29.975	1	29.975	63.983	0.000
Error					
Level 1 vs Later	31.061	146	0.213		
Level 2 vs Later	28.684	146	0.196		
Level 3 vs Later	28.609	146	0.196		
Level 4 vs Later	40.365	146	0.276		
Level 5 vs Level 6	68.399	146	0.468		

Output 2.13d Results of a GLM for repeated measures to analyse the development over time in cholesterol with a repeated contrast

Within-subject contrasts

Source	Sum of squares	df	Mean square	F	Sig.
Level 1 vs Level 2	1.830	1	1.830	8.345	0.004
Level 2 vs Level 3	0.480	1	0.480	2.242	0.136
Level 3 vs Level 4	1.258	1	1.258	8.282	0.005
Level 4 vs Level 5	36.242	1	36.242	125.877	0.000
Level 5 vs Level 6	29.975	1	29.975	63.983	0.000
Error					
Level 1 vs Level 2	32.010	146	0.219		
Level 2 vs Level 3	31.260	146	0.214		
Level 3 vs Level 4	22.182	146	0.152		
Level 4 vs Level 5	42.036	146	0.288		
Level 5 vs Level 6	68.399	146	0.468		

this is not the case. With a simple contrast for instance, the groups are compared to a certain reference group, and with a repeated contrast each group is compared to the next group (dependent on the coding of the group variable). The advantage of contrasts in performing post-hoc procedures is when an adjustment for particular covariates is applied. In that situation, the traditional post-hoc procedures cannot be performed, while with contrasts, the adjusted difference between groups can be obtained. Again, it is important to realise that the post-hoc procedures for group differences performed with different contrasts are only suitable (as the traditional post-hoc procedures) for analysing the between-subjects effect.

2.9 Non-parametric Equivalent of GLM for Repeated Measures

When the assumptions of a GLM for repeated measures are violated, an alternative non-parametric method can be applied. This non-parametric equivalent of a GLM for repeated measures is called the Friedman test and can only be used in a one-within design. Like any other non-parametric test, the Friedman test does not make any assumptions about the distribution of the outcome variable under study. To perform the Friedman test, for each subject the outcome variable at T time-points is ranked from 1 to T. The Friedman test statistic is based on these rankings. In fact, the mean rankings (averaged over all subjects) at each time-point are compared to each other. The idea behind the Friedman test is that the observed rankings are compared to the expected

rankings, assuming there is no change over time. The Friedman test statistic can be calculated according to Equation 2.6:

$$H = \frac{12\sum_{t=1}^{T} R_t^2}{NT(T+1)} - 3N(T+1) \tag{2.6}$$

where H is the Friedman test statistic, R_t is the sum of the ranks at time-point t, N is the number of subjects, and T is the number of repeated measurements.

To illustrate this non-parametric test, consider again the hypothetical dataset presented earlier in Table 2.4. In Table 2.9 the ranks of this dataset are presented.

Applied to the (simple) longitudinal dataset the Friedman test statistic (H) is equal to:

$$\frac{12 \times (15.5^2 + 16^2 + 8.5^2 + 20^2)}{6 \times 4 \times 5} - 3 \times 6 \times 5 = 6.85$$

This value follows a Chi-square distribution with $T - 1$ degrees of freedom. The corresponding p-value is 0.077. When this p-value is compared to the value obtained from a GLM for repeated measures (see Output 2.4) it can be seen that they are almost the same. That the p-value from the non-parametric test is slightly higher than the p-value from the parametric test has to do with the fact that non-parametric tests are in general less powerful than the parametric equivalents.

Table 2.9 Absolute values and ranks (between brackets) of the hypothetical dataset presented in Table 2.4

Id	Y_{t1}(rank)	Y_{t2}(rank)	Y_{t3}(rank)	Y_{t4}(rank)
1	31 (4)	29 (3)	15 (1)	26 (2)
2	24 (2)	28 (3)	20 (1)	32 (4)
3	14 (1)	20 (2)	28 (3)	30 (4)
4	38 (4)	34 (2.5)	30 (1)	34 (2.5)
5	25 (1.5)	29 (3.5)	25 (1.5)	29 (3.5)
6	30 (3)	28 (2)	16 (1)	34 (4)
Total rank	15.5	16	8.5	20

Output 2.14 Results of a non-parametric Friedman test to analyse the development over time in cholesterol

Friedman two-way ANOVA

Mean rank	Variable	
3.49	cholt1	cholesterol at t1
2.93	choltt2	cholesterol at t2
2.79	cholt3	cholesterol at t3
2.32	cholt4	cholesterol at t4
4.23	cholt5	cholesterol at t5
5.24	cholt6	cholesterol at t6

Cases	Chi-Square	DF	Significance
147	244.1535	5	0.0000

2.9.1 Example

Because the number of subjects in the example dataset is reasonably high (i.e. 147), in practice the Friedman test will not be used in the example dataset. However, for educational purposes the non-parametric Friedman test will be used to answer the question of whether there is a development over time in cholesterol. Output 2.14 shows the result of this analysis.

From Output 2.14 it can be seen that there is a significant difference between the measurements at different time-points. The Chi-square statistic is 244.1535, and with five degrees of freedom (the number of repeated measurements minus one) this value is highly significant, i.e. a similar result to that found with the GLM for repeated measures. The Friedman test statistic gives no direct information about the direction of the development, although from the mean rankings it can be seen that a decrease from the second to the fourth measurement is followed by an increase at the fifth and sixth measurement.

Chapter 3

Continuous Outcome Variables: Regression-based Methods

3.1 Introduction

With a paired *t*-test and a generalised linear model (GLM) for repeated measures it is possible to investigate changes in a continuous variable over time and to compare the development of a continuous outcome over time between different groups. These methods, however, are not suitable for analysis of the longitudinal relationship between a continuous outcome and several covariates. Before the development of longitudinal regression methods such as mixed model analysis and generalised estimating equations (GEE analysis), traditional methods were used to analyse longitudinal data. The general idea of these traditional methods was to reduce the longitudinal problem into a cross-sectional problem by, for instance, analysing the average values of both the outcome and the covariates (Twisk, 2013). However, nowadays these (limited) methods are never used in practice and therefore, they will not be discussed any further.

3.2 Longitudinal Regression Methods

With the development of longitudinal regression methods, such as mixed model analysis and GEE analysis, it has become possible to analyse longitudinal relationships using all available longitudinal data, without summarising the longitudinal development of each subject into one value. The longitudinal relationship between a continuous outcome and one or more covariate(s) can be described by Equation 3.1:

$$Y_{it} = \beta_0 + \beta_1 X_{it} + \varepsilon_{it} \qquad (3.1)$$

where Y_{it} are observations of the outcome for subject i at time t, β_0 is the intercept, X_{it} are observations of the covariate for subject i at time t, β_1 is the regression coefficient for the covariate X and ε_{it} is the error for subject i at time t.

This model is almost the same as a cross-sectional linear regression model, except for the subscripts t. These subscripts indicate that the outcome variable is repeatedly measured on the same subject, and that the covariate(s) also can be repeatedly measured on the same subject. In this model the coefficient of interest is β_1, because this regression coefficient shows the magnitude of the longitudinal relationship between the outcome variable and the covariate.

Based on a long data structure (see Table 1.3), the regression coefficient for a covariate can be estimated with a cross-sectional linear regression analysis. However, one of the assumptions of a cross-sectional linear regression analysis is that the observations are independent of each other. In a longitudinal dataset, the observations performed on the same subject are highly dependent and therefore a cross-sectional linear regression analysis cannot be used to estimate the regression coefficients of Equation 3.1. Because of the dependency of the repeated observations within the subject, the relationship between the continuous outcome and the covariate must be adjusted for the subject (Equation 3.2):

$$Y_{it} = \beta_0 + \beta_1 X_{it} + \beta_2 id_{number} + \varepsilon_{it} \qquad (3.2)$$

where Y_{it} are observations of the outcome for subject i at time t, β_0 is the intercept, X_{it} are observations of the covariate for subject i at time t, β_1 is the regression coefficient for the covariate X, β_2 is the regression coefficient for the variable representing subject i, id_{number} is the variable representing subject i and ε_{it} is the error for subject i at time t.

When the id_{number} is added as a discrete or continuous variable to the regression model, the regression coefficient (β_2) has a very strange interpretation; i.e. when the id_{number} differs with one unit, the outcome variable differs with β_2 units. This assumes a linear relationship between the

id_{number} and the outcome variable, which is rather strange. The problem is that the variable id_{number} is not a discrete or continuous variable, but it is a categorical one. When a categorical variable is added to a regression model, it should be represented by dummy variables. In the example dataset, there are 147 subjects, so when this method is performed on the example dataset, 146 dummy variables are needed to adjust for the subject (Equation 3.3):

$$Y_{it} = \beta_0 + \beta_1 X_{it} + \beta_2 id_{number2} + \beta_3 id_{number3} + \cdots$$
$$+ \beta_{147} id_{number147} + \varepsilon_{it} \qquad (3.3)$$

where Y_{it} are observations of the outcome for subject i at time t, β_0 is the intercept, X_{it} are observations of the covariate for subject i at time t, β_1 is the regression coefficient for the covariate X, β_2 is the regression coefficient for the dummy variable representing subject 2, β_3 is the regression coefficient for the dummy variable representing subject 3, β_{147} is the regression coefficient for the dummy variable representing subject 147, and ε_{it} is the error for subject i at time t.

Using so many dummy variables in a cross-sectional linear regression model is a very inefficient way to adjust for the subject. Especially because the magnitude of the differences in the outcome variable between the subjects (which is the interpretation for the regression coefficients belonging to the dummy variables representing the subjects) is neither interesting nor informative. In fact, because of this problem, i.e. the id_{number} cannot be added to the model as a continuous/discrete variable, but it can also not be represented by dummy variables, longitudinal data analysing methods are developed. The general idea behind a longitudinal data analysing method is that the adjustment for the subject is performed in a very efficient way. The different regression methods that are available for the analyses of longitudinal data differ from each other in the way they perform this adjustment.

It should be noted that the regression models with the efficient adjustment for the subject are basically the same as cross-sectional regression models. This means that the covariates can be either continuous, dichotomous or categorical. For the latter, the same method as in cross-sectional linear regression analysis has to be followed, i.e. dummy variables must be created

for each of the categories. In the following sections the two most commonly used longitudinal regression methods (mixed model analysis and GEE analysis) will be discussed in great detail. Both methods are highly suitable for estimation of the regression coefficients of the general model given in Equation 3.1. Besides that, also the adjustment for covariance method will be briefly discussed.

3.3 Mixed Model Analysis

3.3.1 Introduction

Mixed model analysis was initially developed in the social sciences, more specifically for educational research. Investigating the performance of pupils in schools, researchers realised that the performance of pupils within the same class are not independent, i.e. their performance is more or less correlated. Similarly, the performance of classes within the same school can be dependent on each other. This type of study design is characterised by a hierarchical structure. Students are nested within classes, and classes are nested within schools. Because various levels can be distinguished, mixed model analysis is also known as multilevel analysis (Laird and Ware, 1982; Longford, 1993; Goldstein, 1995; Twisk, 2006; Twisk, 2019). Because the performance of pupils within a class are not independent of each other, an adjustment should be made for this dependency in the analysis of the performance of the pupils. Mixed model analysis is developed to adjust for this dependency, for instance by allowing different regression coefficients for different classes. As this technique is suitable for correlated observations, it is obvious that it is also suitable for use in longitudinal studies. In longitudinal studies the observations within a subject over time are correlated, so the observations over time are nested within the subject.

3.3.2 Mixed Models for Longitudinal Data Analysis

As for all longitudinal data analyses, the general idea behind a mixed model analysis is that the adjustment for the subject is performed in a very efficient way. To understand the general idea behind a mixed model analysis, it should be realised that within regression analysis an adjustment for a certain variable means that different intercepts are estimated for the different values of that particular variable. For instance, when in a cross-sectional regression analysis, an adjustment is made for gender, for males and females, different intercepts are calculated. In other words, when an adjustment is made for the subject (i.e. the *id_number*), a different intercept is calculated for each subject. In the model in which the *id_number* is treated as a categorical variable and represented by dummy variables (see Equation 3.3), the different intercepts for each subject can be calculated by β_0 + the regression coefficient for the dummy variable representing that subject. However, it has already been mentioned that adding all the dummy variables to the model is not a very efficient way to adjust for the subject. Nevertheless, the first step in a mixed model analysis is the estimation of different intercepts for all subjects. In the next step within a mixed model analysis a normal distribution is drawn around the intercepts and in the third step the variance of that normal distribution is estimated. That variance is added to the longitudinal regression model in order to adjust for the subject. This adjustment is very efficient because only one additional parameter (i.e. the variance of the normal distribution around the intercepts) is added to the model. Because this variance is known as the random intercept, mixed model analysis is also known as random coefficient analysis. The corresponding statistical model is given in Equation 3.4:

$$Y_{it} = \beta_{0i} + \beta_1 X_{it} + \varepsilon_{it} \qquad (3.4)$$

where Y_{it} are observations of the outcome for subject i at time t, β_{0i} is the random intercept, X_{it} are observations of the covariate for subject i at time t, β_1 is the regression coefficient for the covariate X, and ε_{it} is the error for subject i at time t.

It should be noted that the general idea behind a mixed model analysis is the same as the general idea behind a GLM for repeated measures. In Section 2.3.1 the individual sum of squares was introduced in order to take into account that the measurements over time were performed in the same subject. The individual sum of squares was in fact an estimation of the differences between the mean values over time between the subjects. The latter is actually the same as the differences

between the intercepts of each subject. In this way, a mixed model analysis can be seen as an extension of a GLM for repeated measures.

In a model with a random intercept the intercepts are allowed to differ between the subjects, but the regression coefficient for a particular covariate is the same for all subjects. In a longitudinal study it is not uncommon that besides the intercepts also the regression coefficients for a particular covariate differ between the subjects. When the regression coefficients for a particular covariate differ between subjects, there is basically an interaction between the covariate and the subject. As for the adjustment for the subject, also the interaction with the subject has to be added to a cross-sectional regression model with dummy variables; i.e. for each dummy variable, an interaction term has to be created. In the example dataset with 147 subjects, for each of the 146 dummy variables representing the subjects, an interaction term has to be created. This means that in total 292 additional coefficients must be estimated, which is far from efficient. Within a mixed model analysis, the solution for this inefficiency is the same as the solution for the different intercepts. Again, in the first step the regression coefficients for all subjects are estimated, Then, in the second step, a normal distribution is drawn around the different regression coefficients and from that normal distribution the variance is estimated. This variance is then added to the regression model. Analogue to the random intercept, the variance around the different regression coefficients is known as a random slope. The corresponding statistical model is given in Equation 3.5:

$$Y_{it} = \beta_{0i} + \beta_{1i} X_{it} + \varepsilon_{it} \qquad (3.5)$$

where Y_{it} are observations of the outcome for subject i at time t, β_{0i} is the random intercept, X_{it} are observations of the covariate for subject i at time t, β_{1i} is the random regression coefficient for the covariate X, and ε_{it} is the error for subject i at time t.

The idea behind a mixed model analysis can be effectively illustrated with an example in which the development over time is analysed. In Figure 3.1, there are different intercepts for each subject, but the slopes (i.e. the developments over time) are equal. In Figure 3.2 the development over time is also different for each subject. It should be realised that a random slope can only be added to

arbitrary value

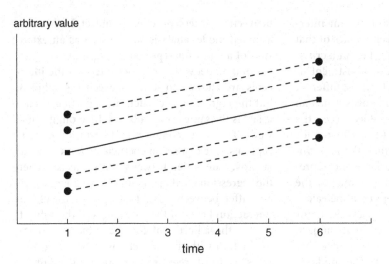

time

Figure 3.1 Development over time of a continuous outcome; different intercepts for different subjects (■ ---- population, • – – – subjects 1 to *n*).

arbitrary value

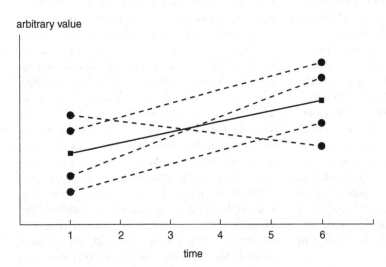

time

Figure 3.2 Development over time of a continuous outcome; different intercepts and different slopes for different subjects (■ —— population, • – – – subjects 1 to *n*).

the mixed model analysis when the covariate is time-dependent. When the covariate is time-independent, there is no regression coefficient for an individual subject. This is due to the fact that each individual subject has only one value for the particular covariate. When there is no regression coefficient for each individual subject, there is no random slope.

It should be realised that the assumption of mixed model analysis is that the intercepts (and slopes) of different subjects are normally distributed. Although the assumption of normality is quite sufficient in many situations, sometimes the individual intercepts (and/or slopes) are not normally distributed. This problem is mostly caused by skewness of the outcome variable of interest and can be solved by a proper transformation of the outcome variable. However, some software packages provide the possibility of modelling (to some extent) the distribution of the variation in the regression coefficients (see for instance Rabe-Hesketh et al., 2001a). However, the use of different distribution for the variation in the regression coefficients is not much used in practice.

3.3.3 Example

To illustrate the use of the longitudinal regression methods, the longitudinal relationship between cholesterol and the sum of skinfolds is analysed (see Section 1.5). Both variables were measured six times and Output 3.1 shows the result of a linear mixed model analysis to analyse the relationship between cholesterol and the sum of

Output 3.1 Results of a linear mixed model analysis with only a random intercept to analyse the relationship between cholesterol and the sum of skinfolds

```
Mixed-effects ML regression              Number of obs     =       882
Group variable: id                       Number of groups  =       147

                                         Obs per group:
                                                       min =         6
                                                       avg =       6.0
                                                       max =         6

                                         Wald chi2(1)      =    103.88
Log likelihood = -830.19309              Prob > chi2       =    0.0000

-----------------------------------------------------------------------
     chol |     Coef.    Std. Err.      z     P>|z|   [ 95% Conf. Interval]
----------+------------------------------------------------------------
    skinf |   .1871179    .018359    10.19   0.000   .1511349   .2231008
    _cons |   3.799312   .0838674    45.30   0.000   3.634935   3.963689
-----------------------------------------------------------------------


-----------------------------------------------------------------------
Random-effects Parameters | Estimate  Std. Err.   [ 95% Conf. Interval]
--------------------------+--------------------------------------------
id: Identity              |
             var(_cons)   | .293719   .0397034     .2253571 .3828185
--------------------------+--------------------------------------------
           var(Residual)  | .2755989  .0143773     .2488127 .3052687
-----------------------------------------------------------------------
LR test vs. linear model: chibar2(01)  =  345.41   Prob >= chibar2 = 0.0000
```

skinfolds in which a random intercept is modelled (Equation 3.4).

The first line of Output 3.1 refers to the fact that a mixed model analysis has been performed. Furthermore, it is mentioned that it is a ML regression analysis. ML stands for maximum likelihood, which is the default estimation method for a linear mixed model analysis in STATA. In other software programmes, a restricted maximum likelihood estimation method is used by default. In Section 3.3.5 the difference between maximum likelihood and restricted maximum likelihood will be further discussed.

In the last line of the first part of the output, the log likelihood value of the model is given (-830.19309). The log likelihood is an indication of the adequacy (or fit) of the model. The value by itself is useless, but can be used in the likelihood ratio test. This likelihood ratio test used within mixed model analyses is exactly the same as known from, for instance, logistic regression analysis (Hosmer and Lemeshow, 1989; Kleinbaum, 1994) and can be used to compare different models with each other.

In the right column of the first part of the output, some general information of the model is given. It shows the number of observations (882), the number of subjects (147) and the average minimum and maximum number of observations within a subject. From these numbers it can be seen that there is no missing data in the example dataset. The Chi-square test shown in the last line of the right column is a test to evaluate the significance of the whole model. In other words, it is a test to evaluate the importance of all covariate(s) in the model, which is basically not very interesting. The second part of the output shows the regression coefficients. This part of the output is known as the fixed part of the model. For the sum of skinfolds, the output gives the regression coefficient, the standard error, the z-statistic (which is obtained by dividing the regression coefficient by its standard error), the corresponding p-value and the 95% confidence interval around the regression coefficient. The latter is calculated in the usual way (i.e. the regression coefficient ±1.96 times the standard error). Besides the regression coefficient for the sum of skinfolds, in the fixed part of the output also the constant (i.e. the average intercept value) is given.

The last part of the output shows the random part of the model. In general, the idea of a mixed model analysis is that the overall error (or residual) variance is divided into different parts. In this example, the overall error variance is divided into two parts, one which is related to the random variation around the intercept (i.e. var(_cons)), and one which is the remaining error variance (i.e. var(Residual)). Besides the variances (0.293719 and 0.2755989 respectively), also the standard errors and 95% confidence intervals around the variances are given. Because the variance is skewed to the right, the 95% confidence intervals around the variances are not symmetric. However, both the standard errors and 95% confidence intervals around the random variances are not very informative. Based on the random variation around the intercept (i.e. the differences between the subjects), the so-called intraclass correlation coefficient (ICC) can be calculated. The ICC is an indication of the within-subjects dependency (Twisk, 2019) and can be calculated by the variance around the intercept divided by the total variance. In this example the ICC is equal to 0.293719 / (0.293719 + 0.2755989) = 52%.

The last line of the output gives the result of a likelihood ratio test. This likelihood ratio test is related to the random part of the model, and for this test, the −2 log likelihood of the presented model is compared to the −2 log likelihood which would have been found if the same analysis was performed without a random intercept. Apparently, the difference in −2 log likelihood between the two models is 345.41, which follows a Chi-square distribution with one degree of freedom; one degree of freedom, because the difference in estimated parameters between the two models is one (i.e. the random variation around the intercept). This value is highly significant

(Prob > chi2 = 0.0000), which indicates that in this situation a model with a random intercept is significantly better than a model without a random intercept. Not a very surprising finding, because in the case of a longitudinal mixed model analysis, adding a random intercept to the model is a theoretical necessity. It has already been mentioned that in the random part of the output in which the two variance components are given, the standard error is also given for each variance. It is very tempting to use the z-statistic of the random variation around the intercept to evaluate the importance of considering a random intercept. However, one must realise that the z-statistic is a normal approximation which is not very valid in the evaluation of variance parameters because the variance is skewed to the right. In other words, it is advised to use the likelihood ratio test to evaluate the importance of allowing random coefficients.

For illustrative purposes, Output 3.2 shows the result of an analysis in which no random intercept is considered (i.e. a naive cross-sectional linear regression analysis).

First of all, it can be seen that the total error variance (i.e. 0.5690835) is comparable to the sum of the random intercept variance and the remaining error variance shown in Output 3.1. Secondly, the log likelihood of this model is −1002.8997. Performing the likelihood ratio test between the model with and without a random intercept gives (as expected from Output 3.1) a value of 348.63, which is highly significant.

Again, it should be realised that the likelihood ratio test performed to evaluate whether or not a random intercept must be considered is not very useful in a longitudinal study. Not adding a random intercept to the model is theoretically wrong, because such a model ignores the dependency of repeated observations within the subject. Or in other words, a model without a random intercept ignores the longitudinal nature of the data.

In the two models considered, the regression coefficient for the sum of skinfolds is considered to be fixed (i.e. not assumed to vary between individuals). The next step in the modelling process can be to add a random slope for the sum of skinfolds to the model, i.e. to allow the regression coefficients to vary among subjects (see Equation 3.2). As has been mentioned before, adding a random slope to the model is only possible for

Output 3.2 Results of a linear mixed model analysis without a random intercept to analyse the relationship between cholesterol and the sum of skinfolds

```
Mixed-effects ML regression                    Number of obs   =      882

                                               Wald chi2(1)    =   140.84
Log likelihood = -1002.8997                    Prob > chi2     =   0.0000


        chol |    Coef.    Std. Err.     z    P>|z|   [ 95% Conf. Interval]
-------------+----------------------------------------------------------
       skinf |  .1971277   .0166107   11.87   0.000   .1645713   .2296841
       _cons |  3.761841   .0671691   56.01   0.000   3.630192   3.89349



Random-effects Parameters |   Estimate  Std. Err. [ 95% Conf. Interval]
--------------------------+---------------------------------------------
           var(Residual)  |   .5690835  .0270992   .5183733   .6247545
```

covariates that change over time. Because in the present example, the sum of skinfolds is a time-dependent covariate, a random slope for the sum of skinfolds can be added to the model. The result of a linear mixed model analysis with both a random intercept and a random slope for the sum of skinfolds is shown in Output 3.3.

Output 3.3 looks more or less the same as the output of a linear mixed model analysis with only a random intercept (Output 3.1). The important information in the first part of the output is the log likelihood (i.e. −828.92752). This is the likelihood value related to the total model, including the regression coefficients (the fixed part) and the variance components (the random part). This value can be used to evaluate the importance of the inclusion of a random slope for the sum of skinfolds in the model. Therefore, the −2 log likelihood of this model must be compared to the −2 log likelihood of the model without a random slope for the sum of skinfolds. The difference between the -2 log likelihoods is 1660.4 − 1657.9 = 2.5. This value follows a Chi-square distribution with a number of degrees of freedom equal to the difference in the number of parameters estimated by the two models. Although only a random slope is added to the model it can be seen from the output that two additional parameters are estimated. Obviously, one of the estimated

parameters is the variance of the slopes (var (skinf)), and the other (not so obviously) is the covariance between the random intercept and the random slope (cov(skinf,_cons)). The magnitude and direction of the covariance between the random intercept and the random slope give information about the interaction between random intercept and slope. When a negative covariance is found, subjects with a high intercept have a low slope. When a positive covariance is found, subjects with a high intercept also have a high slope (see Figure 3.3).

Because the covariance between the random intercept and random slope is also added to the random part of the model, the model with a random slope has two more parameters than the model with only a random intercept. So, the value calculated earlier with the likelihood ratio test (i.e. 2.5) follows a Chi-square distribution with two degrees of freedom. This value is not statistically significant because the critical value of the Chi-square distribution with two degrees of freedom is 5.99 (the actual p-value of the likelihood ratio test is 0.28), so in this situation a random slope for the sum of skinfolds does not seem to be important. So, the best linear mixed model to analyse the longitudinal relationship between cholesterol and the sum of skinfolds is a model with only a random intercept.

Output 3.3 Results of a linear mixed model analysis with both a random intercept and a random slope for the sum of skinfolds to analyse the relationship between cholesterol and the sum of skinfolds

```
Mixed-effects ML regression                Number of obs     =      882
Group variable: id                         Number of groups  =      147

                                           Obs per group:
                                                         min =        6
                                                         avg =      6.0
                                                         max =        6

                                           Wald chi2(1)      =    84.22
Log likelihood = -828.92752                Prob > chi2       =   0.0000

-------------------------------------------------------------------------
     chol  |    Coef.    Std. Err.     z    P>|z|    [ 95% Conf. Interval]
-----------+-------------------------------------------------------------
     skinf | .1919554    .0209166    9.18   0.000    .1509597    .2329511
     _cons | 3.790025    .0927074   40.88   0.000    3.608322    3.971729
-------------------------------------------------------------------------


-------------------------------------------------------------------------
Random-effects Parameters | Estimate  Std. Err.   [ 95% Conf. Interval]
--------------------------+----------------------------------------------
id: Unstructured          |
             var(skinf)   | .0094033    .00713    .0021274    .0415627
             var(_cons)   | .4729297  .1540841    .2497288    .8956214
        cov(skinf,_cons)  | -.0413358 .0309756   -.1020469    .0193753
--------------------------+----------------------------------------------
           var(Residual)  | .2656575  .0151428    .237576    .2970582
-------------------------------------------------------------------------
LR test vs. linear model: chi2(3) = 347.94         Prob > chi2 = 0.0000
```

3.3.4 Interpretation of the Regression Coefficient

Basically, the regression coefficient β_1 for a particular covariate relates the vector of the outcome over time to the vector of the covariate over time:

$$\begin{bmatrix} Y_1 \\ Y_2 \\ Y_3 \\ Y_4 \\ Y_5 \\ Y_6 \end{bmatrix} = \beta_0 + \beta_1 \begin{bmatrix} X_1 \\ X_2 \\ X_3 \\ X_4 \\ X_5 \\ X_6 \end{bmatrix} + \ldots$$

Unfortunately, there is no simple straightforward interpretation of the regression coefficient β_1. In fact, the mixed model analysis based on the model presented here includes a pooled analysis of longitudinal and cross-sectional relationships; or in other words, it combines a between-subjects relationship with a within-subjects relationship, resulting in one single regression coefficient. Although the interpretation of the regression coefficient seems to be different from the interpretation of a regression coefficient in a cross-sectional regression analysis, this is not the case. The regression coefficient derived from a cross-sectional regression analysis is interpreted as the difference in the outcome variable when the covariate differs with one unit. This is further simplified by comparing two subjects who differ one unit in the covariate. In a longitudinal data analysis, only the latter is not the case, because the

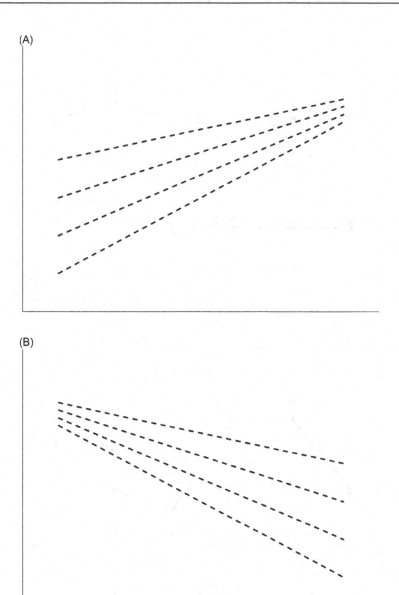

Figure 3.3 (A) Negative covariance between random slope and random intercept. (B) Positive covariance between random slope and random intercept.

difference between two observations in a longitudinal dataset with a long data structure (see Table 1.3) can be either between-subjects or within-subjects. This double interpretation has the following implications for the interpretation of the regression coefficient derived from a longitudinal regression analysis. Suppose that for a particular subject the value of an outcome variable is relatively high at each repeated measurement, and that this value does not change much over time. Suppose further that for that subject

the value of a particular covariate is also relatively high at each repeated measurement, and also does not change much over time. This indicates a longitudinal between-subjects relationship between the outcome variable and the covariate. Suppose that for another subject the value of the outcome variable increases rapidly along the longitudinal period, and suppose that for the same subject this pattern is also found for the covariate. This indicates a within-subjects relationship between the outcome variable and the covariate. Both relationships are

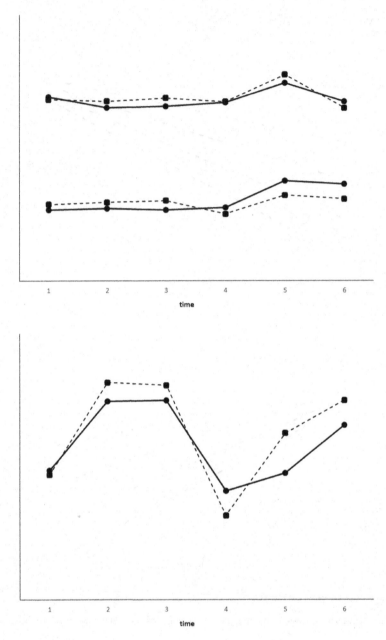

Figure 3.4 Illustration of the relationship between two continuous variables. (A) The between-subjects relationship and (B) the within-subjects relationship (■ – – – outcome variable, •——covariate).

part of the overall longitudinal relationship between the outcome variable and the particular covariate, so both should be taken into account in the analysis of the longitudinal relationship. The regression coefficient β_1 estimated with a longitudinal regression analysis combines the two possible relationships into one regression coefficient. Both phenomena are illustrated in Figure 3.4.

The interpretation of the regression coefficient for the sum of skinfolds in the example dataset is, therefore, twofold: (1) the between-subjects interpretation indicates that a difference between two subjects of 1 unit in the sum of skinfolds is associated with a difference of 0.187 units in cholesterol; (2) the within-subjects interpretation indicates that a change of 1 unit in the sum of skinfolds within a subject is associated with a change of

0.187 units in cholesterol. The real interpretation is a weighted average of both relationships.

It should be realised that this double interpretation of the regression coefficient of a longitudinal regression analysis only holds for time-dependent covariates. For time-independent covariates (i.e. covariates that do not change over time), such as gender, the regression coefficient reflects only the between-subjects relationship.

In Chapter 5, alternative models will be discussed with which it is possible to disentangle the between-subjects and within-subjects relationships.

3.3.5 Comments

In the first line of the output of a linear mixed model analysis it was indicated that a maximum likelihood estimation method had been performed. There is some debate in the literature about whether maximum likelihood or restricted maximum likelihood is the best way to estimate the regression coefficients in a linear mixed model analysis. It is sometimes argued that a maximum likelihood estimation is more suitable for the estimation of the fixed effects (i.e. for the estimation of the regression coefficients), while restricted maximum likelihood estimation is more suitable for the estimation of the different variance components (Harville, 1977; Laird and Ware, 1982; Pinheiro and Bates, 2000). To illustrate the difference between the two estimation methods, Output 3.4 shows the result of a linear mixed model analysis with only a random intercept, to analyse the relationship between cholesterol and the sum of skinfolds, performed with a restricted maximum likelihood estimation method.

From Output 3.4 it can be seen that all the estimated parameters (i.e. regression coefficients, standard errors, log likelihood and random variances) of a linear mixed model analysis with only a random intercept estimated with restricted

Output 3.4 Results of a linear mixed model analysis with only a random intercept estimated with restricted maximum likelihood to analyse the relationship between cholesterol and the sum of skinfolds

```
Mixed-effects REML regression              Number of obs     =      882
Group variable: id                         Number of groups  =      147

                                           Obs per group:
                                                         min =        6
                                                         avg =      6.0
                                                         max =        6

                                           Wald chi2(1)      =   103.56
Log restricted-likelihood = -835.38517     Prob > chi2       =   0.0000
```

chol	Coef.	Std. Err.	z	P>|z|	[95% Conf. Interval]	
skinf	.1870887	.0183847	10.18	0.000	.1510553	.223122
_cons	3.799421	.0840631	45.20	0.000	3.63466	3.964182

Random-effects Parameters	Estimate	Std. Err.	[95% Conf. Interval]	
id: Identity				
var(_cons)	.2965547	.0401821	.2273893	.3867583
var(Residual)	.2758851	.0143979	.249061	.3055982

```
LR test vs. linear model: chibar2(01) = 346.89      Prob >= chibar2 = 0.0000
```

maximum likelihood are slightly different from the parameters estimated with a maximum likelihood estimation method (see Output 3.1). However, the differences are very small.

3.4 Generalised Estimating Equations

3.4.1 Introduction

As has been mentioned before, the different longitudinal regression methods differ from each other in the way the adjustment for the dependency of the repeated observations within the subject is performed. Within mixed model analysis, the adjustment was performed by modelling the differences between the subjects by estimating a random intercept variance and (if necessary) a random slope variance. Within GEE analysis the adjustment is performed by modelling directly the correlation between the repeated observations within the subject. Besides the difference in adjusting for the dependency of the repeated observations within the subject, GEE analysis also uses quasi-likelihood instead of maximum or restricted maximum likelihood to estimate the regression coefficients (Liang and Zeger, 1986; Zeger and Liang, 1986; Zeger et al., 1988; Zeger and Liang, 1992; Liang and Zeger, 1993; Lipsitz et al., 1994a). An extensive explanation of the details of quasi-likelihood goes beyond the scope of this book, but it can be found in several other publications (McCullagh, 1983; Nelder and Pregibon, 1987; Zeger and Qaqish, 1988; Nelder and Lee, 1992).

3.4.2 Correlation Structures

It has already been mentioned that within GEE analysis, the adjustment for the dependency of the observations within the subject is performed to model directly the correlation between the repeated measurements. This is done by assuming a priori a certain (working) correlation structure for the repeated measurements of the outcome variable. Depending on the software package, there is a choice between various correlation structures. The first possibility is an independent structure. With this structure the correlations between subsequent measurements are assumed to be zero. In fact, this option is counterintuitive because a special method is being used to adjust for the

Table 3.1 Illustration of an independent correlation structure

	Y_{t1}	Y_{t2}	Y_{t3}	Y_{t4}	Y_{t5}	Y_{t6}
Y_{t1}	—	0	0	0	0	0
Y_{t2}		—	0	0	0	0
Y_{t3}			—	0	0	0
Y_{t4}				—	0	0
Y_{t5}					—	0
Y_{t6}						—

Table 3.2 Illustration of an exchangeable correlation structure

	Y_{t1}	Y_{t2}	Y_{t3}	Y_{t4}	Y_{t5}	Y_{t6}
Y_{t1}	—	ρ	ρ	ρ	ρ	ρ
Y_{t2}		—	ρ	ρ	ρ	ρ
Y_{t3}			—	ρ	ρ	ρ
Y_{t4}				—	ρ	ρ
Y_{t5}					—	ρ
Y_{t6}						—

dependency of the observations and this correlation structure assumes independence of the observations. In the correlation structures shown in the next tables, a longitudinal study with six repeated measurements is assumed (i.e. comparable to the example dataset used throughout the book). Table 3.1 shows an independent correlation structure.

A second possible choice for a correlation structure is an exchangeable structure. In this structure the correlations between subsequent measurements are assumed to be the same, irrespective of the length of the time interval, which means that one (average) correlation coefficient is estimated (see Table 3.2).

A third possible correlation structure, the so-called (stationary) m-dependent structure assumes that the correlations t measurements apart are equal, the correlations $t + 1$ measurements apart are equal, and so on for $t = 1$ to $t = m$. Correlations more than m measurements apart are assumed to be zero. When, for instance, a 2-dependent correlation structure is assumed, all correlations one measurement apart are assumed to be the same, all

Table 3.3 Illustration of a 2-dependent correlation structure

	Y_{t1}	Y_{t2}	Y_{t3}	Y_{t4}	Y_{t5}	Y_{t6}
Y_{t1}	—	ρ_1	ρ_2	0	0	0
Y_{t2}		—	ρ_1	ρ_2	0	0
Y_{t3}			—	ρ_1	ρ_2	0
Y_{t4}				—	ρ_1	ρ_2
Y_{t5}					—	ρ_1
Y_{t6}						—

Table 3.5 Illustration of an autoregressive correlation structure

	Y_{t1}	Y_{t2}	Y_{t3}	Y_{t4}	Y_{t5}	Y_{t6}
Y_{t1}	—	ρ^1	ρ^2	ρ^3	ρ^4	ρ^5
Y_{t2}		—	ρ^1	ρ^2	ρ^3	ρ^4
Y_{t3}			—	ρ^1	ρ^2	ρ^3
Y_{t4}				—	ρ^1	ρ^2
Y_{t5}					—	ρ^1
Y_{t6}						—

Table 3.4 Illustration of a 5-dependent correlation structure

	Y_{t1}	Y_{t2}	Y_{t3}	Y_{t4}	Y_{t5}	Y_{t6}
Y_{t1}	—	ρ_1	ρ_2	ρ_3	ρ_4	ρ_5
Y_{t2}		—	ρ_1	ρ_2	ρ_3	ρ_4
Y_{t3}			—	ρ_1	ρ_2	ρ_3
Y_{t4}				—	ρ_1	ρ_2
Y_{t5}					—	ρ_1
Y_{t6}						—

Table 3.6 Illustration of an unstructured correlation structure

	Y_{t1}	Y_{t2}	Y_{t3}	Y_{t4}	Y_{t5}	Y_{t6}
Y_{t1}	—	ρ_1	ρ_2	ρ_3	ρ_4	ρ_5
Y_{t2}		—	ρ_6	ρ_7	ρ_8	ρ_9
Y_{t3}			—	ρ_{10}	ρ_{11}	ρ_{12}
Y_{t4}				—	ρ_{13}	ρ_{14}
Y_{t5}					—	ρ_{15}
Y_{t6}						—

correlations two measurements apart are assumed to be the same, and the correlations more than two measurements apart are assumed to be zero (see Table 3.3).

It should be noted that in a longitudinal study with six repeated measurements, it makes a lot of sense to use a 5-dependent structure (see Table 3.4), because the correlations between the repeated measurements are in general quite high, even if the time intervals between the repeated measurements are long.

A fourth possibility is an autoregressive correlation structure, i.e. the correlations one measurement apart are assumed to be ρ; correlations two measurements apart are assumed to be ρ^2; correlations t measurements apart are assumed to be ρ^t (see Table 3.5).

The least restrictive correlation structure is the unstructured correlation structure. With this structure, all correlations are assumed to be different (see Table 3.6).

In the literature it is assumed that GEE analysis is robust against a wrong choice of the correlation structure (i.e. it does not matter which correlation structure is chosen, the results of the GEE analyses will be more or less the same). This robustness has

to do with the fact that within a GEE-analysis the Huber-White sandwich estimator is used for the estimation of the parameters of the model (Liang and Zeger, 1986; Zeger and Liang, 1986). However, this is only the case when there is no missing data and when the model correctly specifies the mean. So, when the results of analyses with different correlation structures on real data are compared to each other, they can differ remarkably (Twisk, 1997; Twisk, 2013). It is therefore important to realise which correlation structure is most appropriate for the analysis. Unfortunately, within GEE analysis there is no straightforward way to determine which correlation structure should be used. One of the possibilities is to analyse the within-subjects correlation structure of the observed data to find out which possible structure is the best approximation of the real correlation structure. Furthermore, the simplicity of the correlation structure has to be taken into account when choosing a certain correlation structure. The number of parameters (in this case correlation coefficients) that need to be estimated differs for each of the various correlation structures. For instance, for an exchangeable correlation structure only one correlation coefficient has to be estimated, while for a stationary 5-dependent correlation structure, five correlation coefficients must be estimated. Assuming an unstructured correlation structure in a longitudinal study with six repeated measurements, 15 correlation coefficients must be estimated. As a result, the efficiency of the statistical analysis is influenced by the choice of a certain structure. Basically, the best choice is the simplest correlation structure which fits the data well. It should be realised that, in fact, GEE analysis adjusts for correlated residuals. The correlated residuals are caused by the correlated observations, but they are not exactly the same. Adding covariates to the longitudinal regression model, for instance, can lead to another correlation structure in the residuals than the one approximated by the within-subjects correlation structure of the observed data.

In order to enhance insight in GEE analysis, the estimation method can be seen as follows. First a naive linear regression analysis is carried out, assuming the observations within the subject are independent. Then, based on the residuals of this analysis, the parameters of the correlation structure are calculated. The last step is to re-estimate the regression coefficients, adjusting for the dependency of the observations. Although the whole method is slightly more complicated (i.e. the estimation process alternates between steps two and three, until the estimates of the regression coefficients and standard errors stabilise), it basically consists of the three above-mentioned steps (Burton et al., 1998).

In GEE analysis, the within-subjects correlation structure is treated as a nuisance variable (i.e. as a sort of confounder). So, in principle, the way in which GEE analysis adjusts for the dependency of observations within the subject is the way that has been shown in Equation 3.6:

$$Y_{it} = \beta_0 + \beta_1 X_{it} + corr_t + \varepsilon_{it} \qquad (3.6)$$

where Y_{it} are observations of the outcome for subject i at time t, β_0 is the intercept, X_{it} are observations of the covariate for subject i at time t, β_1 is the regression coefficient for the covariate X, $corr_t$ is the correlation structure, and ε_{it} is the error for subject i at time t.

3.4.3 Example

Before carrying out a GEE analysis, the correlation structure must be chosen. As mentioned before, a possible choice for this correlation structure can be based on the correlation structure of the observed data. Output 3.5 shows the observed correlation structure for the outcome variable of the example dataset, i.e. cholesterol.

The first correlation structure that should be considered is an independent structure; i.e. all correlations are assumed to be zero. From Output 3.5 it can be seen that the lowest correlation coefficient is 0.59, i.e. far from zero, so an independent correlation structure does not appear to fit the observed data. The second possibility is an exchangeable structure, i.e. all correlations are assumed to be the same. The correlation coefficients range from 0.59 to 0.85. They are not equal, but they are generally of the same magnitude. Another possible correlation structure to consider is an m-dependent structure. With six repeated measurements, the highest order for an m-dependent structure is a 5-dependent structure (five time intervals). A lower-order-dependent structure does not appear to fit, because it implies that there are correlations close to zero, which is not the case in this particular situation. A 5-dependent correlation structure indicates that

Output 3.5 Within-subjects correlation structure for the outcome variable cholesterol

	cholt1	cholt2	cholt3	cholt4	cholt5	cholt6
cholt1	1.0000					
cholt2	0.7557	1.0000				
cholt3	0.7040	0.7741	1.0000			
cholt4	0.6703	0.7790	0.8468	1.0000		
cholt5	0.6369	0.6675	0.7134	0.7437	1.0000	
cholt6	0.5863	0.5909	0.6284	0.6528	0.6896	1.0000

all correlations one measurement apart are equal, all correlations two measurements apart are equal, etc. Looking at the observed correlation structure, the correlations one measurement apart range from 0.69 to 0.85, the correlations two measurements apart range between 0.65 and 0.78, the correlations three measurements apart range between 0.63 and 0.67, and the correlations four measurements apart range between 0.59 and 0.64. In other words, a 5-dependent correlation structure fits the observed data quite well. From Output 3.5 it can be seen that an autoregressive correlation structure is less appropriate than a 5-dependent correlation structure. An autoregressive correlation structure assumes a steep decrease in correlation coefficients when the time interval between measurements increases. From Output 3.5 it can be seen that there is only a marginal decrease in the magnitude of the correlation coefficients with an increasing time interval. In every situation the unstructured correlation structure fits the data best, but it is questionable whether in this particular situation the loss of efficiency due to the estimation of 15 correlation coefficients is worthwhile – probably not. Another issue that should be taken into account is the fact that an unstructured correlation structure is highly data driven. Because of that, in real life practice, an

unstructured correlation structure is almost never used.

So, neither an exchangeable structure nor a 5-dependent structure are perfect, but both seem to fit the observed data well. In such a situation, the correlation structure for which the least number of parameters need to be estimated is the best choice. Therefore, in the example, GEE analysis with an exchangeable correlation structure is chosen.

Output 3.6 shows the result of a linear GEE analysis with an exchangeable correlation structure to analyse the relationship between cholesterol and the sum of skinfolds.

The output is short, simple and straightforward. The left column of the first part of the output indicates that a linear GEE analysis was performed, i.e. a GEE analysis with a continuous outcome variable. This is indicated by the link function (i.e. identity) and the family (i.e. Gaussian). Furthermore, it is indicated that an exchangeable correlation structure is chosen. In this part of the output also the scale parameter is given. The scale parameter is an indication of the unexplained variance of the model and can be used to obtain an indication of the explained variance of the model. To obtain this indication, Equation 3.7 must be applied:

Output 3.6 Results of a linear GEE analysis with an exchangeable correlation structure to analyse the relationship between cholesterol and the sum of skinfolds

```
GEE population-averaged model          Number of obs      =     882
Group variable:                    id  Number of groups =     147
Link:                        identity  Obs per group:
Family:                      Gaussian                   min =       6
Correlation:             exchangeable                   avg =     6.0
                                                        max =       6
                                       Wald chi2(1)       =   86.10
Scale parameter:              .5693178  Prob > chi2      = 0.0000

                         (Std. Err. adjusted for clustering on id)
------------------------------------------------------------------
             |              Robust
       chol|    Coef.    Std. Err.      z   P>|z| [ 95% Conf. Interval]
------------+-----------------------------------------------------
      skinf |  .1871179   .0201657    9.28  0.000   .1475938   .226642
      _cons |  3.799312   .0907438   41.87  0.000   3.621457  3.977166
------------------------------------------------------------------
```

Output 3.7 Descriptive information of the data used in the example

Variable	Obs	Mean	Std. Dev.	Min	Max
chol	882	4.498141	.811115	2.4	7.46
skinf	882	1.975476	.2188769	1.45625	2.525831

$$R^2 = 1 - \left(\frac{S_{model}}{S_Y^2} \right) \qquad (3.7)$$

where R^2 is percentage of explained variance, S_{model} is the variance of the model (given as Scale parameter in the GEE output), and S_Y^2 is the variance of the outcome variable Y, calculated over all available data.

The standard deviation of the outcome variable cholesterol can be found in the descriptive information of the data, which is shown in Output 3.7.

From Output 3.7 it can be seen that the standard deviation of cholesterol is 0.811. Applying Equation 3.7 to the result of the GEE analysis leads to an explained variance of $1 - (0.565)/(0.811)^2 = 14.1\%$. So, 14.1% of the variance in cholesterol is explained by the sum of skinfolds.

The right column of the first part of the output of the GEE analysis (Output 3.6) is exactly the same as has been shown in the output of the mixed model analysis. It shows the number of observations (i.e. 882), the number of subjects (i.e. 147), the average number of observations for each subject as well as the minimum and maximum number of observations. Here, it can be seen that there is no missing data in the example dataset. The last part of the right column shows a Chi-square value and a corresponding p-value. The test performed here is an overall test of all covariates in the model, which is not very interesting.

The second part of the output contains the most important part of the output, i.e. the regression coefficient for the sum of skinfolds, the standard error, the z-statistic (which is obtained by dividing the regression coefficient by its standard error), the corresponding p-value and the 95% confidence interval around the regression coefficient. The latter can be obtained by taking the regression coefficient ± 1.96 times the standard error.

The interpretation of the magnitude of the regression coefficient for a particular covariate is exactly the same as has been mentioned for mixed model analysis, i.e. twofold: (1) the between-subjects

interpretation indicates that a difference between two subjects of 1 unit in the sum of skinfolds is associated with a difference of 0.187 units in cholesterol; (2) the within-subjects interpretation indicates that a change within a subject of 1 unit in the sum of skinfolds is associated with a change of 0.187 units in cholesterol. Again, the real interpretation of the regression coefficient is a combination (i.e. a weighted average) of both relationships.

It should be noted that the estimated standard errors are called robust. It was already mentioned that the parameters of a GEE model are estimated with the Huber-White sandwich estimator. In the output this is indicated by a robust estimation of the standard error.

3.4.3.1 Different Correlation Structures

Based on the observed correlation structure presented in Output 3.5, an exchangeable correlation structure was found to be the most appropriate choice in this particular situation. It has already been discussed in Section 3.4.2 that in the literature it is assumed that the GEE method is robust against a wrong choice of the correlation structure. To verify this, the example dataset was reanalysed using different correlation structures. Output 3.8 shows the results of the GEE analyses with different correlation structures. In the first column of the output the correlation structure is given; i.e. an independent structure, a stationary 5-dependent structure, an autoregressive structure and an unstructured structure.

Table 3.7 summarises the results of the analyses with different correlation structures. From Table 3.7 it can be seen that, although the conclusions based on p-values are the same, there are differences in the magnitude of the regression coefficients. This is important, because it is far more interesting to estimate the magnitude of the relationship by means of the regression coefficients and the 95% confidence intervals than just estimating p-values. Based on the results of Table 3.7, it is obvious that it is important to choose a suitable correlation structure before a GEE analysis is performed.

Output 3.8 Results of a linear GEE analysis with different correlation structures to analyse the relationship between cholesterol and the sum of skinfolds

```
GEE population-averaged model            Number of obs    =       882
Group variable:                    id    Number of groups =       147
Link:                        identity    Obs per group:
Family:                      Gaussian                   min =         6
Correlation:              independent                   avg =       6.0
                                                        max =         6
                                         Wald chi2(1)     =     70.87
Scale parameter:            .5690835     Prob > chi2      =    0.0000

Pearson chi2(882):           501.93      Deviance         =    501.93
Dispersion (Pearson):       .5690835     Dispersion       = .5690835

                           (Std. Err. adjusted for clustering on id)
- - - - - - - - - - - - - - - - - - - - - - - - - - - - - - - - - - - - -
           |              Robust
     chol  |    Coef.    Std. Err.     z    P>|z|  [ 95% Conf. Interval]
- - - - - -+- - - - - - - - - - - - - - - - - - - - - - - - - - - - - - -
    skinf  |  .1971277  .0234164    8.42   0.000   .1512324   .243023
    _cons  | 3.761841   .1028083   36.59   0.000   3.56034    3.963341
- - - - - - - - - - - - - - - - - - - - - - - - - - - - - - - - - - - - -



GEE population-averaged model            Number of obs    =       882
Group and time vars:             id time Number of groups =       147
Link:                        identity    Obs per group:
Family:                      Gaussian                   min =         6
Correlation:            stationary(5)                   avg =       6.0
                                                        max =         6
                                         Wald chi2(1)     =     70.75
Scale parameter:            .5713592     Prob > chi2      =    0.0000

                           (Std. Err. adjusted for clustering on id)
- - - - - - - - - - - - - - - - - - - - - - - - - - - - - - - - - - - - -
           |              Robust
     chol  |    Coef.    Std. Err.     z    P>|z|  [ 95% Conf. Interval]
- - - - - -+- - - - - - - - - - - - - - - - - - - - - - - - - - - - - - -
    skinf  |  .1685182  .0200345    8.41   0.000   .1292514   .207785
    _cons  | 3.887956   .0928468   41.87   0.000   3.705979   4.069932
- - - - - - - - - - - - - - - - - - - - - - - - - - - - - - - - - - - - -



GEE population-averaged model            Number of obs    =       882
Group and time vars:             id time Number of groups =       147
Link:                        identity    Obs per group:
Family:                      Gaussian                   min =         6
Correlation:                    AR(1)                   avg =       6.0
                                                        max =         6
                                         Wald chi2(1)     =     53.97
Scale parameter:             .587524     Prob > chi2      =    0.0000
```

Output 3.8 *(cont.)*

```
                                  (Std. Err. adjusted for clustering on id)
    - - - - - - - - - - - - - - - - - - - - - - - - - - - - - - - - - - - - -
            |           Robust
     chol |    Coef.    Std. Err.      z    P>|z|    [ 95% Conf. Interval]
    - - - - - -+- - - - - - - - - - - - - - - - - - - - - - - - - - - - - - -
     skinf |  .1451045   .0197525    7.35   0.000     .1063903   .1838187
     _cons |  4.066639   .0962832   42.24   0.000     3.877927   4.25535
    - - - - - - - - - - - - - - - - - - - - - - - - - - - - - - - - - - - - -
```

```
GEE population-averaged model            Number of obs      =        882
Group and time vars:            id time   Number of groups   =        147
Link:                          identity   Obs per group:
Family:                        Gaussian                      min =        6
Correlation:               unstructured                      avg =      6.0
                                                             max =        6
                                          Wald chi2(1)       =      55.13
Scale parameter:               .5867011   Prob > chi2        =     0.0000
```

```
                                  (Std. Err. adjusted for clustering on id)
    - - - - - - - - - - - - - - - - - - - - - - - - - - - - - - - - - - - - -
            |           Robust
     chol |    Coef.    Std. Err.      z    P>|z|    [ 95% Conf. Interval]
    - - - - - —+- - - - - - - - - - - - - - - - - - - - - - - - - - - - - - -
     skinf |  .1397279   .0188181    7.43   0.000     .102845    .1766108
     _cons |  4.076277   .0943363   43.21   0.000     3.891381   4.261172
    - - - - - - - - - - - - - - - - - - - - - - - - - - - - - - - - - - - - -
```

Table 3.7 Regression coefficients and standard errors for the sum of skinfolds estimated by a linear GEE analysis with different correlation structures

Correlation structure	Regression coefficient (se)
Exchangeable	0.187 (0.020)
Independent	0.197 (0.023)
Stationary 5-dependent	0.169 (0.020)
Autoregressive	0.145 (0.020)
Unstructured	0.140 (0.019)

3.5 Comparison between Mixed Model Analysis and GEE Analysis

In the preceding sections the general ideas behind mixed model analysis and GEE analysis have been discussed. Both methods are highly suitable for the analysis of longitudinal data, because in both methods an adjustment is made for the dependency of the observations within the subject in a very efficient way: within mixed model analysis, by allowing the regression coefficients to vary between subjects, and within GEE analysis, by assuming a certain correlation structure. The question then arises: Which of the two methods should be used? Theoretically, GEE analysis with an exchangeable correlation structure is the same as a mixed model analysis with only a random intercept. The adjustment for the dependency of observations with an exchangeable correlation structure is the same as allowing subjects to have different intercepts. When an exchangeable correlation structure is not appropriate, GEE analysis with a different correlation structure can be used and when there is significant and relevant random variation in the regression coefficients of one or more covariates, mixed model analysis has the additional possibility of allowing these regression coefficients to vary between subjects. The latter

Output 3.9 Results of a linear GEE analysis without a robust estimation of the standard error to analyse the relationship between cholesterol and the sum of skinfolds

```
GEE population-averaged model      Number of obs      =        882
Group variable:               id   Number of groups   =        147
Link:                   identity   Obs per group:
Family:                 Gaussian                       min =          6
Correlation:        exchangeable                       avg =        6.0
                                                        max =          6
                                   Wald chi2(1)        =     103.88
Scale parameter:        .5693178   Prob > chi2         =     0.0000

- - - - - - - - - - - - - - - - - - - - - - - - - - - - - - - - - - - - -
     chol |    Coef.   Std. Err.     z    P>|z|    [ 95% Conf. Interval]
- - - - -+- - - - - - - - - - - - - - - - - - - - - - - - - - - - - - - -
    skinf |  .1871179   .018359   10.19   0.000   .1511349   .2231008
    _cons |  3.799312   .0838674  45.30   0.000   3.634935   3.963689
- - - - - - - - - - - - - - - - - - - - - - - - - - - - - - - - - - - - -
```

makes mixed model analysis slightly more flexible compared to GEE analysis. Especially because the necessity of random slopes can be statistically evaluated with the likelihood ratio test.

It should be noted that the standard errors derived from the two analyses were different. Because within GEE analysis the standard errors are estimated in a robust way, the standard errors obtained from a GEE analysis were higher than the ones obtained from a mixed model analysis. However, when the standard errors within a GEE analysis would have been estimated in a non-robust way, the standard errors would have been exactly the same as the ones obtained from the mixed model analysis. To illustrate this, Output 3.9 shows the results of a linear GEE analysis to analyse the relationship between cholesterol and the sum of skinfolds without estimating the standard error in a robust way.

It is very important to realise that the differences and commonalities between GEE analysis and mixed model analysis described in this section only hold for continuous outcome variables and for datasets without missing data. For dichotomous and categorical outcome variables, the situation is different (see Chapters 7 and 8) as well as for datasets with missing data (see Chapter 11). In Chapter 11 it will be shown that mixed model analysis deals better with missing data than GEE analysis. In fact, that is the most important reason why mixed model analysis is preferred above GEE analysis when a

continuous outcome variable is analysed in a longitudinal study.

To facilitate the discussion, all the models have been restricted to simple linear models, i.e. no squared terms, no interactions between covariates, etc. This does not mean that it is not possible to use more complicated models. In fact, both GEE analysis and mixed model analysis with a continuous outcome variable are extensions of cross-sectional linear regression analysis. This means that for instance confounding and effect modification can be investigated with mixed model analysis and GEE analysis in exactly the same way as in cross-sectional linear regression analysis.

3.6 The Adjustment for Covariance Method

Besides using mixed model analysis or GEE analysis, the adjustment for the correlated observations within the subject can also be performed with the adjustment for covariance method. This method is comparable to a GEE analysis, but instead of using a correlation matrix, a covariance matrix is used to adjust for the correlated observations within the subject. The covariance between two measurements is a combination of the correlation between the two measurements and the variances (i.e. standard deviations) of the two measurements (Equation 3.8):

$$cov(Y_t, Y_{t+1}) = corr(Y_t, Y_{t+1}) \times sd(Y_t) \times sd(Y_{t+1})$$
$$(3.8)$$

where $cov(Y_t, Y_{t+1})$ is the covariance between Y_t and Y_{t+1}, $corr(Y_t, Y_{t+1})$ is the correlation between Y_t and Y_{t+1}, $sd(Y_t)$ is the standard deviation of Y_t and $sd(Y_{t+1})$ is the standard deviation of Y_{t+1}.

Comparable to the adjustment for the correlation between the repeated measurements used in GEE analysis, there are many different possibilities for the adjustment for covariance between repeated measurements. Again, basically the adjustment is made for the covariance of the residuals, which is equal to the observed covariance of the repeated measurements in an analysis without any covariates. The general idea behind this method is to select a priori a certain covariance structure, which is used in the estimation of the regression coefficients. It is not surprising that the possible choice of structures is comparable to the choice of correlation structures for GEE analysis (see Section 3.4.2). As in GEE analysis, one possibility is the exchangeable covariance structure, which assumes equal correlations (irrespective of the time interval between the repeated measurements), and equal

variances of the repeated measurements. An exchangeable covariance structure for a longitudinal study with six repeated measurements is shown in Table 3.8.

The most extensive covariance structure is an unstructured covariance structure (see Table 3.9).

Although the unstructured covariance structure is obviously the best choice for the covariance structure, it can be seen that, when using this structure in a study with six repeated measurements, 21 parameters must be calculated (six variance parameters and 15 correlation coefficients). As in GEE analysis, it is worthwhile to choose the least complicated covariance structure, which fits the data well. It has already been mentioned that for GEE analysis there was no indication of the fit of the longitudinal model which could be used to evaluate the different correlation structures. In the adjustment for covariance method, however, the regression coefficients are estimated with maximum likelihood or restricted maximum likelihood, so models with different covariance structures can be compared with each other by using the likelihood ratio test.

3.6.1 Example

Output 3.10 shows the result of an adjustment for covariance analysis with an exchangeable covariance structure to analyse the relationship between cholesterol and the sum of skinfolds.

The output of the adjustment for covariance analysis looks similar to the output of the linear mixed model analysis. This is due to the fact that the adjustment for covariance analysis is performed within the mixed model environment. This can also be seen from the random part of the model: no random intercept is estimated. This makes sense because the adjustment for the dependency of the repeated measurements is performed by an

Table 3.8 Illustration of an exchangeable covariance structure

	Y_{t1}	Y_{t2}	Y_{t3}	Y_{t4}	Y_{t5}	Y_{t6}
Y_{t1}	σ^2	$\sigma^2\rho$	$\sigma^2\rho$	$\sigma^2\rho$	$\sigma^2\rho$	$\sigma^2\rho$
Y_{t2}		σ^2	$\sigma^2\rho$	$\sigma^2\rho$	$\sigma^2\rho$	$\sigma^2\rho$
Y_{t3}			σ^2	$\sigma^2\rho$	$\sigma^2\rho$	$\sigma^2\rho$
Y_{t4}				σ^2	$\sigma^2\rho$	$\sigma^2\rho$
Y_{t5}					σ^2	$\sigma^2\rho$
Y_{t6}						σ^2

Table 3.9 Illustration of an unstructured covariance structure

	Y_{t1}	Y_{t2}	Y_{t3}	Y_{t4}	Y_{t5}	Y_{t6}
Y_{t1}	σ_1^2	$\rho_{12}\sigma_1\sigma_2$	$\rho_{13}\sigma_1\sigma_3$	$\rho_{14}\sigma_1\sigma_4$	$\rho_{15}\sigma_1\sigma_5$	$\rho_{16}\sigma_1\sigma_6$
Y_{t2}		σ_2^2	$\rho_{23}\sigma_2\sigma_3$	$\rho_{24}\sigma_2\sigma_4$	$\rho_{25}\sigma_2\sigma_5$	$\rho_{26}\sigma_2\sigma_6$
Y_{t3}			σ_3^2	$\rho_{34}\sigma_3\sigma_4$	$\rho_{35}\sigma_3\sigma_5$	$\rho_{36}\sigma_3\sigma_6$
Y_{t4}				σ_4^2	$\rho_{45}\sigma_4\sigma_5$	$\rho_{46}\sigma_4\sigma_6$
Y_{t5}					σ_5^2	$\rho_{56}\sigma_5\sigma_6$
Y_{t6}						σ_6^2

Output 3.10 Results of an adjustment for covariance analysis with an exchangeable covariance structure to analyse the relationship between cholesterol and the sum of skinfolds

```
Mixed-effects ML regression              Number of obs       =        882
Group variable: id                       Number of groups    =        147

                                         Obs per group:
                                                         min =          6
                                                         avg =        6.0
                                                         max =          6

                                         Wald chi2(1)        =     103.88
Log likelihood = -830.19309              Prob > chi2         =     0.0000

-------------------------------------------------------------------------
    chol |      Coef.    Std. Err.      z     P>|z|    [ 95% Conf. Interval]
---------+---------------------------------------------------------------
   skinf |    .1871179    .018359    10.19    0.000     .1511349    .2231008
   _cons |    3.799312    .0838674   45.30    0.000     3.634935    3.963689
-------------------------------------------------------------------------


-------------------------------------------------------------------------
 Random-effects Parameters |  Estimate  Std. Err.  [ 95% Conf. Interval]
---------------------------+---------------------------------------------
id:            (empty)     |
---------------------------+---------------------------------------------
Residual: Exchangeable     |
                  var(e) |  .5693177   .0413985     .493695    .6565241
                  cov(e) |  .2937188   .0397033    .2159017    .3715359
-------------------------------------------------------------------------
LR test vs. linear model: chi2(1) = 345.41              Prob > chi2 = 0.0000
```

adjustment for covariance and not by the estimation of a random intercept. From Output 3.10 it can further be seen that with an exchangeable covariance structure only two covariance parameters are estimated (var(e) and cov(e)). It should be noted that the value for cov(e) is exactly the same as the random intercept variance obtained from a linear mixed model analysis with only a random intercept (see Output 3.1). Besides that, it can also be seen that all the other values are exactly the same as in the mixed model analysis with only a random intercept. This holds for the -2 log likelihood as well as for the regression coefficient for the sum of skinfolds and its standard error.

One of the advantages of the use of the adjustment for covariance method is that the parameters are estimated with maximum likelihood. Therefore, in the output the log likelihood is provided, and based on the log likelihood the likelihood ratio test can be performed. With the likelihood ratio test, different models can be compared to each other. To illustrate this, Output 3.11 shows the result of an adjustment for covariance analysis with an unstructured covariance structure to analyse the relationship between cholesterol and the sum of skinfolds.

From Output 3.11 it can be seen that in this analysis 21 parameters are estimated to adjust for the dependency of the observations within the subject. Six variance parameters (var(e1) to var (e6)) and 15 covariance parameters (cov(e1,e6) to cov(e5,e6)).

The likelihood ratio test can be used to decide which covariance structure is to be preferred in the analysis. Therefore, the difference between the -2 log likelihoods of both models has to be calculated. This difference follows a Chi-square distribution with 19 degrees of freedom. Again,

Output 3.11 Results of an adjustment for covariance analysis with an unstructured covariance structure to analyse the relationship between cholesterol and the sum of skinfolds

```
Mixed-effects ML regression              Number of obs     =      882
Group variable: id                       Number of groups  =      147

                                         Obs per group:
                                                            min =        6
                                                            avg =      6.0
                                                            max =        6

                                         Wald chi2(1)      =    48.39
Log likelihood = -680.74451              Prob > chi2       =   0.0000

- - - - - - - - - - - - - - - - - - - - - - - - - - - - - - - - - - - - - -
    chol |    Coef.    Std. Err.     z     P>|z|    [ 95% Conf. Interval]
- - - - -+- - - - - - - - - - - - - - - - - - - - - - - - - - - - - - - - -
   skinf | .1216995   .0174956    6.96    0.000    .0874088   .1559903
   _cons | 3.920117   .0791613   49.52    0.000    3.764964   4.07527
- - - - - - - - - - - - - - - - - - - - - - - - - - - - - - - - - - - - - -


- - - - - - - - - - - - - - - - - - - - - - - - - - - - - - - - - - - - - -
Random-effects Parameters | Estimate  Std. Err.   [ 95% Conf. Interval]
- - - - - - - - - - - - - -+- - - - - - - - - - - - - - - - - - - - - - - -
id:                (empty) |
- - - - - - - - - - - - - -+- - - - - - - - - - - - - - - - - - - - - - - -
Residual: Unstructured     |
              var(e1) |  .4571604   .0566516   .3585808    .582841
              var(e2) |  .4091829   .047744    .3255353    .514324
              var(e3) |  .4423262   .0536723   .3487041   .5610845
              var(e4) |  .4586168   .0628011   .350663    .599805
              var(e5) |  .5641309   .0769756   .4317511   .7370998
              var(e6) |  1.255289   .1860593   .9388117   1.678453
           cov(e1,e2) |  .3194199   .0452447   .2307421   .4080978
           cov(e1,e3) |  .2910988   .0442932   .2042857   .377912
           cov(e1,e4) |  .2550142   .0439305   .168912    .3411164
           cov(e1,e5) |  .3089937   .0565647   .198129    .4198585
           cov(e1,e6) |  .3964422   .0962182   .2078579   .5850265
           cov(e2,e3) |  .3195029   .0446176   .2320539   .4069518
           cov(e2,e4) |  .3163264   .0474911   .2232456   .4094073
           cov(e2,e5) |  .2854775   .0496163   .1882314   .3827236
           cov(e2,e6) |  .3042992   .0849226   .137854    .4707445
           cov(e3,e4) |  .3663268   .0535731   .2613255   .4713282
           cov(e3,e5) |  .2960743   .0496323   .1987968   .3933518
           cov(e3,e6) |  .29401     .082363    .1325815   .4554385
           cov(e4,e5) |  .2725047   .0481962   .1780419   .3669675
           cov(e4,e6) |  .2000177   .0765935   .0498971   .3501383
           cov(e5,e6) |  .5614837   .1142978   .3374641   .7855033
- - - - - - - - - - - - - - - - - - - - - - - - - - - - - - - - - - - - - -
 LR test vs. linear model: chi2(20) = 644.31        Prob > chi2 = 0.0000
```

Output 3.12 Results of an adjustment for covariance analysis with a Toeplitz 5 covariance structure to analyse the relationship between cholesterol and the sum of skinfolds

```
Mixed-effects ML regression              Number of obs     =        882
Group variable: id                       Number of groups  =        147

                                         Obs per group:
                                                       min =          6
                                                       avg =        6.0
                                                       max =          6

                                         Wald chi2(1)      =      56.59
Log likelihood = -781.9781               Prob > chi2       =     0.0000


- - - - - - - - - - - - - - - - - - - - - - - - - - - - - - - - - - - - - - -
     chol |    Coef.   Std. Err.     z   P>|z|       [ 95% Conf. Interval]
- - - - - - +- - - - - - - - - - - - - - - - - - - - - - - - - - - - - - - -
    skinf | .1465355  .0194787   7.52  0.000        .1083579    .184713
    _cons | 4.023712  .0879447  45.75  0.000        3.851343    4.19608
- - - - - - - - - - - - - - - - - - - - - - - - - - - - - - - - - - - - - - -


- - - - - - - - - - - - - - - - - - - - - - - - - - - - - - - - - - - - - - -
Random-effects Parameters | Estimate  Std. Err.   [ 95% Conf. Interval]
- - - - - - - - - - - - - - - - +- - - - - - - - - - - - - - - - - - - - - -
id:                   (empty) |
- - - - - - - - - - - - - - - - +- - - - - - - - - - - - - - - - - - - - - -
Residual: Toeplitz(5)         |
                        cov1 | .4214187  .0461136    .3310378    .5117997
                        cov2 | .3085257  .0449446    .2204359    .3966155
                        cov3 | .2515171  .0440767    .1651285    .3379058
                        cov4 | .2246511  .0457451    .1349924    .3143098
                        cov5 | .2276423  .0483785    .1328221    .3224624
                      var(e) | .6053248  .0464042    .5208772    .7034636
- - - - - - - - - - - - - - - - - - - - - - - - - - - - - - - - - - - - - - -
LR test vs. linear model: chi2(5) = 441.84          Prob > chi2 = 0.0000
- - - - - - - - - - - - - - - - - - - - - - - - - - - - - - - - - - - - - - -
```

the number of degrees of freedom is based on the difference in the number of parameters estimated with each analysis. With the unstructured covariance structure 21 variance and covariance parameters were estimated, while for the exchangeable covariance structure only two parameters were estimated. The difference between the −2 log likelihoods (i.e. 298.9) is highly significant or, in other words, the model with an unstructured covariance structure is statistically better than the model with an exchangeable covariance structure. Because there are other possible covariance structures that can be considered with less parameters to be estimated than with the unstructured covariance structure, the data were reanalysed with a 5-dependent (i.e. Toeplitz (5)) covariance structure. Output 3.12 shows the result of this analysis.

Output 3.13 Correlation matrix of the residuals after a linear mixed model analysis with only a random intercept to analyse the relationship between cholesterol and the sum of skinfolds

	res1	res2	res3	res4	res5	res6
res1	1.0000					
res2	0.1887	1.0000				
res3	-0.1155	0.0054	1.0000			
res4	-0.2176	0.0510	0.1815	1.0000		
res5	-0.2757	-0.3023	-0.2314	-0.1567	1.0000	
res6	-0.3085	-0.3983	-0.2150	-0.2922	-0.0059	1.0000

Based on the result of the likelihood ratio test comparing the different models with each other, it is obvious that an unstructured covariance structure seems to be the most appropriate in this particular situation. However, it is questionable whether the choice for a particular model should only be based on the fit of the model (i.e. on the result of the likelihood ratio test). For instance, using an unstructured covariance structure is highly data driven and it is debatable whether a highly data driven choice is the best option. Besides that, when the model becomes too complex it can lead to overfitting, which leads to considerable uncertainty of the scientific importance of the result (Baybak, 2004). Therefore, in actual use, a simpler covariance structure is generally employed to adjust for the dependency of the observations. This is a strategy which was also used for the choice of the correlation structure within GEE analysis (see Section 3.4.3).

3.6.2 Extension of Mixed Model Analysis

It is sometimes argued that a linear mixed model analysis must be extended by adding an additional adjustment to the model. The reason for this argument is that adding only a random intercept to the model is not enough to take into account the dependency of the repeated observations within the subject. The additional adjustment is than basically an additional adjustment for covariance. It is, however, highly questionable whether this additional adjustment is necessary. To illustrate this, Output 3.13 shows the correlation matrix of the residuals from the example dataset after a linear mixed model analysis with only a random intercept to analyse the relationship between cholesterol and the sum of skinfolds.

From Output 3.13 it can be seen that there are no strong positive correlations between residuals at the different time-points. So, in the example an additional adjustment for the correlated residuals is not necessary. A situation which is very common in real life data. So, again, it is highly questionable whether this additional adjustment is necessary.

3.6.3 Comments

In the previous sections it has often been mentioned that special longitudinal methods are needed to adjust for correlated observations within the subject. However, it has already been stated that the adjustment in longitudinal data analysis is carried out for correlated residuals. When there are no covariates in the model, the magnitude of the within-subjects correlation in the observations is equivalent to the magnitude of the within-subjects correlation in the residuals. It is possible that by adding particular covariates to the model (part of) the within-subjects correlation is explained. Because of this, in the literature it is sometimes argued that there are correlated observations given the covariates in the statistical model. This issue can be illustrated by comparing the observed correlation structure for cholesterol (see Output 3.5) with the estimated within-subjects correlation structure derived from a linear GEE analysis with an exchangeable correlation structure. Output 3.14 shows the estimated within-subjects correlation matrix derived from a linear GEE analysis to evaluate the longitudinal relationship between cholesterol and the sum of skinfolds.

Output 3.14 Correlation matrix derived from a linear GEE analysis (with an exchangeable correlation structure) to analyse the relationship between cholesterol and the sum of skinfolds

```
Estimated within-id correlation matrix R:

            c1           c2           c3           c4           c5           c6
r1      1.0000
r2      0.5163       1.0000
r3      0.5163       0.5163       1.0000
r4      0.5163       0.5163       0.5163       1.0000
r5      0.5163       0.5163       0.5163       0.5163       1.0000
r6      0.5163       0.5163       0.5163       0.5163       0.5163       1.0000
```

From Output 3.14 it is obvious that the estimated within-subjects correlation is much lower than the average observed within-subjects correlation in the data. This indicates that in the example, part of the within-subjects correlation in cholesterol is explained by the sum of skinfolds.

The Modelling of Time

4.1 Growth Curve Analysis

In Chapter 2, the generalised linear model (GLM) for repeated measures was introduced as a way to analyse the development over time in a continuous outcome variable. With the regression-based methods introduced in Chapter 3, i.e. mixed model analysis, generalised estimating equations (GEE) analysis and the adjustment for covariance method, it is also possible to analyse the development over time. To do so, the longitudinal regression analysis has to be performed with the time variable as covariate of interest. The simplest way of analysing the development over time in a continuous outcome variable is to assume a linear development. Using the example dataset, Output 4.1 shows the result of a linear mixed model analysis in which the linear development over time is analysed for cholesterol. This analysis is also known as a (linear) growth curve mixed model analysis.

From Output 4.1 it can be seen that there is a significant increase over time in cholesterol. Because time is coded as yearly intervals (1, 2, 3, 4, 5 and 6) this increase is with 0.1252128 units per year. The same analysis can also be performed with a linear GEE analysis (see Output 4.2).

As expected, the magnitude of the regression coefficient for time is exactly the same as the one estimated with a linear mixed model analysis with only a random intercept. The difference between the two analyses is the standard error of the regression coefficient, which is a bit higher for the coefficient estimated with the GEE analysis. This is caused by the robust estimation of the standard error within GEE analysis (see Section 3.4.3). Because it is known that a linear mixed model analysis is preferred above a linear GEE analysis for a longitudinal analysis of a continuous outcome variable (see Section 3.5), in the remaining part of this chapter, linear mixed model analysis will be used for the analyses.

The next step in the linear mixed model analysis is to add a random slope for time to the model. Output 4.3 shows the result of that analysis.

It was already mentioned that within mixed model analysis, the likelihood ratio test can be used to evaluate whether or not it is necessary to add a random slope to the model. Therefore, the -2 log likelihood of the model with only a random intercept (Output 4.1) can be compared to the -2 log likelihood of the model with both a random intercept and a random slope for time (Output 4.3). The difference between the two -2 log likelihoods follows a Chi-square distribution with (in this case) two degrees of freedom. Two degrees of freedom, because besides the variance of the slopes, also the covariance between the random intercept and the random slope is estimated. In the example, the difference between the two -2 log likelihoods is equal to 18. On a Chi-square distribution with two degrees of freedom, this is highly significant; i.e. the model with both a random intercept and a random slope for time is significantly better than the model with only a random intercept.

One of the disadvantages of the analyses performed to investigate the development over time in cholesterol so far is that a linear development is assumed, while the data suggests a more quadratic development over time (see Chapter 2). Within the regression-based methods, this can be done by adding a quadratic term to the models. In statistical terms, this means that a second order polynomial function with time is modelled. Output 4.4 shows the result of the linear mixed model analysis including a quadratic term for time (i.e. time squared).

The question that should be answered now is whether this model (assuming a quadratic development over time) is better than the model assuming a linear development over time. This can be done by evaluating the importance of the quadratic term in the model, which is normally done by looking at the significance level of the

Output 4.1 Results of a linear mixed model analysis with only a random intercept to analyse the linear development over time for cholesterol

```
Mixed-effects ML regression              Number of obs    =      882
Group variable: id                       Number of groups =      147

                                         Obs per group:
                                                       min =        6
                                                       avg =      6.0
                                                       max =        6

                                         Wald chi2(1)     =   165.59
Log likelihood = -804.40727              Prob > chi2      =   0.0000
```

```
------------------------------------------------------------------
     chol |    Coef.  Std. Err.      z    P>|z|   [ 95% Conf. Interval]
------+-----------------------------------------------------------
     time | .1262974 .0098147   12.87   0.000    .1070609   .1455338
    _cons | 4.057732 .062835    64.58   0.000    3.934578   4.180887
------------------------------------------------------------------
```

```
------------------------------------------------------------------
Random-effects Parameters | Estimate Std. Err.  [ 95% Conf. Interval]
--------------------------+---------------------------------------
id: Identity              |
           var(_cons)     | .3656268  .0475139    .283415   .4716862
--------------------------+---------------------------------------
          var(Residual)   | .247804   .0129265   .2237208   .2744799
------------------------------------------------------------------
LR test vs. linear model: chibar2(01) = 463.17    Prob >= chibar2 = 0.0000
```

Output 4.2 Results of a linear GEE analysis with an exchangeable correlation structure to analyse the linear development over time for cholesterol

```
GEE population-averaged model            Number of obs    =      882
Group variable:               id         Number of groups =      147
Link:                   identity         Obs per group:
Family:                 Gaussian                       min =        6
Correlation:        exchangeable                       avg =      6.0
                                                       max =        6
                                         Wald chi2(1)     =   127.92
Scale parameter:         .6134308        Prob > chi2      =   0.0000

                         (Std. Err. adjusted for clustering on id)
------------------------------------------------------------------
          |             Robust
     chol |    Coef.  Std. Err.      z    P>|z|   [ 95% Conf. Interval]
------+-----------------------------------------------------------
     time | .1262974 .0111668   11.31   0.000    .1044108    .148184
    _cons | 4.057732 .0563626   71.99   0.000    3.947264   4.168201
------------------------------------------------------------------
```

Output 4.3 Results of a linear mixed model analysis with both a random intercept and a random slope for time to analyse the linear development over time for cholesterol

```
Mixed-effects ML regression              Number of obs     =        882
Group variable: id                       Number of groups  =        147

                                         Obs per group:
                                                          min =          6
                                                          avg =        6.0
                                                          max =          6

                                         Wald chi2(1)      =     128.79
Log likelihood = -795.2782               Prob > chi2       =     0.0000


- - - - - - - - - - - - - - - - - - - - - - - - - - - - - - - - - - - - - - - -
    chol |    Coef.    Std. Err.      z    P>|z|     [ 95% Conf. Interval]
- - - - -+- - - - - - - - - - - - - - - - - - - - - - - - - - - - - - - - - - -
    time | .1262974   .0111288   11.35    0.000     .1044853    .1481094
   _cons | 4.057732   .0561706   72.24    0.000      3.94764    4.167825
- - - - - - - - - - - - - - - - - - - - - - - - - - - - - - - - - - - - - - - -


- - - - - - - - - - - - - - - - - - - - - - - - - - - - - - - - - - - - - - - -
Random-effects Parameters |  Estimate  Std. Err.   [ 95% Conf. Interval]
- - - - - - - - - - - - - - - +- - - - - - - - - - - - - - - - - - - - - - - - -
id: Unstructured          |
              var(time) | .0050572   .0022578     .0021081    .012132
             var(_cons) | .2643811   .0553354     .1754174    .3984632
        cov(time,_cons) | .0060351   .0086904    -.0109977    .0230679
- - - - - - - - - - - - - - - +- - - - - - - - - - - - - - - - - - - - - - - - -
           var(Residual) | .230104    .0134199     .205249     .2579688
- - - - - - - - - - - - - - - - - - - - - - - - - - - - - - - - - - - - - - - -
LR test vs. linear model: chi2(3) = 481.43           Prob > chi2 = 0.0000
```

regression coefficient for the quadratic term. From Output 4.4 it can be seen that the p-value belonging to the quadratic term is very low, i.e. highly significant and therefore it can be concluded that the development over time can better be described with a quadratic function instead of a linear one. In the next step of the modelling process, a random slope can also be added for the quadratic term for the time variable. In addition, all covariances have to be added, i.e. the covariance between the random intercept and the random slope for the quadratic term for time and the covariance between the random slope for time and the random slope for the quadratic term for time. Output 4.5 shows the result of this analysis.

With the likelihood ratio test, it can be evaluated whether the model with a random slope for the quadratic term for the time variable is better than the model without that random slope. The difference between the two -2 log likelihoods is equal to 32.6. This difference follows a Chi-square distribution with three degrees of freedom, which is highly significant. There are three degrees of freedom because, besides the random slope for the quadratic term for the time variable, two covariances were also added to the model.

In Chapter 2, it has already been shown that the development over time for cholesterol was quadratic (see Figure 2.3), so it is not really necessary to model the development over time with more complicated functions, such as a cubic S-shaped function (i.e. a third degree polynomial). However, the method to evaluate a higher order function is exactly the same as has been described for a quadratic function.

Output 4.4 Results of a linear mixed model analysis with both a random intercept and a random slope for time to analyse the quadratic development over time in cholesterol

```
Mixed-effects ML regression              Number of obs    =       882
Group variable: id                       Number of groups =       147

                                         Obs per group:
                                                        min =         6
                                                        avg =       6.0
                                                        max =         6

                                         Wald chi2(2)     =    417.57
Log likelihood = -677.81693              Prob > chi2      =    0.0000

      chol |    Coef.    Std. Err.      z    P>|z|  [ 95% Conf. Interval]
-------+-------------------------------------------------------------
      time | -.5044849   .0387514   -13.02  0.000  -.5804363  -.4285335
     time2 |  .0901118   .0053027    16.99  0.000   .0797186   .1005049
     _cons |  4.898775   .0748638    65.44  0.000   4.752045   5.045506

Random-effects Parameters |   Estimate  Std. Err.[ 95% Conf. Interval]
--------------------------+------------------------------------------
id: Unstructured          |
              var(time)   |  .0093879   .002185   .0059492   .0148143
              var(_cons)  |  .3300639   .0546587  .2385826   .4566224
         cov(time,_cons)  | -.0091225   .0084592 -.0257023   .0074573
-----------+--------------------------------------------------------
           var(Residual)  |  .1543161   .0089999  .1376474   .1730033
--------------------------------------------------------------------
LR test vs. linear model: chi2(3) = 640.54            Prob > chi2 = 0.0000
```

The use of a mathematical function to model the development over time always assumes a particular shape of the development over time. An elegant solution is to model time as a categorical variable instead of a continuous one. With time as a categorical variable, the development over time is modelled without assuming a certain shape of the development. Table 4.1 illustrates part of the example dataset with time as a categorical variable.

A limitation of the use of time as a categorical variable is the fact that this is only possible when the time intervals between the repeated measurements are the same for each subject. In other words, the measurements have to be fixed. It is obvious that with unequal time intervals between subjects (i.e. when the measurements are not fixed), the dummy coding goes wrong. On the other hand, the time intervals between the fixed time-points do not have to be the same over the whole longitudinal measurement period, a situation which is not uncommon in longitudinal studies.

In the examples presented in this chapter, each subject was assumed to be measured at the same time-points. Time was simply coded as [1, 2, 3, 4, 5, 6]. However, with the regression-based methods it is also possible to model the actual time of each measurement. For instance, the number of days or weeks after at the first measurement can be used as a time indicator (see Table 4.2). This is sometimes more realistic, because subjects are almost never measured at exactly the same time. For each subject this indicates that a different time sequence of the measurements is modelled, which directly implies that time cannot be modelled as a categorical variable, represented by dummy variables. In that case, only a mathematical function can be used to analyse the development over time.

Output 4.6 shows the result of a linear mixed model analysis with only a random intercept to analyse the development over time in cholesterol, with time treated as a categorical variable, represented by five dummy variables.

Output 4.5 Results of a linear mixed model analysis with both a random intercept and random slopes for time and time squared to analyse the quadratic development over time in cholesterol

```
Mixed-effects ML regression              Number of obs    =       882
Group variable: id                       Number of groups =       147

                                         Obs per group:
                                                        min =         6
                                                        avg =       6.0
                                                        max =         6

                                         Wald chi2(2)     =    252.64
Log likelihood = -661.47223              Prob > chi2      =    0.0000


- - - - - - - - - - - - - - - - - - - - - - - - - - - - - - - - - - - -
   chol |     Coef.    Std. Err.      z     P>|z|    [ 95% Conf. Interval]
- - - - - -+- - - - - - - - - - - - - - - - - - - - - - - - - - - - - - -
   time | -.5044849   .0433872   -11.63    0.000    -.5895222   -.4194477
  time2 |  .0901118   .0064676    13.93    0.000     .0774354    .1027881
  _cons |  4.898775   .0764881    64.05    0.000     4.748862    5.048689
- - - - - - - - - - - - - - - - - - - - - - - - - - - - - - - - - - - -


- - - - - - - - - - - - - - - - - - - - - - - - - - - - - - - - - - - -
Random-effects Parameters |  Estimate  Std. Err.   [ 95% Conf. Interval]
- - - - - - - - - - - - - - -+- - - - - - - - - - - - - - - - - - - - - -
id: Unstructured          |
             var(time) |   .0997162   .0344086    .0507044    .1961038
            var(time2) |   .0026875   .0007542    .0015505    .0046582
            var(_cons) |   .4464672   .1041104    .2826834    .7051454
        cov(time,time2) |  -.0157557   .0050116   -.0255783   -.0059331
        cov(time,_cons) |  -.1089017   .0528508   -.2124874   -.005316
       cov(time2,_cons) |   .0176128   .0075938    .0027292    .0324963
- - - - - - - - - - - - - - -+- - - - - - - - - - - - - - - - - - - - - -
          var(Residual) |   .1292332    .008703    .1132534    .1474678
- - - - - - - - - - - - - - - - - - - - - - - - - - - - - - - - - - - -
LR test vs. linear model: chi2(6) = 673.23            Prob > chi2 = 0.0000
```

The regression coefficients of the five dummy variables (time 2 to 6) can be interpreted as follows: compared to the first measurement (which is the reference category), there is a decrease in cholesterol at the second measurement of 0.1115646. At the third measurement the decrease continues (the regression coefficient for the second dummy variable (i.e. -0.1687075) represents the difference between the third measurement and the first measurement), and at the fourth measurement the lowest point is reached. At the fifth and the sixth measurements the value of cholesterol is higher than at the first measurement, indicating a (steep) increase during the last two measurements. In

theory it is possible to add random slopes for the five dummy variables to the model, but this leads to a very complicated model with the risk of overfitting. Moreover, in most situations, these complicated models will not converge, which means that the modelling will not lead to a proper solution. Therefore, in models treating time as a categorical variable, generally, random slopes are not considered.

4.2 Comparing Groups

In Chapter 2 it was mentioned that with a GLM for repeated measures, it is possible to compare

Table 4.1 Example dataset with time as a continuous variable and as a categorical variable with dummy variable coding

Id	Time (continuous)	Time (categorical) Dummy1	Dummy2	Dummy3	Dummy4	Dummy5
1	1	0	0	0	0	0
1	2	1	0	0	0	0
1	3	0	1	0	0	0
1	4	0	0	1	0	0
1	5	0	0	0	1	0
1	6	0	0	0	0	1
2	1	0	0	0	0	0
2	2	1	0	0	0	0
2	3	0	1	0	0	0
2	4	0	0	1	0	0
2	5	0	0	0	1	0
2	6	0	0	0	0	1

Table 4.2 Example of a dataset with four repeated measurements *(N = 3)* with time as a continuous variable with equal measurement points and time as the actual date of measurement

Id	Time (continuous)	Time (in days)
1	1	0
1	2	20
1	3	45
1	4	100
2	1	0
2	2	30
2	3	40
2	4	80
3	1	0
3	2	25
3	3	50
3	4	70

the development over time in a continuous outcome variable between two (or more) groups. With regression-based methods, it is also possible to compare the development over time between two (or more) groups. Therefore, the interaction between the time variable and the group variable must be added to the model. In the example dataset, sex is a dichotomous time-independent covariate (i.e. males versus females) and this variable is used to illustrate this analysis. Output 4.7 shows the result of a linear mixed model analysis to analyse the difference in development over time in cholesterol between males and females.

From Output 4.7 it can be seen that the interaction between sex and time is statistically significant (the z-value equals 4.03 and the p-value is less than 0.001). This indicates that the linear development over time is significantly different for males and females. For males (coded 0 in the example dataset) there is a yearly increase of 0.0847205 units per year, while for females (coded 1 in the example dataset) there is a yearly increase of 0.0847205 + 0.0783564 = 0.1630769 units per year.

It should be noted that this analysis assumes a linear development over time, while in Section 4.1 it was already shown that the development over time in cholesterol could be better described with a quadratic development over time, or could be better analysed with time as a categorical variable, represented by dummy variables. The latter in particular is very popular these days and especially in intervention studies in which the effect of an intervention is evaluated at different time-points (see

Output 4.6 Results of a linear mixed model analysis with only a random intercept to analyse the development over time in cholesterol with time treated as a categorical variable, represented by five dummy variables

```
Mixed-effects ML regression               Number of obs    =      882
Group variable: id                        Number of groups =      147

                                          Obs per group:
                                                        min =        6
                                                        avg =      6.0
                                                        max =        6

                                          Wald chi2(5)     =   506.57
Log likelihood = -686.40878               Prob > chi2      =   0.0000


         chol |    Coef.   Std. Err.    z    P>|z|  [ 95% Conf. Interval]
--------------+--------------------------------------------------------------
         time |
            2 | -.1115646  .0494525  -2.26  0.024  -.2084897  -.0146396
            3 | -.1687075  .0494525  -3.41  0.001  -.2656325  -.0717824
            4 | -.2612245  .0494525  -5.28  0.000  -.3581495  -.1642994
            5 |  .2408163  .0494525   4.87  0.000   .1438913   .3377414
            6 |  .6911565  .0494525  13.98  0.000   .5942314   .7880815
              |
         _cons|  4.434694  .0615402  72.06  0.000   4.314077   4.55531


 Random-effects Parameters | Estimate  Std. Err.   [ 95% Conf. Interval]
---------------------------+-------------------------------------------------
id: Identity               |
             var(_cons)    |  .3769695  .0474907   .2944907   .4825483
---------------------------+-------------------------------------------------
           var(Residual)   |  .1797477  .0093764   .1622786   .1990973
---------------------------+-------------------------------------------------
LR test vs. linear model: chibar2(01) = 613.60    Prob >= chibar2 = 0.0000
```

Chapter 10). Output 4.8 shows the result of a linear mixed model analysis to analyse the difference in quadratic development over time between males and females.

From Output 4.8 it can be seen that both the interaction between sex and time and the interaction between sex and time squared are statistically significant, which indicates that the difference in quadratic development over time between males and females is statistically significant. However, the interpretation of the regression coefficients of this analysis is rather complicated. Therefore, if

possible, time is better treated as a categorical variable, represented by dummy variables. Output 4.9 shows the result of a linear mixed model analysis with time as a categorical variable to analyse the difference in development over time between males and females.

Although Output 4.9 looks a bit complicated, the regression coefficients can be interpreted in a straightforward way. The regression coefficients of the dummy variables have the same interpretation as in Output 4.6, although they now represent the development over time in cholesterol for

Output 4.7 Results of a linear mixed model analysis with only a random intercept to analyse the difference in linear development over time between two groups

```
Mixed-effects ML regression                Number of obs     =       882
Group variable: id                         Number of groups  =       147

                                           Obs per group:
                                                         min =         6
                                                         avg =       6.0
                                                         max =         6

                                           Wald chi2(3)      =    191.95
Log likelihood = -793.21116                Prob > chi2       =    0.0000
```

chol	Coef.	Std. Err.	z	P>|z|	[95% Conf. Interval]
time	.0847205	.01417	5.98	0.000	.0569478	.1124931
sex	-.011557	.1236147	-0.09	0.926	-.2538374	.2307234
time#sex	.0783564	.0194527	4.03	0.000	.0402298	.1164831
_cons	4.063865	.0900448	45.13	0.000	3.88738	4.240349

Random-effects Parameters	Estimate	Std. Err.	[95% Conf. Interval]
id: Identity				
var(_cons)	.3493319	.0455091	.2706127	.4509499
var(Residual)	.2424519	.0126473	.2188888	.2685516

```
LR test vs. linear model: chibar2(01) = 453.88    Prob >= chibar2 = 0.0000
```

males (sex coded zero). For females (sex coded 1), the difference between the second and first measurement is equal to: $-0.2043478 + 0.1748607 = -0.0294871$, indicating a small decrease between the first and the second measurement. In the same way the difference between the other measurements and the first measurement for females can be calculated. For instance, the difference between the third and first measurement is equal to: $-0.3884058 + 0.4140468 = 0.025641$. So, for females there is a slight increase in cholesterol between the first and the third measurement, while for males there is a (sharp) decrease (i.e. -0.3884058). It should be noted that with this analysis, only for the group which is coded 0, the significance level for the change over time

can be directly derived from the output. For the group which is coded 1, this is not directly possible. Therefore, the group variable should be recoded and a new analysis with the recoded variable should be performed. Output 4.10 shows the same result of the mixed model analysis reported in Output 4.9, only with sex recoded (i.e. females coded as 0 and males coded as 1).

From Output 4.10 it can, for instance, be seen that the difference between the first and second measurement for females is equal to -0.0294871. This number was already known from the analysis reported in Output 4.9. However, from Output 4.10, it can now be seen that the p-value which belongs to this difference is equal to 0.655.

Output 4.8 Results of a linear mixed model analysis with only a random intercept to analyse the difference in quadratic development over time between two groups

```
Mixed-effects ML regression                      Number of obs    =       882
Group variable: id                               Number of groups =       147

                                                 Obs per group:
                                                             min =         6
                                                             avg =       6.0
                                                             max =         6

                                                 Wald chi2(5)     =    524.94
Log likelihood = -679.73704                      Prob > chi2      =    0.0000
```

chol	Coef.	Std. Err.	z	P>|z|	[95% Conf. Interval]
time	-.7134679	.0594487	-12.00	0.000	-.8299853 -.5969505
sex	-.4322185	.1593614	-2.71	0.007	-.7445611 -.1198758
time#sex	.3938525	.081612	4.83	0.000	.2338959 .5538091
time2	.1140269	.0083136	13.72	0.000	.0977325 .1303213
time2#sex	-.0450709	.0114131	-3.95	0.000	-.0674401 -.0227017
_cons	5.128116	.1160839	44.18	0.000	4.900596 5.355636

Random-effects Parameters	Estimate	Std. Err.	[95% Conf. Interval]
id: Identity			
var(_cons)	.3600665	.0454866	.2810942 .4612259
var(Residual)	.1780439	.0092875	.1607404 .1972102

```
LR test vs. linear model: chibar2(01) = 596.97    Prob >= chibar2 = 0.0000
```

4.3 Adjustment for Time

In Chapter 3, the longitudinal relationship between cholesterol and the sum of skinfolds was investigated. In all analyses the time variable was not included in the model. A major point of discussion in all longitudinal analyses is how to deal with the time variable in a situation when the analysis of the development over time is not the main purpose of the study. In some studies, an a priori adjustment for time is performed, while in other studies (as in the examples in Chapter 3) the time variable is ignored. In most studies, however, it is not clear whether or not a time variable is part of the statistical model. In this section, the influence of the time variable in a longitudinal data analysis will be discussed. For this purpose, a different example dataset will be used. The dataset is also taken from the Amsterdam Growth and Health Longitudinal Study (AGAHLS), but in this example a selection is made of three repeated measurements performed over a period of 10 years. The purpose of the example was to investigate the relationship

Output 4.9 Results of a linear mixed model analysis with only a random intercept to analyse the difference in development over time for cholesterol between males and females with time treated as a categorical variable, represented by five dummy variables

```
Mixed-effects ML regression              Number of obs     =        882
Group variable: id                       Number of groups  =        147

                                         Obs per group:
                                                        min =          6
                                                        avg =        6.0
                                                        max =          6

                                         Wald chi2(11)     =     581.72
Log likelihood = -663.45381              Prob > chi2       =     0.0000
```

chol	Coef.	Std. Err.	z	P>|z|	[95% Conf. Interval]
time					
2	-.2043478	.070264	-2.91	0.004	-.3420627	-.066633
3	-.3884058	.070264	-5.53	0.000	-.5261206	-.250691
4	-.5130435	.070264	-7.30	0.000	-.6507583	-.3753286
5	-.0246377	.070264	-0.35	0.726	-.1623525	.1130772
6	.5101449	.070264	7.26	0.000	.3724301	.6478598
sex					
females	-.0547937	.1205069	-0.45	0.649	-.290983	.1813955
time#sex					
2#females	.1748607	.0964593	1.81	0.070	-.014196	.3639174
3#females	.4140468	.0964593	4.29	0.000	.2249901	.6031035
4#females	.4745819	.0964593	4.92	0.000	.2855252	.6636386
5#females	.5002787	.0964593	5.19	0.000	.3112219	.6893354
6#females	.3411371	.0964593	3.54	0.000	.1520804	.5301939
_cons	4.463768	.087781	50.85	0.000	4.29172	4.635816

Random-effects Parameter	Estimate	Std. Err.	[95% Conf. Interval]
id: Identity			
var(_cons)	.3613526	.0454844	.2823503	.46246
var(Residual)	.1703274	.008885	.1537738	.1886629

```
LR test vs. linear model: chibar2(01) = 618.93   Prob >= chibar2 = 0.0000
```

Output 4.10 Results of a linear mixed model analysis with only a random intercept to analyse the difference in development over time for cholesterol between males and females with time treated as a categorical variable, represented by five dummy variables

```
Mixed-effects ML regression                  Number of obs     =        882
Group variable: id                           Number of groups  =        147

                                             Obs per group:
                                                          min =          6
                                                          avg =        6.0
                                                          max =          6

                                             Wald chi2(11)     =     581.72
Log likelihood = -663.45381                  Prob > chi2       =     0.0000
---------------------------------------------------------------------------
       chol |     Coef.   Std. Err.      z   P>|z|    [ 95% Conf. Interval]
------------+--------------------------------------------------------------
       time |
          2 | -.0294871   .0660861   -0.45   0.655    -.1590135    .1000392
          3 |   .025641   .0660861    0.39   0.698    -.1038853    .1551673
          4 | -.0384615   .0660861   -0.58   0.561    -.1679878    .0910648
          5 |   .475641   .0660861    7.20   0.000     .3461147    .6051673
          6 |  .8512821   .0660861   12.88   0.000     .7217557    .9808084
            |
        sex |
      males |  .0547937   .1205069    0.45   0.649    -.1813955    .290983
            |
   time#sex |
    2#males | -.1748607   .0964593   -1.81   0.070    -.3639174    .014196
    3#males | -.4140468   .0964593   -4.29   0.000    -.6031035   -.2249901
    4#males | -.4745819   .0964593   -4.92   0.000    -.6636386   -.2855252
    5#males | -.5002787   .0964593   -5.19   0.000    -.6893354   -.3112219
    6#males | -.3411371   .0964593   -3.54   0.000    -.5301939   -.1520804
            |
      _cons |  4.408974   .0825616   53.40   0.000     4.247157    4.570792
---------------------------------------------------------------------------


---------------------------------------------------------------------------
  Random-effects Parameters |  Estimate  Std. Err.   [ 95% Conf. Interval]
----------------------------+----------------------------------------------
id: Identity                |
               var(_cons)   |  .3613526   .0454844     .2823504     .46246
----------------------------+----------------------------------------------
             var(Residual)  |  .1703274    .008885     .1537738   .1886629
---------------------------------------------------------------------------
LR test vs. linear model: chibar2(01) = 618.93    Prob >= chibar2 = 0.0000
```

Table 4.3 Means and standard deviations (between brackets) of cholesterol and body weight at three repeated measurements

	Measurement		
	1	2	3
Number of subjects	437	379	338
Cholesterol (mmol/l)	4.4 (0.9)	5.0 (0.9)	5.5 (0.8)
Body weight (kg)	72.7 (12.3)	75.4 (13.1)	77.6 (13.6)

between cholesterol as the outcome variable and body weight as the time-dependent covariate. Table 4.3 shows descriptive information regarding the data used in this example.

In the first analysis, a linear mixed model analysis with only a random intercept was performed without an adjustment for time. In the second analysis, time (a continuous variable coded 1 to 3) was added to the model and the same mixed model analysis was performed. Output 4.11 and Output 4.12 show the results of the two analyses.

The results of the mixed model analyses show that the regression coefficient for body weight decreases by about 40% when time is added to the model. So obviously, adding time to the model has a huge influence on the magnitude of the regression coefficient of interest. It is therefore important to address the question which of the two results gives the real longitudinal relationship between cholesterol and body weight?

In Chapter 3 it has already been mentioned that one of the most difficult parts of longitudinal data analysis is the interpretation of the regression coefficient, especially the interpretation of a regression coefficient of a time-dependent covariate, as in this example. It has previously been discussed that when both the outcome variable and the covariate are time-dependent, the regression coefficient has to be interpreted as a combination of a between-subjects and a within-subjects relationship (see Section 3.3.4). It is often suggested that when the time variable is added to the longitudinal model, the interpretation of the regression coefficient of a time-dependent covariate is limited to the within-subjects interpretation (i.e. a change of one unit in the time-dependent covariate is associated with a change of regression coefficient units in the outcome variable). This is, however, not true. An adjustment

for time only leads to a more relative interpretation of the regression coefficient. Figure 4.1 shows an (extreme) example, which illustrates the impact of an adjustment for time in a longitudinal data analysis.

From Figure 4.1 it can be seen that both the outcome variable and the covariate increase over time. Furthermore, it can be seen that at each time-point, both variables are hardly related. A longitudinal analysis between the Y- and X-variable without adjusting for time would reveal a strong positive relationship. Adjustment for time will attenuate the relationship enormously. In fact, in an adjusted analysis, no relationship would be found between Y and X. Theoretically, by adding time to the model, the variance between the time-points is removed from the statistical model. In the example, time can be seen as a huge confounder in the longitudinal relationship between the outcome variable and the covariate. From the results reported in Output 4.11 and Output 4.12 it can be seen that in the cholesterol and body weight example more or less the same phenomenon occurs; both variables increase over time, which causes the crude analysis to reveal a much stronger relationship than the time-adjusted analysis.

The same idea can be achieved by performing an analysis with time-specific z-scores (calculated at each time-point separately by subtracting the mean value from the observed value and divided by the standard deviation) of the outcome variable and the covariate instead of the observed values. Basically, using time-specific z-scores also removes the variance between the time-points. In longitudinal studies, the use of time-specific z-scores is quite common, for instance, when there is a change in measurement equipment over time. To illustrate the effect of using time-specific z-scores, Output 4.13 shows the result of a linear mixed model analysis to analyse the relationship between time-specific z-scores of cholesterol and body weight.

Although the regression coefficient and standard error for body weight are different from the earlier analyses reported in Output 4.12 (which is due to the fact that the scale of both variables has changed), the test statistic (z-value) is almost equal to the test statistic obtained from the time-adjusted analysis which shows that both analyses are similar.

It is important to realise that the potential confounding effect of time only holds for covariates that

Output 4.11 Results of a linear mixed model analysis to analyse the relationship between cholesterol and body weight

```
Mixed-effects ML regression              Number of obs     =      1,148
Group variable: id                       Number of groups  =        468

                                         Obs per group:
                                                        min =          1
                                                        avg =        2.5
                                                        max =          3

                                         Wald chi2(1)      =     100.93
Log likelihood = -1491.0945              Prob > chi2       =     0.0000

- - - - - - - - - - - - - - - - - - - - - - - - - - - - - - - - - - - - - -
     chol |    Coef.    Std. Err.     z    P>|z|      [ 95% Conf. Interval]
- - - - - +- - - - - - - - - - - - - - - - - - - - - - - - - - - - - - - - -
   weight | .0272757   .002715   10.05   0.000      .0219543    .032597
    _cons | 2.873453   .206916   13.89   0.000      2.467905    3.279001
- - - - - - - - - - - - - - - - - - - - - - - - - - - - - - - - - - - - - -


- - - - - - - - - - - - - - - - - - - - - - - - - - - - - - - - - - - - - -
Random-effects Parameters |  Estimate  Std. Err.   [ 95% Conf. Interval]
- - - - - - - - - - - - - -+- - - - - - - - - - - - - - - - - - - - - - - -
id: Identity              |
              var(_cons)  | .4624268   .0495219    .3748751    .5704261
- - - - - - - - - - - - - -+- - - - - - - - - - - - - - - - - - - - - - - -
            var(Residual) | .4874143   .0274546    .4364682    .544307
- - - - - - - - - - - - - - - - - - - - - - - - - - - - - - - - - - - - - -
LR test vs. linear model: chibar2(01) = 184.51     Prob >= chibar2 = 0.0000
```

are time-dependent. When the longitudinal relationship is analysed with covariates that are time-independent, an adjustment for time is not necessary. This has to do with the definition of a confounder: a variable can only be a confounder in a particular relationship when the possible confounder is related to both the outcome and the covariate. Because time is not associated with a time-independent covariate, time cannot be a confounder in such a relationship.

So, although it depends on the research question, time should be treated as a potential confounder and therefore, it is recommended to report both the results (i.e. with and without an adjustment for time), and interpret the possible differences between the two results. However, again this only holds for time-dependent covariates.

4.3.1 Time versus Age

In the example dataset, the subjects started the longitudinal study exactly at the same age. So, the adjustment for time is exactly the same as the adjustment for age. In this situation time and age are collinear. In many other longitudinal studies, however, subjects do not start the longitudinal study at the same age. In those situations, age and time can play a different role in the analysis. There are a few options to deal with this problem. In most studies, age at the start of the study is treated as a time-independent covariate and the time variable is treated as the time-dependent covariate. In that case, the two influences of age at the start of the study and the time development are disentangled. In other studies

Output 4.12 Results of a linear mixed model analysis to analyse the relationship between cholesterol and body weight adjusted for time

```
Mixed-effects ML regression          Number of obs     =     1,148
Group variable: id                   Number of groups  =       468

                                     Obs per group:
                                                   min =         1
                                                   avg =       2.5
                                                   max =         3

                                     Wald chi2(2)      =    961.91
Log likelihood = -1226.0798          Prob > chi2       =    0.0000
- - - - - - - - - - - - - - - - - - - - - - - - - - - - - - - - - - -
     chol |    Coef.   Std. Err.    z    P>|z|    [ 95% Conf. Interval]
- - - - - -+- - - - - - - - - - - - - - - - - - - - - - - - - - - - - -
   weight | .0164721  .0025331   6.50   0.000     .0115074   .0214368
     time | .5263038  .0193273  27.23   0.000     .4884229   .5641847
    _cons | 2.698839  .1863636  14.48   0.000     2.333573   3.064105
- - - - - - - - - - - - - - - - - - - - - - - - - - - - - - - - - - -


- - - - - - - - - - - - - - - - - - - - - - - - - - - - - - - - - - -
Random-effects Parameters | Estimate  Std. Err.   [ 95% Conf. Interval]
- - - - - - - - - - - - - - -+- - - - - - - - - - - - - - - - - - - - -
id: Identity              |
             var(_cons) | .5167684  .0421184    .4404739   .606278
- - - - - - - - - - - - - - -+- - - - - - - - - - - - - - - - - - - - -
          var(Residual) | .2378124  .0130311    .2135957   .2647748
- - - - - - - - - - - - - - - - - - - - - - - - - - - - - - - - - - -
LR test vs. linear model: chibar2(01) = 450.73    Prob >= chibar2 = 0.0000
```

age is treated as a time-dependent covariate and therefore, the influence of age at the start of the study and the time development are combined into one variable. For applied researchers, it is very important to realise what an adjustment for age and/or time actually means.

4.4 Interaction with Time

In Section 4.2 the development over time between different groups was compared. To do so, the interaction between the time variable and a group variable was added to the linear mixed model. In the example, the development of cholesterol was compared between males and females. So, the research question was related to the development over time in the outcome variable. It is also possible that the research question of interest is not

related to the development over time, but related to the question whether the longitudinal relationship of interest is different over time. To answer that question, an interaction with time must also be added to the linear mixed model. In the example dataset, the longitudinal relationship between cholesterol and the sum of skinfolds was investigated. The regression coefficient of the linear mixed model analysis indicated the relationship between the two variables on average over time. In some situations, it can be interesting to investigate whether the relationship between the two variables is different over time. Output 4.14 shows the result of the linear mixed model analysis with cholesterol as the continuous outcome variable and including sum of skinfolds, time and the interaction between time and the sum of skinfolds as covariates.

Y-variable

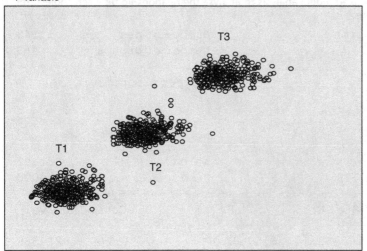

Figure 4.1 Example of the influence of an adjustment for time in a longitudinal data analysis.

X-variable

From Output 4.14 it can be seen that the interaction between the sum of skinfolds and time is highly significant. It can also be seen that the regression coefficient for the interaction term is positive, which indicates that the relationship between cholesterol and the sum of skinfolds is stronger when time has a higher value (i.e. stronger at the end of the longitudinal period than at the beginning). In this analysis time was treated as a continuous variable. For the interaction this means that the strength of the relationship between cholesterol and the sum of skinfolds linearly changes over time. At each time-point the relationship is estimated to be 0.0487617 stronger. It is, however, highly questionable whether the interaction with time is linear. Therefore, in studies where the time-points are fixed, it is probably better to treat time as a categorical variable (i.e. by using dummy variables) and investigate the interaction with time with the dummy variables. Output 4.15 shows the results of the linear mixed model analysis with cholesterol as the continuous outcome variable and including the sum of skinfolds, five dummy variables for time and the interaction between the five dummy variables for time and the sum of skinfolds as covariates.

The regression coefficient for the sum of skinfolds in Output 4.15 (-0.0262909) reflects the relationship between cholesterol and the sum of skinfolds at the first measurement. At the second measurement, the relationship between cholesterol and the sum of skinfolds can be calculated by the regression coefficient for the sum of skinfolds (-

0.0262909) plus the regression coefficient for the interaction between the sum of skinfolds and the dummy variable for the second measurement (0.0656557) which equals 0.04. The strength of the relationship between cholesterol and the sum of skinfolds at the other measurements can be calculated in the same way. From Output 4.15 it is clear that the interaction between the sum of skinfolds and time is almost linear from the third to the last measurement. The differences in strength of the relationship between the first and the third measurement are slightly higher.

It should be realised that the interaction with time is not very interesting within an observational longitudinal study. In intervention studies, however, the analysis of the interaction with time is one of the main purposes of the analysis. In Chapter 10, this will be further explained and illustrated.

4.5 Classification of Subjects with Different Growth Trajectories

Although the analysis of the development over time is of great interest, researchers are often interested in dividing the population under study into groups of subjects with comparable developments over time, i.e. comparable growth trajectories. Firstly, as a tool to describe the population under study, and secondly as a first step to study either the determinants of different growth trajectories or the consequences of different growth trajectories. Although the division into subgroups

Output 4.13 Results of a linear mixed model analysis to analyse the relationship between the time-specific z-scores for cholesterol and body weight

```
Mixed-effects ML regression              Number of obs     =      1,148
Group variable: id                       Number of groups  =        468

                                         Obs per group:
                                                        min =          1
                                                        avg =        2.5
                                                        max =          3

                                         Wald chi2(1)      =      43.57
Log likelihood = -1378.7805              Prob > chi2       =     0.0000

-----------------------------------------------------------------------
    z_chol |      Coef.  Std. Err.      z   P>|z|    [ 95% Conf. Interval]
-----------+-----------------------------------------------------------
  z_weight |   .2474249  .0374823    6.60   0.000      .173961    .3208888
     _cons |   .0015724  .0416811    0.04   0.970    -.0801211    .0832658
-----------------------------------------------------------------------


-----------------------------------------------------------------------
Random-effects Parameters | Estimate  Std. Err.    [ 95% Conf. Interval]
--------------------------+--------------------------------------------
id: Identity              |
             var(_cons)   |  .6700243  .0547364      .570891    .7863718
--------------------------+--------------------------------------------
            var(Residual) |  .3112846  .0170621     .2795771    .3465882
-----------------------------------------------------------------------
LR test vs. linear model: chibar2(01) = 447.99    Prob >= chibar2 = 0.0000
```

can be done in many different ways, most methods are based on structural equation modelling (Duncan et al., 1999), a fairly complex statistical method particularly popular in psychology and social science, but not so much in medical science. The general idea behind structural equation modelling is that the development over time in a particular outcome variable is captured by so-called latent or unobserved variables. In a longitudinal study these latent variables are the growth curve parameters. When a linear development over time is modelled, there are two growth curve parameters, i.e. the intercept and the slope. Figure 4.2 is a typical illustration of a structural equation model, in which, in this case, a linear growth curve example for a longitudinal study with six repeated measurements is shown. The six repeated measurements of the outcome variable are the observed variables and they are summarised into two latent

growth curve parameters; the intercept and the slope.

It should be noted that in a situation when one is interested in the development over time for a particular continuous outcome variable, the result of a structural equation model is exactly the same as the result from a linear mixed model analysis. This not only holds for the regression coefficients of the growth parameters, but also for the variances and covariances of the random intercept and random slope. To illustrate this, Output 4.16 shows the result of the structural equation model to analyse the linear development over time for cholesterol.

From Output 4.16 it can be seen that the numbers are exactly the same as has been shown in Output 4.3 in which the result of a comparable linear mixed model analysis with both a random intercept and a random slope for time was shown.

Output 4.14 Results of a linear mixed model analysis to analyse the relationship between cholesterol and the sum of skinfolds with an interaction with time

```
Mixed-effects ML regression                Number of obs    =      882
Group variable: id                         Number of groups =      147

                                           Obs per group:
                                                        min =        6
                                                        avg =      6.0
                                                        max =        6

                                           Wald chi2(3)     =   266.58
Log likelihood = -763.68628               Prob > chi2       =   0.0000
```

```
       chol |      Coef.   Std. Err.       z    P>|z|     [ 95% Conf. Interval]
------------+----------------------------------------------------------------
      skinf | -.0982397   .0352536    -2.79   0.005     -.1673355   -.0291439
       time | -.0721294    .026779    -2.69   0.007     -.1246153   -.0196435
            |
     skinf#|
       time |  .0487617   .0069353     7.03   0.000      .0351688    .0623546
            |
      _cons |  4.450081   .1316748    33.80   0.000      4.192003    4.708159
------------+----------------------------------------------------------------
```

```
Random-effects Parameters |  Estimate  Std. Err.  [ 95% Conf. Interval]
--------------------------+--------------------------------------------
id: Identity              |
             var(_cons) |  .3296508  .0437366    .2541678    .427551
--------------------------+--------------------------------------------
           var(Residual) |  .2263944  .0118544    .2043126   .2508628
--------------------------+--------------------------------------------
LR test vs. linear model: chibar2(01) = 431.09    Prob >= chibar2 = 0.0000
```

When one is interested in the classification of subjects with different growth trajectories, the structural equation model shown in Figure 4.2 is extended with another latent variable, i.e. a categorical variable defining the different classes of growth trajectories. This classification is based on the intercepts and slopes for the individual growth curve parameters (see Figure 4.3).

Within this structural equation framework, two methods are often used to classify subjects with the same growth trajectories, i.e. latent class growth analysis (LCGA) and latent class growth mixture modelling (LCGMM). LCGMM can be seen as an extension of LCGA. The difference between LCGA and LCGMM has to do with the assumptions regarding the individual growth trajectories within a certain class. Looking at the development over time from an LCGA perspective, the population under study consists of a number of classes, each of which has their own growth trajectory. The classes differ in trajectory shape, but within the classes the individuals are assumed to have a similar growth trajectory (there is no within-class variation). Looking at the development over time from an LCGMM perspective, the interpretation of the classes is similar, but within the classes, individuals are allowed to differ in growth trajectory (so there can be within-class variation). This indicates that subjects with slightly different growth parameters are classified

Output 4.15 Results of a linear mixed model analysis to analyse the relationship between cholesterol and the sum of skinfolds with an interaction with time as a categorical variable

```
Mixed-effects ML regression              Number of obs      =       882
Group variable: id                       Number of groups   =       147

                                         Obs per group:
                                                      min =         6
                                                      avg =       6.0
                                                      max =         6

                                         Wald chi2(11)      =    611.80
Log likelihood = -653.10108              Prob > chi2        =    0.0000

------------------------------------------------------------------------
      chol |     Coef.  Std. Err.      z   P>|z|    [95% Conf. Interval]
-----------+------------------------------------------------------------
     skinf | -.0262909  .0327509   -0.80  0.422    -.0904816   .0378998
           |
      time |
         2 | -.3296897  .1325698   -2.49  0.013    -.5895217  -.0698577
         3 | -.5391874  .1321692   -4.08  0.000    -.7982343  -.2801406
         4 | -.7114043  .1335746   -5.33  0.000    -.9732056   -.449603
         5 | -.3892849  .1371759   -2.84  0.005    -.6581447  -.1204251
         6 | -.0306268  .1384165   -0.22  0.825    -.3019181   .2406646
           |
 time#skinf|
         2 |  .0656557  .0373826    1.76  0.079    -.0076128   .1389242
         3 |  .1060974   .036363    2.92  0.004     .0348273   .1773676
         4 |  .1231961  .0360044    3.42  0.001     .0526288   .1937635
         5 |  .1513956   .035241    4.30  0.000     .0823244   .2204667
         6 |   .179339  .0362157    4.95  0.000     .1083576   .2503205
           |
      _cons|  4.520411  .1217846   37.12  0.000     4.281718   4.759105
------------------------------------------------------------------------


------------------------------------------------------------------------
Random-effects Parameters | Estimate  Std. Err.   [95% Conf. Interval]
--------------------------+---------------------------------------------
id: Identity              |
              var(_cons)  | .3363173  .0431409    .2615544   .4324506
--------------------------+---------------------------------------------
           var(Residual)  | .1678476  .0087807    .1514906   .1859708
------------------------------------------------------------------------
LR test vs. linear model: chibar2(01) = 563.22   Prob >= chibar2 = 0.0000
```

more easily to the same class within LCGMM compared to LCGA.

There is some discussion about the use of LCGA or LCGMM (Connell and Frye, 2006a, 2006b; Hoeksma and Kelderman, 2006; Muthén, 2006). The LCGA methodology is developed by Nagin and colleagues (Nagin, 1999; Nagin and Tremblay, 2001) and implemented in the SAS procedure Traj (Jones et al., 2001), whereas the LCGMM methodology is developed by Muthén

Output 4.16 Results of a structural equation model to analyse the linear development over time for cholesterol

```
Structural equation model                    Number of obs   =    147
Estimation method = ml
Log likelihood      = -795.2782
-----------+-----------------------------------------------
  mean(Inter~t)|  4.057732  .0561706  72.24  0.000    3.94764   4.167825
    mean(Slope)|  .1262974  .0111288  11.35  0.000   .1044853   .1481094
-----------+-----------------------------------------------
   var(e.chol1)|  .230104   .0134199                 .205249    .2579688
   var(e.chol2)|  .230104   .0134199                 .205249    .2579688
   var(e.chol3)|  .230104   .0134199                 .205249    .2579688
   var(e.chol4)|  .230104   .0134199                 .205249    .2579688
   var(e.chol5)|  .230104   .0134199                 .205249    .2579688
   var(e.chol6)|  .230104   .0134199                 .205249    .2579688
  var(Interc~t)|  .2643809  .0553353                .1754173    .3984629
     var(Slope)|  .0050572  .0022578                .0021081    .012132
-----------+-----------------------------------------------
  cov(Inter~t,|
        Slope)|  .0060351  .0086904   0.69  0.487  -.0109977   .0230679
-----------+-----------------------------------------------
LR test of model vs. saturated: chi2(21) =   352.65, Prob > chi2 = 0.0000
```

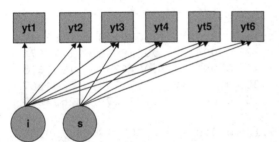

Figure 4.2 Schematic representation of the latent variable modelling framework. The six repeated measurements are represented by squares and the latent growth curve parameters (i and s) are represented by circles.

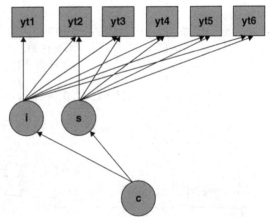

Figure 4.3 Schematic representation of the latent variable modelling framework. The six repeated measurements are represented by squares and the latent growth curve parameters (i and s) and the latent class variable (c) are represented by circles.

and colleagues (Muthén and Shedden, 1999; Muthén and Muthén, 2000; Muthén, 2004) and implemented in the Mplus software programme. As has been mentioned before, LCGMM can be seen as an extension of LCGA. The difference between the two methods has to do with the variation within a certain class. With LCGA this variation is set to zero, while for LCGMM this is not the case. This implies that the (optimal) number of classes derived from LCGA is always bigger than the (optimal) number of classes derived from LCGMM. Within LCGA, subjects with slightly different growth parameters are

sooner defined to a different class compared to LCGMM in which the growth parameters within a class are allowed to differ. To find the optimal number of classes, various methods are available. Probably the best way is a forward classifying method which starts with a one class solution (i.e. there are no subgroups; all individuals follow the same growth trajectory), then adding additional classes one at a time to investigate whether or not model fit becomes better due to the additional class. This method ends the moment the model fit does not improve any more. However, with this method, one has to be very careful. It could be that the solution that statistically optimally describes the data is a solution with one (or more) clinically uninterpretable classes, or with (a) class(es) with very few subjects. Both issues should be kept in mind when analysing the data with these classification methods.

Within medical science, creating groups with the same growth trajectory is increasingly popular these days. It is mostly used as a descriptive tool, but the trajectories are also used either as a determinant for future (health) outcomes or as an outcome variable in order to investigate potential predictors of these trajectories. However, it should be realised that both additional questions can be answered with different methods as well. Regarding the investigation of potential predictors for the development over time

in a certain outcome, it is not necessary to classify the population under study into several groups. The outcome variable itself can be analysed with a mixed model analysis. Regarding the relationship between different developments over time and future (health) outcomes, it is also not necessary to classify the population under study into several groups. Instead of using the categorical group variable as a determinant for future (health) outcomes, it is also possible to use the individual growth parameters as determinants. In general, it should be realised that classifying growth trajectories is mostly not the only solution to answer certain research questions (Twisk and Hoekstra, 2012; Twisk, 2014).

For detailed insight into the (complicated) mathematical background of the methods used to classify subjects with different growth trajectories one is referred to several fundamental papers (Muthén and Shedden, 1999; Nagin, 1999; Muthén and Muthén, 2000 ;Muthén, 2004; Jung and Wickrama, 2008; Muthén and Asparouhov, 2008; Feldman et al., 2009).

Chapter 5

Models to Disentangle the Between- and Within-subjects Relationship

5.1 Introduction

In Chapter 3, regression-based methods were introduced to analyse the longitudinal relationship between a continuous outcome variable and several covariates. One of the most difficult parts of longitudinal regression analysis is the interpretation of the regression coefficient. In Section 3.3.4 it was explained that the regression coefficient derived from longitudinal regression method is a weighted average of a between-subjects and a within-subjects relationship. Although this is an important strength of the analysis, it also limits the interpretation of the result in such a way that no separation can be made between the two aspects of the longitudinal relationship. In this chapter, a few alternative models will be discussed which aim to disentangle the between-subjects and the within-subjects part of the relationship or which aim to estimate only the within-subjects part of the relationship.

5.2 Hybrid Models

Hybrid models, which are also known as between-within models, are used to disentangle the between-subjects and within-subjects part of the longitudinal relationship (Curren and Bauer, 2001). The between-subjects part of the relationship can be estimated with the relationship between the mean value of the particular covariate for each subject and the repeatedly measured outcome variable (Equation 5.1). To obtain the within-subjects part of the relationship, the covariate can be centred around the mean of the particular subject (Equation 5.2). The difference between the observations at each time-point and the individual mean value is known as the deviation score. To obtain both the between- and within-subjects part of the relationship, a combination of Equation 5.1 and Equation 5.2 can be applied (Equation 5.3):

$$Y_{it} = \beta_0 + \beta_b \overline{X}_i + \varepsilon_{it} \tag{5.1}$$

$$Y_{it} = \beta_0 + \beta_w (X_{it} - \overline{X}_i) + \varepsilon_{it} \tag{5.2}$$

$$Y_{it} = \beta_0 + \beta_b \overline{X}_i + \beta_w (X_{it} - \overline{X}_i) + \varepsilon_{it} \tag{5.3}$$

where Y_{it} are observations of the outcome for subject i at time t, β_0 is the intercept, X_{it} are observations of the covariate for subject i at time t, β_b is the regression coefficient for the between-subjects part of the relationship, $\overline{X}_i$ is the mean value of the covariate for subject i, β_w is the regression coefficient for the within-subjects part of the relationship, and ε_{it} is the error for subject i at time t.

Because the mean value over time within a subject is not correlated with the subjects deviation score (the correlation equals zero) the regression coefficient reflecting the between-subjects relationship (Equation 5.1) and the regression coefficient reflecting the within-subjects relationship (Equation 5.2) are exactly the same as the comparable regression coefficients obtained from Equation 5.3.

5.2.1 Example

To apply the hybrid model to the example dataset (i.e. the longitudinal relationship between cholesterol and the sum of skinfolds), the mean value over time for the sum of skinfolds for each subject and the deviation score at each time-point for the sum of skinfolds has to be calculated (see Table 5.1).

Output 5.1 shows the result of the linear mixed model analysis between cholesterol and the individual mean value of the sum of skinfolds in order to obtain the between-subjects part of the relationship.

From Output 5.1 it can be seen that the between-subjects part of the relationship between cholesterol and the sum of skinfolds is somewhat higher than the overall relationship. The regression coefficient for the between-subjects part equals 0.2042728, while the overall regression coefficient (see Output 3.1) was equal to 0.1871179. In Chapter 3 it has already been mentioned that the overall regression coefficient is a weighted average of the between-subjects and within-subjects part of the relationship. This directly implies that the within-subjects part of the relationship must be less strong than the overall regression coefficient.

Table 5.1 Data structure needed for performing a hybrid model analysis

Id	Time	Covariate X	Mean_X	Deviation_X
1	1	3	5	−2
1	2	4	5	−2
1	3	5	5	0
1	4	5	5	0
1	5	6	5	1
1	6	7	5	2

Output 5.2 shows the result of the linear mixed model analysis between cholesterol and the deviation score of the sum of skinfolds in order to obtain the within-subjects part of the relationship.

From Output 5.2 it can indeed be seen that the within-subjects part of the relationship is slightly lower than the between-subjects part of the relationship, but that they are both very close to the overall relationship. This is, however, not always the case. There are examples in which the between-subjects part of the relationship has a different sign than the within-subjects part of the relationship. To illustrate that the variables reflecting the between-subjects part and the within-subjects part of the relationship are uncorrelated, Output 5.3 shows the result of the linear mixed model analysis between cholesterol and both the individual mean value and the deviation score of the sum of skinfolds.

Output 5.1 Results of a linear mixed model analysis to analyse the relationship between cholesterol and the individual mean value of the sum of skinfolds

```
Mixed-effects ML regression              Number of obs      =       882
Group variable: id                       Number of groups   =       147

                                         Obs per group:
                                                         min =         6
                                                         avg =       6.0
                                                         max =         6

                                         Wald chi2(1)       =     29.61
Log likelihood = -862.49535              Prob > chi2        =    0.0000

- - - - - - - - - - - - - - - - - - - - - - - - - - - - - - - - - - - - - - -
        chol |    Coef.   Std. Err.     z    P>|z|    [ 95% Conf. Interval]
- - - - - - - - - - - - - - - - - - - - - - - - - - - - - - - - - - - - - - -
  mean_skinf | .2042728   .037537    5.44   0.000    .1307017   .2778439
       _cons | 3.733461  .1484745   25.15   0.000    3.442456   4.024466
- - - - - - - - - - - - - - - - - - - - - - - - - - - - - - - - - - - - - - -


- - - - - - - - - - - - - - - - - - - - - - - - - - - - - - - - - - - - - - -
 Random-effects Parameters | Estimate Std. Err.   [ 95% Conf. Interval]
- - - - - - - - - - - - - - - - - - - -+- - - - - - - - - - - - - - - - - - -
id: Identity               |
              var(_cons)   |     .2878542 .0395184 .2199452  .3767304
- - - - - - - - - - - - - - - - - - - -+- - - - - - - - - - - - - - - - - - -
            var(Residual)  |     .3012036  .015712 .2719306  .3336279
- - - - - - - - - - - - - - - - - - - - - - - - - - - - - - - - - - - - - - -
LR test vs. linear model: chibar2(01) = 311.24    Prob >= chibar2 = 0.0000
```

Output 5.2 Results of a linear mixed model analysis to analyse the relationship between cholesterol and the deviation score of the sum of skinfolds

```
Mixed-effects ML regression            Number of obs     =        882
Group variable: id                     Number of groups  =        147

                                       Obs per group:
                                                         min =          6
                                                         avg =        6.0
                                                         max =          6

                                       Wald chi2(1)      =      74.31
Log likelihood = -840.58997            Prob > chi2       =     0.0000

- - - - - - - - - - - - - - - - - - - - - - - - - - - - - - - - - - - - - - -
      chol |    Coef.   Std. Err.      z    P>|z|   [ 95% Conf. Interval]
- - - - - - - - - - - - - - - - - - - - - - - - - - - - - - - - - - - - - - -
  dev_skinf | .1806347  .0209543    8.62    0.000   .1395651   .2217043
     _cons | 4.498141   .0525641   85.57    0.000   4.395117   4.601164
- - - - - - - - - - - - - - - - - - - - - - - - - - - - - - - - - - - - - - -


- - - - - - - - - - - - - - - - - - - - - - - - - - - - - - - - - - - - - - -
Random-effects Parameters |  Estimate  Std. Err.  [ 95% Conf. Interval]
- - - - - - - - - - - - - - - -+- - - - - - - - - - - - - - - - - - - - - - -
id: Identity              |
             var(_cons)   | .3605675   .047435    .2786157   .4666246
- - - - - - - - - - - - - - - -+- - - - - - - - - - - - - - - - - - - - - - -
         var(Residual)    | .2735468   .0142693   .2469617   .3029938
- - - - - - - - - - - - - - - - - - - - - - - - - - - - - - - - - - - - - - -
LR test vs. linear model: chibar2(01) = 420.05    Prob >= chibar2 = 0.0000
```

From Output 5.3 it can be seen that the regression coefficients from the analysis with both variables are exactly the same as the regression coefficients obtained from the two separate analyses.

The hybrid model can be extended with a random slope, but this can only be done for the within-subjects part of the relationship (i.e. the deviation score). The variable reflecting the between-subjects part of the relationship (i.e. the individual mean value) is not changing over time and therefore measured on subject level. Because of that, it is not possible to add a random slope for the individual mean value to the model. Output 5.4 shows the result of a hybrid model including a random slope for the deviation score.

As with all mixed model analyses, the necessity of the random slope for the deviation score can be evaluated by comparing the −2 log likelihood of the model with only a random intercept with the −2 log likelihood of the model with a random intercept, a random slope for the deviation score and the covariance between the random intercept and random slope. This difference equals 10.7, which is statistically significant on a Chi-square distribution with two degrees of freedom. So, the final result of this (hybrid) analysis can be derived from the analysis with a random intercept and a random slope for the deviation score shown in Output 5.4.

5.2.2 Direct Estimation of the Hybrid Model

It was already mentioned that the between-subjects part of the relationship is basically nothing more than the relationship between the mean value of the particular covariate for each subject and the time dependent outcome variable. To obtain the within-subjects part of the relationship, the covariate has to be centred around the mean of the

Output 5.3 Results of a linear mixed model analysis to analyse the relationship between cholesterol and both the individual mean value and the deviation score of the sum of skinfolds

```
Mixed-effects ML regression              Number of obs     =        882
Group variable: id                       Number of groups  =        147

                                         Obs per group:
                                                       min =          6
                                                       avg =        6.0
                                                       max =          6

                                         Wald chi2(2)      =     103.93
Log likelihood = -827.10007              Prob > chi2       =     0.0000

- - - - - - - - - - - - - - - - - - - - - - - - - - - - - - - - - - - - -
       chol |     Coef.   Std. Err.      z   P>|z|   [ 95% Conf. Interval]
- - - - - - - - - - - - - - - - - - - - - - - - - - - - - - - - - - - - -
 mean_skinf | .2042728    .037537    5.44   0.000    .1307017   .2778439
  dev_skinf | .1806347   .0209543    8.62   0.000    .1395651   .2217043
      _cons | 3.733461   .1484745   25.15   0.000    3.442456   4.024466
- - - - - - - - - - - - - - - - - - - - - - - - - - - - - - - - - - - - -


- - - - - - - - - - - - - - - - - - - - - - - - - - - - - - - - - - - - -
Random-effects Parameters | Estimate  Std. Err.  [ 95% Conf. Interval]
- - - - - - - - - - - - - - - - - -+- - - - - - - - - - - - - - - - - - -
id: Identity              |
            var(_cons) | .2924636  .0395032      .2244397  .3811044
- - - - - - - - - - - - - - - - - -+- - - - - - - - - - - - - - - - - - -
          var(Residual) | .2735468  .0142693      .2469617  .3029938
- - - - - - - - - - - - - - - - - - - - - - - - - - - - - - - - - - - - -
LR test vs. linear model: chibar2(01) = 346.82    Prob >= chibar2 = 0.0000
```

particular subject. The difference between the observations at each time-point and the individual mean value is known as the deviation score and reflects the within-subjects part of the longitudinal relationship. In Section 5.2.1 both variables were calculated and analysed with a linear mixed model analysis. In STATA it is, however, also possible to obtain the between- and within-subjects part of the longitudinal relationship directly with the *xtreg* procedure. Basically, the *xtreg* procedure is a linear mixed model analysis with only a random intercept. When *fe* is added to the *xtreg* procedure, the within-subjects part of the relationship is estimated, while with *be*, the *xtreg* procedure provides the between-subjects part of the relationship. It should be noted that *fe* stands for fixed effect. This is rather confusing, because in Section 3.3.3 it was mentioned that within mixed model analysis a distinction is made between the fixed part of the

regression model and the random part of the regression model. The fixed part of the regression model is the part in which the regression coefficients are given, while the random part of the model contains the random variances and the residual variance. It should be realised that in other research fields, such as econometrics, the fixed effect model refers to a model in which the within-subjects part of the longitudinal relationship is estimated (Imlach Gunasekara et al., 2014).

To illustrate the use of the *xtreg* procedures, the example used in Section 5.2.1 (i.e. the longitudinal relationship between cholesterol and sum of skinfolds) will be reanalysed with the *xtreg* procedure. Output 5.5 shows the result of the *xtreg* procedure to analyse the between-subjects part of the relationship, while Output 5.6 shows the result of the *xtreg* procedure to analyse the within-subjects part of the relationship.

Output 5.4 Results of a linear mixed model analysis to analyse the relationship between cholesterol and both the individual mean value and the deviation score of the sum of skinfolds with a random slope for the deviation score

```
Mixed-effects ML regression          Number of obs     =      882
Group variable: id                   Number of groups  =      147

                                     Obs per group:
                                                   min =        6
                                                   avg =      6.0
                                                   max =        6

                                     Wald chi2(2)      =    77.30
Log likelihood = -821.74781          Prob > chi2       =   0.0000
-------------------------------------------------------------------
      chol |      Coef.   Std. Err.      z    P>|z|   [ 95% Conf. Interval]
-----------+-------------------------------------------------------
mean_skinf |   .2086209   .0374826    5.57   0.000    .1351564   .2820854
 dev_skinf |    .193318   .0278516    6.94   0.000    .1387299   .2479061
     _cons |   3.717184   .1482824   25.07   0.000    3.426556   4.007812
-------------------------------------------------------------------


-------------------------------------------------------------------
Random-effects Parameters |  Estimate  Std. Err.   [ 95% Conf. Interval]
--------------------------+----------------------------------------
  id: Unstructured        |
            var(dev_sk~f) |   .029545   .0129097    .0125473   .0695692
             var(_cons)   |  .2961119   .0395121    .2279683   .3846247
     cov(dev_sk~f, _cons) |  .0108371   .0166647   -.0218251   .0434993
--------------------------+----------------------------------------
            var(Residual) |  .2518422   .0143999    .2251429   .2817077
-------------------------------------------------------------------
 LR test vs. linear model: chi2(3) = 357.53         Prob > chi2 = 0.0000
```

From Output 5.5 and Output 5.6, it can be seen that the two regression coefficients are exactly the same as the regression coefficients obtained from the hybrid mixed model analysis shown in Output 5.4. The standard errors, however, are slightly different between the two procedures as well as the random intercept variance and the residual variance. It can further be seen that the *xtreg* procedure provides some additional information which is not provided by the standard linear mixed model analyses with the mean value and the deviation score. This additional information includes the explained variances of the between-subjects part and the within-subjects part of the relationship, an estimation of the residual standard deviation and the correlation

between the regression coefficient for the within-subjects part of the relationship and the corresponding random effect. However, this additional information is not very relevant for a proper interpretation of the result.

5.2.3 Hybrid Models with Categorical Time-dependent Covariates

In the example used in this chapter, the sum of skinfolds was the continuous time-dependent covariate of interest. It has been shown that in this case it is relatively easy to calculate the variables used for the hybrid model analysis (i.e. the individual mean value and the deviation score). However, when the covariate of interest is categorical,

Output 5.5 Results of a direct estimation of the between-subjects relationship to analyse the relationship between cholesterol and the sum of skinfolds

```
Between regression (regression on group means)   Number of obs     =    882
Group variable: id                               Number of groups  =    147

R-sq:                                            Obs per group:
  within  = 0.0918                                          min =      6
  between = 0.1677                                          avg =    6.0
  overall = 0.1383                                          max =      6

                                                 F(1,145)          =  29.21
sd(u_i + avg(e_i.)) = .5854208                   Prob > F          = 0.0000

------------------------------------------------------------------------
   chol |      Coef.  Std. Err.      t    P>|t|    [95% Conf. Interval]
--------+---------------------------------------------------------------
  skinf |   .2042728   .037795    5.40   0.000     .1295726   .278973
  _cons |   3.733461   .1494949  24.97   0.000     3.43799   4.028932
------------------------------------------------------------------------
```

the situation is slightly more complex. Especially when the time-dependent covariate of interest consists of more than two groups. In that case, it is not possible to calculate the between- and within-subjects variables and therefore, it is necessary to use the direct estimation of the hybrid model, which was discussed in Section 5.2.2. To illustrate this, the time-dependent covariate used in the earlier examples (sum of skinfolds) is divided into three equally sized groups at each time-point (tertiles) in order to create a time-dependent categorical covariate. First a standard linear mixed model analysis was performed to analyse the overall relationship between cholesterol and tertiles of the sum of skinfolds. Output 5.7 shows the result of this analysis.

From Output 5.7 it can be seen that there are two regression coefficients for the sum of skinfolds. The first one (0.1728317) reflects the difference in cholesterol on average over time between subjects with a sum of skinfolds in the second tertile compared to the subjects with a sum of skinfolds in the first tertile. The second regression coefficient for the sum of skinfolds (0.335043) reflects the difference in cholesterol on average over time between subjects with a sum of skinfolds in the third tertile compared to the subjects with a sum of skinfolds in the first tertile. Because the categorical sum of skinfolds variable is time-dependent, both coefficients are a combination

of the between-subjects part of the relationship and the within-subjects part of the relationship. To estimate both parts of the relationship separately, two direct hybrid model analyses should be performed with the *xtreg* procedure. Output 5.8 shows the result of the linear mixed model analysis to obtain the between-subjects part of the relationship between cholesterol and tertiles of the sum of skinfolds, while Output 5.9 shows the result of the linear mixed model analysis to obtain the within-subjects part of this relationship.

From the two outputs with the between- and within-subjects parts of the relationship it can be seen that the overall relationship between cholesterol and the tertiles of the sum of skinfolds is mostly driven by the between-subjects part of the relationship and less by the within-subjects part of the relationship.

When the time-dependent covariate of interest is dichotomous, it is possible to calculate the two variables used for the hybrid model analysis and use them for estimating the between- and within-subjects part of the relationship. It should, however, be realised that the calculated variables, i.e. the individual mean over time and the deviation score, are not dichotomous anymore (see Table 5.2). Nevertheless, the result obtained from the linear mixed model analysis with the two calculated variables will be identical to the direct estimation of the two regression coefficients with the *xtreg* procedure.

Output 5.6 Results of a direct estimation of the within-subjects relationship to analyse the relationship between cholesterol and the sum of skinfolds

```
Fixed-effects (within) regression        Number of obs     =      882
Group variable: id                       Number of groups  =      147

R-sq:                                     Obs per group:
     within  = 0.0918                                       min =        6
     between = 0.1677                                        avg =      6.0
     overall = 0.1383                                        max =        6

                                          F(1,734)          =    74.21
corr(u_i, Xb)  = 0.0433                   Prob > F          =   0.0000


- - - - - - - - - - - - - - - - - - - - - - - - - - - - - - - - - - - - - - -
      chol |    Coef.   Std. Err.      t    P>|t|    [ 95% Conf. Interval]
- - - - - -+- - - - - - - - - - - - - - - - - - - - - - - - - - - - - - - - -
     skinf | .1806347   .0209685    8.61   0.000    .1394692    .2218001
     _cons | 3.821948   .0804481   47.51   0.000    3.664013    3.979884
- - - - - -+- - - - - - - - - - - - - - - - - - - - - - - - - - - - - - - - -
   sigma_u | .58419889
   sigma_e | .52337321
       rho | .5547529  (fraction of variance due to u_i)
- - - - - - - - - - - - - - - - - - - - - - - - - - - - - - - - - - - - - - -
F test that all u_i=0: F(146, 734) = 7.46              Prob > F = 0.0000
```

5.2.4 Comments

It should be realised that a hybrid model only makes sense when the covariate of interest is time-dependent. When the covariate is time-independent, which is for instance the case for sex in the example used throughout the book, the regression coefficient has only a between-subjects interpretation.

It is argued that the use of hybrid models to disentangle the between- and within-subjects part of the relationship in longitudinal studies only holds when the time-dependent covariate is not increasing or decreasing over time. When the time-dependent covariate is changing over time, it is argued that the deviation score must not be calculated around the individual mean value but that it should be calculated around the individual regression line with time. Furthermore, when the data is unbalanced, i.e. when the time period and the number of repeated measurements is different for different subjects, also the between-subjects part of the relationship should be calculated in a different way, i.e. the between-subjects part of the relationship should be captured with the intercept

of an individual regression line with time when time is centred around the grand mean (Curran and Bauer, 2001). Although the calculation of the individual regression line and the deviation from that line makes sense, a comparable result may be obtained from a hybrid model adjusted for time, which is much easier to perform. See Chapter 4 for a detailed discussion of the use of the time variable in longitudinal data analysis.

5.3 Models to Estimate the Within-subjects Part of the Longitudinal Relationship

5.3.1 Introduction

As mentioned before, the standard longitudinal regression model pools together between-subjects and within-subjects relationships. In Section 5.2, hybrid models were introduced as an elegant way to disentangle the between- and within-subjects part of the relationship. Before hybrid models were introduced within medical science, other alternative models were used. These alternative

Output 5.7 Results of a linear mixed model analysis to analyse the relationship between cholesterol and tertiles of the sum of skinfolds

```
Mixed-effects ML regression              Number of obs      =        882
Group variable: id                       Number of groups  =        147

                                         Obs per group:
                                                         min =          6
                                                         avg =        6.0
                                                         max =          6

                                         Wald chi2(2)      =      20.76
Log likelihood = -866.13569              Prob > chi2       =     0.0000
```

```
----------------------------------------------------------------------
     chol |     Coef.   Std. Err.      z    P>|z|    [ 95% Conf. Interval]
----------+-----------------------------------------------------------
 skinf_ter |
        2 |  .1728317   .0615525    2.81    0.005    .0521911   .2934723
        3 |   .335043   .0735408    4.56    0.000    .1909058   .4791802
          |
     _cons |  4.329033   .0640156   67.62    0.000    4.203565   4.454501
----------------------------------------------------------------------
```

```
----------------------------------------------------------------------
Random-effects Parameters  | Estimate  Std. Err.  [ 95% Conf. Interval]
---------------------------+------------------------------------------
    id: Identity           |
           var(_cons)      | .3111541  .0428257    .2375857   .4075029
---------------------------+------------------------------------------
          var(Residual)    | .3002016  .0157034    .2709487   .3326127
----------------------------------------------------------------------
LR test vs. linear model: chibar2(01) = 322.27   Prob >= chibar2 = 0.0000
```

models did not intend to disentangle the between-subjects and the within-subjects part of the relationship, but rather to estimate only the within-subjects part of the relationship. In the next sections of this chapter, two of those alternative models (i.e. the model of changes and the auto-regressive model) will be discussed.

5.3.2 Model of Changes

With the model of changes, it is not the actual observed values at each time-point that are modelled, but the differences between two consecutive measurements of both the outcome and the covariates (Equation 5.4):

$$(Y_{it} - Y_{it-1}) = \beta_0 + \beta_1(X_{it} - X_{it-1}) + \varepsilon_{it} \quad (5.4)$$

where Y_{it} are observations of the outcome for subject i at time t, Y_{it-1} are observations of the outcome for subject i at time $t-1$, β_0 is the intercept, X_{it} are observations of the covariate for subject i at time t, X_{it-1} are observations of the covariate for subject i at time $t-1$, β_1 is the regression coefficient for the covariate and ε_{it} is the error for subject i at time t.

Table 5.3 shows the data structure needed to perform a model of changes.

5.3.2.1 Example

Output 5.10 shows the result of the model of changes to analyse the relationship between cholesterol and the sum of skinfolds.

From Output 5.10 it can be seen that the regression coefficient for the change in sum of skinfolds

Output 5.8 Results of a direct estimation of the between-subjects relationship to analyse the relationship between cholesterol and tertiles of the sum of skinfolds

```
Between regression (regression on group means) Number of obs    =    882
Group variable: id                              Number of groups =    147

  R-sq:                                         Obs per group:
    within  = 0.0067                                        min =      6
    between = 0.1569                                        avg =    6.0
    overall = 0.0845                                        max =      6

                                                F(2,144)          =  13.40
sd(u_i + avg(e_i.))= .5912291                   Prob > F          = 0.0000

- - - - - - - - - - - - - - - - - - - - - - - - - - - - - - - - - - - - - - - - -
      chol |   Coef.    Std. Err.    t    P>|t|    [ 95% Conf. Interval]
- - - - - -+- - - - - - - - - - - - - - - - - - - - - - - - - - - - - - - - - - -
 skinf_ter |
         2 | .3093071   .1752555   1.76   0.080    -.0370986     .6557128
         3 | .7284806   .1408016   5.17   0.000     .4501757    1.006786
           |
      _cons | 4.152687  .1003059  41.40   0.000     3.954424    4.350949
- - - - - - - - - - - - - - - - - - - - - - - - - - - - - - - - - - - - - - - - -
```

equals 0.0736776. This indicates that for each unit of change in the sum of skinfolds there is (on average over time) a change of 0.0736776 units in cholesterol. Because the coefficient deals with changes in both the outcome and the covariate it is believed that this coefficient only reflects the within-subjects part of the longitudinal relationship between cholesterol and the sum of skinfolds. This is, however, not totally true, because the estimated regression coefficient also has a between-subjects part and a within-subjects part interpretation.

An interesting finding is the magnitude of the random intercept variance, which is shown in the random part of the model of changes. This variance is about zero, which indicates that there is basically no need to adjust for the dependency of the repeated observations within the subject. The reason for this phenomenon is that in the model of changes a different outcome is used, i.e. the changes in cholesterol between subsequent measurements. In most situations, changes between subsequent measurements are not positively correlated with each other and therefore, there is basically no need for using a mixed model analysis. To illustrate this, Output 5.11 shows the observed correlation matrix for the changes between subsequent measurements in cholesterol.

The issue of these non-positive correlations in the outcome also holds for generalised estimating equations (GEE) analysis. In Section 3.4 it was mentioned that within GEE analysis an adjustment is made for the correlated observations by directly estimating the correlation between the repeated measurements. This was done by assuming a priori a certain correlation structure. One of the options to choose from was the independent structure. An independent correlation structure seemed a bit strange, because the general idea of a longitudinal regression method is to adjust for the positive correlations between the repeated observations within the subject. However, when the changes between subsequent measurements are modelled, probably the best option for the GEE analysis is the independent correlation structure. Output 5.12 shows the result of this analysis.

Because there is no missing data in the example dataset, the regression coefficient for the change in sum of skinfolds obtained from the linear GEE analysis is exactly the same as the regression coefficient obtained from the linear mixed model analysis. The difference between the two methods is the higher standard error estimated with the GEE analysis. It has previously been explained in Section 3.4 that this has to do

Output 5.9 Results of a direct estimation of the within-subjects relationship to analyse the relationship between cholesterol and tertiles of the sum of skinfolds

```
Fixed-effects (within) regression          Number of obs     =      882
Group variable: id                         Number of groups  =      147

  R-sq:                                    Obs per group:
    within  = 0.0070                                    min =        6
    between = 0.1555                                    avg =      6.0
    overall = 0.0845                                    max =        6

                                           F(2,733)          =     2.58
corr(u_i, Xb) = 0.2545                     Prob > F          =   0.0768


- - - - - - - - - - - - - - - - - - - - - - - - - - - - - - - - - - - - - - -
     chol |    Coef.    Std. Err.      t  P>|t|    [ 95% Conf. Interval]
- - - - - - - -+- - - - - - - - - - - - - - - - - - - - - - - - - - - - - - - -
skinf_ter |
        2 |  .1041232   .0675186   1.54  0.123   -.0284296    .2366761
        3 |  .1944942   .0857112   2.27  0.024    .0262255    .3627629
          |
    _cons |  4.398704   .0501076  87.79  0.000    4.300332    4.497075
- - - - - - - -+- - - - - - - - - - - - - - - - - - - - - - - - - - - - - - - -
  sigma_u |  .61593675
  sigma_e |  .54764707
      rho |  .55848764    (fraction of variance due to u_i)
- - - - - - - - - - - - - - - - - - - - - - - - - - - - - - - - - - - - - - -
F test that all u_i=0: F(146, 733) = 7.09               Prob > F = 0.0000
```

Table 5.2 Data structure needed for performing a hybrid model analysis with a dichotomous covariate

Id	Time	Covariate X	Mean_X	Deviation_X
1	1	0	0.33	−0.33
1	2	0	0.33	−0.33
1	3	0	0.33	−0.33
1	4	0	0.33	−0.33
1	5	1	0.33	0.67
1	6	1	0.33	0.67

with the robust estimation of the standard error which is used within GEE analysis.

5.3.2.2 Another Example

A very interesting example of the use of the model of changes has been given in a study also based on data from the Amsterdam Growth and Health Longitudinal Study (Twisk et al., 1998). The purpose of that study was to investigate the longitudinal relationship between two lung function parameters: forced vital capacity (FVC) and forced expiratory volume in one second (FEV1) and smoking behaviour. One of the characteristics of these lung function parameters is that, in a relatively healthy population, these parameters are highly influenced by anthropometrics. This indicates that the between-subjects variance of these parameters is high. On the other hand, because the population is relatively healthy, the within-subjects variance is relatively low. The result of the standard longitudinal regression analysis did not show a strong relationship between lung function parameters and smoking behaviour. Thinking about the theoretical relationship between lung function and smoking, finding a weak relationship between these two parameters seems to be very strange. However, taking into account the fact that the between-subjects variance is much higher than the within-subjects variance and also that the between-subjects part of the relationship is much

Table 5.3 Data structure needed for performing a model of changes[1]

Id	Time	Outcome Y	Covariate X	Change Y	Change X
1	1	3	3	1	−1
1	2	4	2	1	0
1	3	5	2	0	2
1	4	5	4	1	0
1	5	6	4	1	2
1	6	7	6	Na	Na

[1] Change is defined as the value at time t minus the value at $t - 1$.
Na = not applicable; these lines are not used in the analysis.

Output 5.10 Results of a linear mixed model analysis to analyse the relationship between the changes in cholesterol and the changes in the sum of skinfolds

```
Mixed-effects ML regression              Number of obs      =       735
Group variable: id                       Number of groups   =       147

                                         Obs per group:
                                                        min =         5
                                                        avg =       5.0
                                                        max =         5

                                         Wald chi2(1)      =     10.73
Log likelihood = -643.91558              Prob > chi2       =    0.0011

- - - - - - - - - - - - - - - - - - - - - - - - - - - - - - - - - - - -
     delchol |      Coef.  Std. Err.     z   P>|z|  [ 95% Conf. Interval]
- - - - - - -+- - - - - - - - - - - - - - - - - - - - - - - - - - - - - -
     delskinf | .0736776  .0224937   3.28  0.001   .0295907   .1177645
       _cons | .1241763   .021809   5.69  0.000   .0814315   .1669212
- - - - - - - - - - - - - - - - - - - - - - - - - - - - - - - - - - - -


- - - - - - - - - - - - - - - - - - - - - - - - - - - - - - - - - - - -
 Random-effects Parameters |  Estimate  Std. Err.  [ 95% Conf. Interval]
- - - - - - - - - - - - - - -+- - - - - - - - - - - - - - - - - - - - - -
id: Identity                |
            var(_cons) |  2.80e-25  1.08e-24    1.46e-28   5.38e-22
- - - - - - - - - - - - - - -+- - - - - - - - - - - - - - - - - - - - - -
           var(Residual)  | .3376566  .0176136    .3048407   .3740052
- - - - - - - - - - - - - - - - - - - - - - - - - - - - - - - - - - - -
LR test vs. linear model: chibar2(01) = 0.00      Prob >= chibar2 = 1.0000
```

weaker than the within-subjects part of the relationship, it is not surprising that the pooled longitudinal regression coefficient is relatively small. It has already been stated that the pooled regression coefficient is a weighted average of the between-subjects relationship and the within-subjects relationship. The weighing of the two coefficients is related to the between-subjects and the within-

Output 5.11 Observed correlation matrix of the changes between subsequent measurements in cholesterol

```
         | delchol1  delchol2  delchol3  delchol4  delchol5
---------+--------------------------------------------------
delchol1 |  1.0000
delchol2 | -0.3473    1.0000
delchol3 |  0.0984   -0.4385    1.0000
delchol4 | -0.1393   -0.0374   -0.2804    1.0000
delchol5 | -0.0420    0.0003   -0.0037   -0.3501    1.0000
```

Output 5.12 Results of a linear GEE analysis with an independent correlation structure to analyse the relationship between the changes in cholesterol and the changes in the sum of skinfolds

```
GEE population-averaged model          Number of obs      =        735
Group variable:                id      Number of groups   =        147
Link:                    identity      Obs per group:
Family:                  Gaussian                              min =          5
Correlation:          independent                              avg =        5.0
                                                               max =          5
                                       Wald chi2(1)       =       6.72
Scale parameter:        .3376566       Prob > chi2        =     0.0095

Pearson chi2(735):        248.18       Deviance           =     248.18
Dispersion (Pearson):   .3376566       Dispersion         =   .3376566

                              (Std. Err. adjusted for clustering on id)
----------------------------------------------------------------------
          |              Robust
  delchol |     Coef.   Std. Err.      z   P>|z|   [ 95% Conf. Interval]
----------+-----------------------------------------------------------
 delskinf | .0736776   .0284147    2.59   0.010    .0179859   .1293693
    _cons | .1241763   .0150948    8.23   0.000    .0945911   .1537616
----------------------------------------------------------------------
```

subjects variances. Regarding lung function in this relatively healthy population, the between-subjects variance is much higher than the within-subjects variance, and the between-subjects part of the relationship is weighted much higher than the within-subjects part of the relationship. Having a very weak between-subjects relationship will lead to a weak overall relationship. So, based on this, it is not surprising that the standard longitudinal regression analysis did not show a strong longitudinal relationship between lung function parameters and smoking behaviour. The next step in the analysis was not to model the actual values of lung function at the different time-points, but rather the changes in lung function between subsequent

measurements. It should be noted that in this model the changes in smoking behaviour were not modelled but smoking behaviour was measured at $t - 1$. Table 5.4 shows the results of both analyses.

From Table 5.4 it can be seen that the model of changes revealed a strong inverse longitudinal relationship between both lung function parameters and smoking behaviour. So, although the values of the lung function parameters were not influenced by smoking behaviour, the changes in lung function parameters over time were highly influenced by smoking behaviour. This example illustrates that the modelling of longitudinal data is more complicated than the modelling of cross-sectional data.

Table 5.4 Standardised regression coefficients and 95% confidence intervals regarding the longitudinal relationship between lung function parameters (forced vital capacity (FVC) and the forced expiratory volume in one second (FEV1)) and smoking behaviour; a comparison between the standard model and the model of changes

	FVC	FEV1
Standard model	− 0.03 (− 0.11 to 0.06)	− 0.01 (− 0.09 to 0.06)
Model of changes	− 0.13 (− 0.22 to − 0.04)**	− 0.14 (− 0.25 to − 0.04)**

** $p < 0.01$.

Table 5.5 Data structure needed for performing an autoregressive model

Id	Time	Outcome Y	Covariate X	Y at t-1	X at t-1
1	1	3	3	Na	Na
1	2	4	2	3	3
1	3	5	2	4	2
1	4	5	4	5	3
1	5	6	4	5	4
1	6	7	6	6	4

Na = not applicable; these lines are not used in the analysis.

5.3.3 Autoregressive Model

Another way in which to remove the between-subjects part of the relationship is to use an autoregressive model. Autoregressive models are also known as Markov models, conditional models or transition models, and an extensive amount of literature has been devoted to these types of models (Rosner et al., 1985; Rosner and Munoz, 1988; Zeger and Qaqish, 1988). The autoregression indicates that the outcome is regressed on the outcome itself, measured one time-point earlier (Equation 5.5):

$$Y_{it} = \beta_0 + \beta_1 X_{it-1} + \beta_2 Y_{it-1} + \varepsilon_{it} \qquad (5.5)$$

where Y_{it} are observations of the outcome for subject i at time t, β_0 is the intercept, X_{it-1} are observations of the covariate for subject i at time $t − 1$, β_1 is the regression coefficient for the covariate, Y_{it-1} are observations of the outcome for subject i at time $t − 1$, β_2 is the autoregression coefficient, and ε_{it} is the error for subject i at time t.

In the autoregressive model shown in Equation 5.5 it can be seen that the value of the outcome variable at time t is related not only to the value of the outcome variable at $t − 1$, but also to the value of the covariate at $t − 1$. This makes sense because basically the autoregressive model deals with the changes in the outcome variable. This can be seen when Y_{it-1} is taken to the other side of the equation. The outcome then becomes $Y_{it} − \beta_2 Y_{it-1}$, which can be seen as a sort of adjusted change in the outcome variable between the two measurements. Knowing this, it makes sense that also the covariate measured at $t − 1$ is used in the analysis. The covariate at $t − 1$ is related to the adjusted change in the outcome variable from $t − 1$ to time t.

The model shown in Equation 5.5 is called a first-order autoregressive model, because the outcome variable at time-point t is only related to the value of the outcome variable at $t − 1$. In a second-order or third-order autoregressive model, the outcome variable at time-point t is also related to the value of the outcome variable at $t − 2$ or $t − 3$. Because the value of an outcome variable at each measurement is primarily influenced by the value of this variable one measurement earlier, in practice the higher order autoregressive models are not much used.

Table 5.5 shows the data structure needed to perform an autoregressive analysis.

5.3.3.1 Example

Output 5.13 shows the result of the autoregressive analysis to analyse the relationship between cholesterol and the sum of skinfolds.

From Output 5.13 it can be seen that in the fixed part of the model there are now two covariates with corresponding regression coefficients. The first one is the regression coefficient for the sum of skinfolds measured at $t − 1$. The second one is the regression coefficient for the outcome variable cholesterol measured at $t − 1$. It has already been mentioned that because an adjustment is made in the autoregressive analysis for the outcome variable measured at $t − 1$, the outcome reflects the (adjusted) change in cholesterol between two subsequent measurements. This is only slightly different from the outcome used in the model of changes, and because of that, the autoregressive model is used to obtain an estimate of the within-subjects part of the relationship between (in this example) cholesterol and the sum of skinfolds. It

Output 5.13 Results of an autoregressive linear mixed model analysis to analyse the relationship between cholesterol and the sum of skinfolds

```
Mixed-effects ML regression            Number of obs     =       735
Group variable: id                     Number of groups  =       147

                                       Obs per group:
                                                    min =         5
                                                    avg =       5.0
                                                    max =         5

                                       Wald chi2(2)      =    940.28
Log likelihood = -607.7352             Prob > chi2       =    0.0000
```

---

chol	Coef.	Std. Err.	z	P>|z|	[95% Conf. Interval]
skinft_1	.1075459	.014569	7.38	0.000	.0789893 .1361025
cholt_1	.7575473	.0301444	25.13	0.000	.6984655 .8166291
_cons	.8040143	.1248782	6.44	0.000	.5592574 1.048771

Random-effects Parameters	Estimate	Std. Err.	[95% Conf. Interval]
id: Identity			
var(_cons)	3.87e-17	1.39e-16	3.38e-20 4.44e-14
var(Residual)	.3059983	.0159622	.2762591 .3389389

```
LR test vs. linear model: chibar2(01) = 2.3e-13   Prob >= chibar2 = 1.0000
```

should be realised, however, that in the present example, it is not the changes in the sum of skinfolds that are added as the covariate of interest, but the value of the sum of skinfolds at $t - 1$. So, the result of the autoregressive model cannot be (directly) compared to the results of the model of changes, which were reported in Section 5.3.2.1.

The random part of the model shows that the random intercept variance of the autoregressive model is almost zero. This seems to be strange, because the outcome variable in the autoregressive model is cholesterol measured at the different time-points. Table 3.1 showed the within-subjects correlations for cholesterol, which are far from zero. The reason why the random intercept variance is almost zero in the autoregressive model has to do with the fact that in longitudinal regression analysis an adjustment is made for the correlated residuals, rather than for the correlated observations. Although in most

situations the structure of the correlation between the observations is comparable to the structure of the correlation between the residuals, for an autoregressive model this is not the case. In an autoregressive model part of the correlation in the observations is explained by the addition of the outcome variable at $t - 1$ to the model. In an autoregressive model, the within-subjects correlation of the residuals is therefore different from the within-subjects correlation of the observations. Because the outcome variable at $t - 1$ is strongly related to the outcome variable at time t, almost all correlations between the observed values are explained by the same variable measured one time-point earlier. As a result, the random intercept variance of the autoregressive model is reduced to almost zero (see Section 3.6.3). This also implies that when an autoregressive model is analysed with GEE analysis an independent

Output 5.14 Results of an autoregressive linear GEE analysis with an independent correlation structure to analyse the relationship between cholesterol and the sum of skinfolds

```
GEE population-averaged model        Number of obs     =       735
Group variable:                 id   Number of groups  =       147
Link:                     identity   Obs per group:
Family:                   Gaussian                 min =         5
Correlation:           independent                 avg =       5.0
                                                    max =         5
                                     Wald chi2(2)      =   1181.72
Scale parameter:         .3059983    Prob > chi2       =    0.0000

Pearson chi2(735):          224.91   Deviance          =    224.91
Dispersion (Pearson):     .3059983   Dispersion        =  .3059983

                         (Std. Err. adjusted for clustering on id)
- - - - - - - - - - - - - - - - - - - - - - - - - - - - - - - - - - -
             |              Robust
      chol |     Coef.   Std. Err.     z   P>|z|   [95% Conf. Interval]
- - - - - - - + - - - - - - - - - - - - - - - - - - - - - - - - - - - -
  skinft_1 |  .1075459   .0150824   7.13  0.000    .0779849   .1371069
   cholt_1 |  .7575473   .0256546  29.53  0.000    .7072652   .8078294
      _cons |  .8040143   .1038861   7.74  0.000    .6004012   1.007627
- - - - - - - - - - - - - - - - - - - - - - - - - - - - - - - - - - -
```

correlation structure can be used. Output 5.14 shows the result of this analysis.

5.3.4 Comments

Although the magnitude of the regression coefficients for the different models cannot be interpreted in the same way, a comparison between the regression coefficients and standard errors of the different models shows directly that the results obtained from the different models are quite different. Using an alternative model (i.e. a model of changes or an autoregressive model) can lead to different conclusions than when using the standard model. On the one hand this is strange, because all analyses attempt to answer the question of whether there is a longitudinal relationship between a continuous outcome and a particular covariate. On the other hand, however, with the different models, different parts of the longitudinal relationships are analysed, and the results of the models should be interpreted in different ways. To obtain the best answer to the question of whether there is a longitudinal relationship between the outcome variable and a covariate, maybe the results of several models should

be combined (Twisk, 1997). In practice, however, this almost never happens: a priori the most appropriate model is chosen (usually the standard model), and only that result is reported.

It is sometimes suggested to use the model fit statistics to decide which model should be used. However, when deciding which model should be used to obtain the best answer to a particular research question, comparing the fit of the models will not provide much interesting information. First of all, in the model of changes and the autoregressive model, less observations are used than in the standard model. The problem is that the number of observations highly influences the likelihood of a particular analysis and therefore all model fit statistics. Secondly, looking at the fit of the models it is obvious that, for instance, an autoregressive model provides a much better fit than a standard model. This is due to the fact that a high percentage of variance of the outcome variable at time t is explained by the value of the outcome variable at $t - 1$. This can, for instance, be seen from the values of the scale parameter presented in the GEE output and the log likelihood presented in the output of the mixed model analysis. Both values are much lower in the autoregressive model than in the standard model. However, this does not mean that the autoregressive model should be used to obtain the best answer to the question of whether there is a longitudinal relationship between the outcome variable and the covariate. In general, it should be realised that it is better to base the choice of a specific longitudinal model on logical considerations instead of statistical ones.

It has already been mentioned that with the model of changes and with the autoregressive model an attempt is made to estimate only the within-subjects part of a relationship. It is therefore surprising that the results of the longitudinal analyses with the model of changes and the autoregressive model are quite different. One reason for the difference in results is that both alternative models use a different model of change. This can be explained by assuming

a longitudinal study with just two measurements. In the autoregressive model, $Y_2 = \beta_0 + \beta_1 Y_1$, while in the model of changes, $Y_2 - Y_1 = \beta_0$ (where β_0 is the difference between subsequent measurements), which is equal to $Y_2 = \beta_0 + Y_1$. The difference between the two equations is the coefficient β_1. In the model of changes the change is a fixed parameter, while in the autoregressive model the change is a function of the value of Y_1. Another reason for the difference in result between the model of changes and the autoregressive model is the different modelling of the covariate. It has already been mentioned that for the model of changes, the changes in the time-dependent covariate were also modelled. In the autoregressive model, however, the covariate measured at $t - 1$ was used. It is obvious that different modelling of the covariates (can) lead to a different result.

Causality in Observational Longitudinal Studies

6.1 Time-lag Models

It is assumed that the greatest advantage of a longitudinal study is that causal relationships can be detected. However, in fact this is only partly true for longitudinal intervention studies (see Chapter 10). In observational longitudinal studies in general, no answer can be given to the question whether a certain relationship is causal or not. With the standard models described in Chapter 3, it is only possible to detect longitudinal relationships between an outcome variable and one (or more) covariate(s). When there is some rationale about possible causation in observational longitudinal studies, these associations are called quasi-causal relationships. In every textbook a list of arguments can be found which can give an indication as to whether or not an observed relationship is causal (see Table 1.1). In Chapter 1, it was already mentioned that only one of these arguments is specific for a longitudinal study: the rule of temporality, i.e. a time sequence between the outcome variable and a particular covariate. With a small change in the standard models described in Chapter 3, this time sequence between the outcome variable and the covariate can be modelled. In this so-called time-lag model the covariate is modelled prior in time to the outcome variable (Equation 6.1):

$$Y_{it} = \beta_0 + \beta_1 X_{it-1} + \varepsilon_{it} \tag{6.1}$$

where Y_{it} are observations of the outcome for subject i at time t, β_0 is the intercept, X_{it-1} are observations of the covariate for subject i at $t - 1$, β_1 is the time-lag regression coefficient for the covariate X, and ε_{it} is the error for subject i at time t.

Table 6.1 shows the data structure needed to perform a time-lag model analysis.

6.1.1 Example

Figure 6.1 shows the path diagram which corresponds with the standard model and the time-lag model assuming six repeated measurements (i.e. comparable to the example dataset). In the example, cholesterol at time t is related to the sum of skinfolds at $t - 1$.

Output 6.1 shows the result of the linear mixed model time-lag analysis to analyse the relationship between cholesterol and the sum of skinfolds.

From the upper part of the output it can be seen that for each subject, five repeated measurements are used in the analysis. For cholesterol, the analysis includes the second to the sixth measurement, while for the sum of skinfolds, the analysis includes the first up to the fifth measurement (see Figure 6.1). In the fixed part of the model, the regression coefficient for the sum of skinfolds (at $t - 1$) is given. Comparable to the standard model explained in Chapter 3, it should be realised that the regression coefficient of a time-lag model also has a double interpretation. The coefficient is a weighted average of the between-subjects and the within-subjects relationship on average over time.

The coefficient obtained from the time-lag model cannot be compared directly with the coefficient obtained from the standard model in order to say something about a possible causal relationship between cholesterol and the sum of skinfolds.

Table 6.1 Data structure needed to perform a time-lag analysis

Id	Time	Outcome Y	Covariate X	X at t-1
1	1	3	3	Na
1	2	4	2	3
1	3	5	2	2
1	4	5	4	2
1	5	6	4	4
1	6	7	6	4

Na = not applicable; these lines are not used in the analysis.

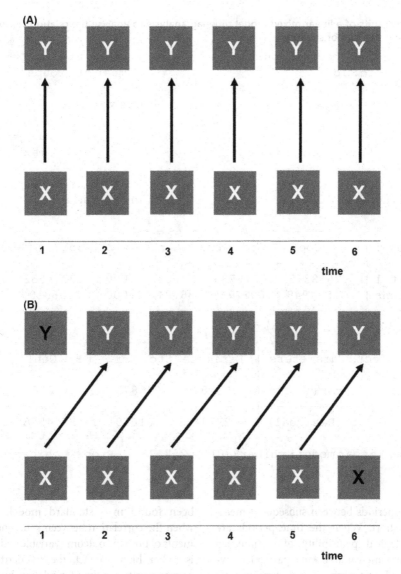

Figure 6.1 Path diagram for (A) a standard model and (B) a time-lag model with six repeated measurements. *Y* stands for the outcome variable and *X* stands for the covariate.

The reason why this direct comparison cannot be made is that in the standard model more observations are included than in the time-lag model. In order to make a proper comparison between the standard and the time-lag model, the standard model should be performed on the data gathered at the second till the sixth measurement for both cholesterol and the sum of skinfolds. Output 6.2 shows the result of this analysis.

From Output 6.2 it can be seen that the regression coefficient obtained from the standard model (only using the second to the sixth measurement) is smaller than the one obtained from the time-lag model (i.e. 0.21 versus 0.26). So, this may suggest

that there is a sort of time sequence in the observed relationship, which may suggest a causal relationship between cholesterol and the sum of skinfolds.

6.1.2 Comments

It has been mentioned before that the only difference between the time-lag model and the standard model is that the time-lag model takes into account the temporal sequence of a possible cause and effect. The question then arises: should a time-lag model be used in every situation in which a causal relationship is suspected? The answer to that question is no! In fact, a time-lag model can only be useful

Output 6.1 Results of a linear mixed model time-lag analysis to analyse the relationship between cholesterol and the sum of skinfolds

```
Mixed-effects ML regression              Number of obs    =      735
Group variable: id                       Number of groups =      147

                                         Obs per group:
                                                        min =        5
                                                        avg =      5.0
                                                        max =        5

                                         Wald chi2(1)     =   149.56
Log likelihood = -706.7596               Prob > chi2      =   0.0000

- - - - - - - - - - - - - - - - - - - - - - - - - - - - - - - - - - - - -
     chol |     Coef.   Std. Err.     z   P>|z|  [ 95% Conf. Interval]
- - - - - +- - - - - - - - - - - - - - - - - - - - - - - - - - - - - - -
 skinft_1 | .2638365  .0215735   12.23   0.000   .2215532   .3061198
    _cons | 3.544948  .0927765   38.21   0.000   3.363109   3.726786
- - - - - - - - - - - - - - - - - - - - - - - - - - - - - - - - - - - - -


- - - - - - - - - - - - - - - - - - - - - - - - - - - - - - - - - - - - -
 Random-effects Parameters |  Estimate  Std. Err.   [ 95% Conf. Interval]
id: Identity               |
            var(_cons) |   .292878   .0408732        .22279   .3850151
- - - - - - - - - - - - - - +- - - - - - - - - - - - - - - - - - - - - - -
          var(Residual) |   .2774438   .016191      .2474576   .3110638
- - - - - - - - - - - - - - - - - - - - - - - - - - - - - - - - - - - - -
LR test vs. linear model: chibar2(01) = 257.78   Prob >= chibar2 = 0.0000
```

when the time periods between subsequent measurements are short. When the time periods are long, the biological plausibility of a time lag between the outcome variable and a particular covariate is doubtful. Furthermore, sometimes a time lag is already taken into account in the way a particular covariate is measured. For instance, when a lifestyle parameter such as dietary intake or physical inactivity is used as covariate in relation to some sort of disease outcome, both lifestyle parameters are often measured by some method of retrospective recall (e.g. measurement of the average amount of dietary intake of a certain nutrient over the previous three months). In other words, when a time lag is included in the method of measuring the covariate, a statistical time-lag model is not necessary. In general, the usefulness of a time-lag model depends on the biological plausibility of a time lag in the relationship analysed.

It is also possible that the result of a time-lag model is a reflection of the result that would have been found in a standard model. This occurs when the correlation between subsequent measurements of both the outcome variable and the covariate is rather high. In fact, the standard relationship carries over to the time-lag relationship through the high correlation of the variables involved in the relationship investigated. Figure 6.2 illustrates this phenomenon.

6.2 Longitudinal Mediation Models

A statistical method often used to get insight into causal processes is mediation analysis. With mediation analysis, the relationship between the outcome and the covariate is decomposed into a direct effect and an indirect effect through a mediating variable. In the example used throughout the book, for example, the relationship between cholesterol and the sum of skinfolds can be mediated by physical fitness. Mediation analysis is therefore an important statistical tool for gaining insight into

Output 6.2 Results of a linear mixed model analysis to analyse the relationship between cholesterol and the sum of skinfolds without using the first measurement

```
Mixed-effects ML regression              Number of obs     =       735
Group variable: id                       Number of groups  =       147

                                         Obs per group:
                                                        min =         5
                                                        avg =       5.0
                                                        max =         5

                                         Wald chi2(1)      =    104.48
Log likelihood = -728.96267              Prob > chi2       =    0.0000


- - - - - - - - - - - - - - - - - - - - - - - - - - - - - - - - - - - -
    chol |    Coef.    Std. Err.     z    P>|z|  [ 95% Conf. Interval]
- - - - - +- - - - - - - - - - - - - - - - - - - - - - - - - - - - - - -
   skinf |  .2070161  .0202528   10.22   0.000   .1673213   .2467109
   _cons |  3.717839  .0918444   40.48   0.000   3.537827   3.897851
- - - - - - - - - - - - - - - - - - - - - - - - - - - - - - - - - - - -


- - - - - - - - - - - - - - - - - - - - - - - - - - - - - - - - - - - -
Random-effects Parameters | Estimate  Std. Err.   [ 95% Conf. Interval]
- - - - - - - - - - - - - - - +- - - - - - - - - - - - - - - - - - - - -
id: Identity              |
            var(_cons) |  .2911511  .0410835    .2208045   .3839096
- - - - - - - - - - - - - - - +- - - - - - - - - - - - - - - - - - - - -
         var(Residual) |  .2986698  .0174195    .2664073   .3348393
- - - - - - - - - - - - - - - - - - - - - - - - - - - - - - - - - - - -
LR test vs. linear model: chibar2(01) = 239.76    Prob >= chibar2 = 0.0000
```

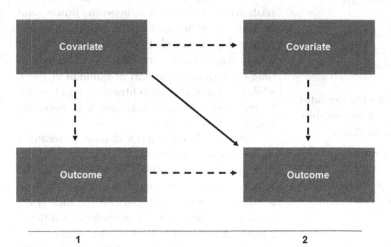

Figure 6.2 A time-lag relationship can be a reflection of the standard relationships when the correlation between subsequent measurements of both the outcome and the covariate is high.

the (causal) mechanisms of a particular relationship. There are a lot of statistical methods available to perform mediation analysis (Rijnhart et al., 2021), but the most simple way is to perform a pair of regression analyses. First, a regression analysis with the outcome and the covariate and second, the same regression analysis with the possible mediator added to the model. The regression coefficient for the covariate in the first analysis can be interpreted as the total effect and the regression coefficient for the covariate in the second analysis can be interpreted as the direct effect. The difference between the total effect and the direct effect can be interpreted as the indirect effect through the particular mediator.

Mediation analysis can be performed in cross-sectional studies, but it is obvious that longitudinal studies are more suitable to investigate mediation. In Section 6.1 the time-lag model was introduced to investigate a possible causal relationship between the outcome and the covariate. Within a longitudinal mediation study, a possible time lag between the covariate and the mediator and a possible time lag between the mediator and the outcome can be added to the longitudinal regression model. Assume a simple longitudinal mediation study, with an outcome variable, one covariate and one mediator. In that situation there are basically four mediation analyses that can be performed:

1. A contemporaneous relationship between the mediator and the covariate and a contemporaneous relationship between the outcome and the mediator.
2. A time-lag relationship between the mediator and the covariate and a contemporaneous relationship between the outcome and the mediator.
3. A contemporaneous relationship between the mediator and the covariate and a time-lag relationship between the outcome and the mediator.
4. A time-lag relationship between the mediator and the covariate and a time-lag relationship between the outcome and the mediator.

Figure 6.3 shows the four possible mediation models for a longitudinal study with six repeated measurements and Tables 6.2 to 6.5 show the data structures needed to analyse the four mediation models.

6.2.1 Example

In the example, the dataset with cholesterol and the sum of skinfolds is extended with a possible mediator, i.e. cardiopulmonary fitness. The fitness variable is measured as maximal oxygen uptake and expressed per kilogram bodyweight. Fitness is a time-dependent variable also measured at the six time-points and is the possible mediator in the relationship between cholesterol and the sum of skinfolds. In the first mediation model no time lags are included in the model, so contemporaneous relationships are modelled between cholesterol, fitness and sum of skinfolds. First the longitudinal relationship between cholesterol and the sum of skinfolds is analysed. This analysis was already performed in Chapter 3 and referred to as the standard model. Output 6.3a shows (again) the result of the linear mixed model analysis to analyse the relationship between cholesterol and the sum of skinfolds. Second, the same longitudinal analysis is performed, but now including fitness in the model. Output 6.3b shows the result of this analysis.

From Outputs 6.3a and 6.3b it can be seen that the regression coefficient for sum of skinfolds decreased from 0.1871179 to 0.0710136 when fitness is added to the model. So, based on these analyses it can be concluded that the total effect of sum of skinfolds on cholesterol equals 0.19 while the direct effect of sum of skinfolds on cholesterol equals 0.07. The indirect effect of sum of skinfolds on cholesterol through fitness can be calculated by the difference between the total effect and the direct effect; $0.19 - 0.07 = 0.12$. Because in the first longitudinal mediation analysis, no time lags are included, all observations of the six repeated measurements are used in the analyses (see Table 6.2).

In the second mediation model, a time-lag relationship is modelled between fitness and the sum of skinfolds, while a contemporaneous relationship is modelled between cholesterol and fitness. Again, in the first analysis, cholesterol at time t is related to the sum of skinfolds at $t - 1$, while in the second analysis fitness at time t is added to the model. Outputs 6.4a and 6.4b show the results of these analyses.

From Outputs 6.4a and 6.4b it can be seen that the regression coefficient for sum of skinfolds decreased from 0.2638365 to 0.1850714 when fitness is added to the model. So, based on these analyses it can be concluded that the total effect of sum of skinfolds at $t - 1$ on cholesterol at time t equals 0.26, while the direct effect of sum of skinfolds at $t - 1$ on cholesterol at time t equals 0.19. The indirect effect of sum of skinfolds at $t - 1$ on cholesterol at time t through fitness at time t can be calculated by the difference between the total effect and the direct effect; $0.26 - 0.19 = 0.07$. Because in the second longitudinal mediation analysis a time

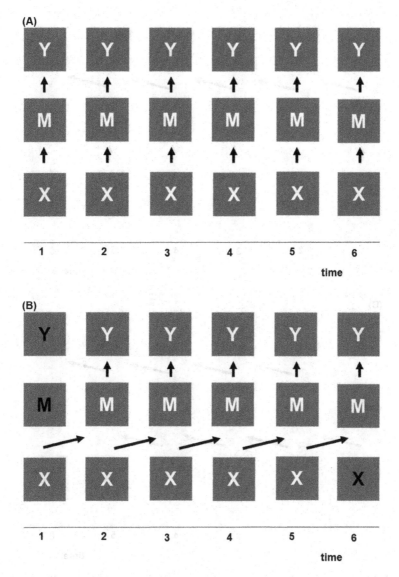

Figure 6.3 Four possible mediation models for a longitudinal study with six repeated measurements; (A) mediation model 1, (B) mediation model 2, (C) mediation model 3 and (D) mediation model 4. Y stands for the outcome, M stands for the mediator and X stands for the covariate.

lag is included for sum of skinfolds, five of the six repeated measurements are used in the analyses (see Table 6.3).

In the third mediation model, a contemporaneous relationship is modelled between fitness and the sum of skinfolds, while a time-lag relationship is modelled between cholesterol and fitness. Again, in the first analysis, cholesterol at time t is related to the sum of skinfolds at $t-1$. This analysis is exactly the same as the first analysis in the second mediation model (see Output 6.4a). The difference between the two mediations models is the

inclusion of the fitness variable. In the second mediation model, fitness at time t was added to the model, while in the third mediation model, in the second analysis fitness at $t-1$ is added to the model. Outputs 6.5a and 6.5b show the results of the two analyses for the longitudinal mediation model 3.

From Outputs 6.5a and 6.5b it can be seen that the regression coefficient for sum of skinfolds decreased from 0.2638365 to 0.1544256 when fitness is added to the model. So, based on these analyses it can be concluded that the total effect of

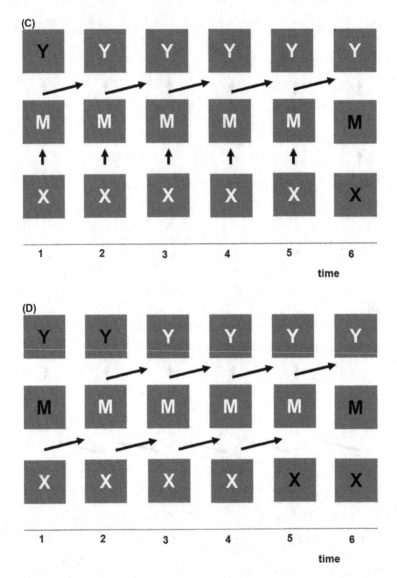

Figure 6.3 (*cont.*)

Table 6.2 Data structure needed to perform mediation model 1

Id	Time	Outcome Y	Covariate X	Mediator M
1	1	3	3	10
1	2	4	2	12
1	3	5	2	10
1	4	5	4	11
1	5	6	4	13
1	6	7	6	13

sum of skinfolds at $t-1$ on cholesterol at time t equals 0.26, while the direct effect of sum of skinfolds at $t-1$ on cholesterol at time t equals 0.15. The indirect effect of sum of skinfolds at $t-1$ on cholesterol at time t through fitness at $t-1$ can be calculated by the difference between the total effect and the direct effect; 0.26 – 0.15 = 0.11. Because in the third longitudinal mediation analysis a time lag is included for fitness, five of the six repeated measurements are used in the analyses (see Table 6.4).

In the fourth and last mediation model, a time-lag relationship is modelled between fitness and the sum of skinfolds, and a time-lag relationship is

Output 6.3a Results of a linear mixed model analysis to analyse the relationship between cholesterol and the sum of skinfolds (mediation model 1)

```
Mixed-effects ML regression              Number of obs      =        882
Group variable: id                       Number of groups   =        147

                                         Obs per group:
                                                        min =          6
                                                        avg =        6.0
                                                        max =          6

                                         Wald chi2(1)       =     103.88
Log likelihood = -830.19309              Prob > chi2        =     0.0000


- - - - - - - - - - - - - - - - - - - - - - - - - - - - - - - - - - - - - - -
      chol |    Coef.    Std. Err.      z   P>|z|     [ 95% Conf. Interval]
- - - - - - - +- - - - - - - - - - - - - - - - - - - - - - - - - - - - - - - -
     skinf |  .1871179   .018359    10.19  0.000      .1511349    .2231008
     _cons |  3.799312   .0838674   45.30  0.000      3.634935    3.963689
- - - - - - - - - - - - - - - - - - - - - - - - - - - - - - - - - - - - - - -


- - - - - - - - - - - - - - - - - - - - - - - - - - - - - - - - - - - - - - -
Random-effects Parameters  |  Estimate  Std. Err. [ 95% Conf. Interval]
- - - - - - - - - - - - - - - - -+- - - - - - - - - - - - - - - - - - - - - -
id: Identity               |
              var(_cons)   |  .293719   .0397034   .2253571    .3828185
- - - - - - - - - - - - - - - - -+- - - - - - - - - - - - - - - - - - - - - -
           var(Residual)   |  .2755989  .0143773   .2488127    .3052687
- - - - - - - - - - - - - - - - - - - - - - - - - - - - - - - - - - - - - - -
LR test vs. linear model: chibar2(01) = 345.41    Prob >= chibar2 = 0.0000
```

modelled between cholesterol and fitness. In this mediation model, in the first analysis, cholesterol at time t is related to the sum of skinfolds at $t - 2$, while in the second analysis fitness at $t - 1$ is added to the model. Outputs 6.6a and 6.6b show the results of the two analyses for the longitudinal mediation model 4.

From Outputs 6.6a and 6.6b it can be seen that the regression coefficient for sum of skinfolds decreased from 0.2762735 to 0.1672743 when fitness is added to the model. So, based on these analyses it can be concluded that the total effect of sum of skinfolds at $t - 2$ on cholesterol at time t equals 0.28, while the direct effect of sum of skinfolds at $t - 2$ on cholesterol at time t equals 0.17. The indirect effect of sum of skinfolds at $t - 2$ on cholesterol at time t through fitness at $t - 1$ can be calculated by the difference between the total effect and the direct effect; 0.28 − 0.17 = 0.11. Because in the fourth longitudinal mediation analysis two

time lags are included, only four of the six repeated measurements are used in the analyses (see Table 6.5).

In Table 6.6, the results of the four longitudinal mediation models are summarised.

Looking at the total effects of the sum of skinfolds on cholesterol, it seems that modelling a time lag between cholesterol and the sum of skinfolds makes sense. In fact, the strongest total effect has been found in the fourth mediation model, in which a double time-lag was modelled between cholesterol and the sum of skinfolds, However, the difference between the total effect of the sum of skinfolds with a single time lag is very small. Furthermore, it can be concluded that the relationship between cholesterol and the sum of skinfolds is strongly mediated by fitness. All indirect effects are relatively strong. Sometimes the indirect effects are expressed as a percentage

Output 6.3b Results of a linear mixed model mediation analysis to analyse the relationship between cholesterol, physical fitness and the sum of skinfolds (mediation model 1)

```
Mixed-effects ML regression                Number of obs      =      882
Group variable: id                         Number of groups   =      147

                                           Obs per group:
                                                         min =        6
                                                         avg =      6.0
                                                         max =        6

                                           Wald chi2(2)       =   187.01
Log likelihood = -791.79549                Prob > chi2        =   0.0000
```

chol	Coef.	Std. Err.	z	P>|z|	[95% Conf. Interval]	
skinf	.0710136	.021954	3.23	0.001	.0279845	.1140427
fitness	-.3271325	.0372392	-8.78	0.000	-.40012	-.2541449
_cons	5.909606	.2537431	23.29	0.000	5.412279	6.406934

Random-effects Parameters	Estimate	Std. Err.	[95% Conf. Interval]	
id: Identity				
var(_cons)	.3378504	.0448049	.2605195	.4381356
var(Residual)	.2429576	.0127082	.2192842	.2691868

```
LR test vs. linear model: chibar2(01) = 410.84    Prob >= chibar2 = 0.0000
```

of the total effect. When this is done in the present example, the percentages range from 27% to 63%. From the results it is not directly clear whether a time lag must be modelled between cholesterol and fitness. The results of the analyses with or without a time lag are more or less the same. By comparing the different models, it should be realised that the number of observations used in the different analyses are not the same. In the first longitudinal mediation model, all six repeated measurements are used in the analysis, in the second and third longitudinal mediation model, five of the six repeated measurements are used, while in the last longitudinal mediation model only four of the six repeated measurements are used. The different number of observations used in the different analyses also complicates the comparison of the models by model fit statistics, such as the Akaike (AIC) and Bayesian (BIC) information

criteria. Both are often used to compare models with each other and both can be seen as adjusted values of the −2 log likelihood, i.e. adjusted for the number of parameters estimated by the particular model (Akaike, 1974; Schwarz, 1978). However, due to the different number of observations used in the different models, a direct comparison of model fit statistics is not possible.

In the table showing an overview of the results (i.e. Table 6.6), only the effect estimates are given. This seems strange, because normally the 95% confidence intervals around the effect estimates and the corresponding *p*-values are also given. This has to do with the fact that for the indirect effects there is some discussion whether the methods that are normally used for estimating the standard errors give valid estimations (Loeys et al., 2015). For the total effect and the direct effect, the 95% confidence intervals can be found

Output 6.4a Results of a linear mixed model mediation analysis to analyse the relationship between cholesterol and the sum of skinfolds (mediation model 2)

```
Mixed-effects ML regression              Number of obs     =       735
Group variable: id                       Number of groups  =       147

                                         Obs per group:
                                                        min =         5
                                                        avg =       5.0
                                                        max =         5

                                         Wald chi2(1)      =    149.56
Log likelihood = -706.7596               Prob > chi2       =    0.0000


- - - - - - - - - - - - - - - - - - - - - - - - - - - - - - - - - - - - - -
        chol |     Coef.  Std. Err.      z   P>|z|  [ 95% Conf. Interval]
- - - - - - -+- - - - - - - - - - - - - - - - - - - - - - - - - - - - - - -
    skinft_1 | .2638365  .0215735   12.23  0.000   .2215532   .3061198
       _cons | 3.544948  .0927765   38.21  0.000   3.363109   3.726786
- - - - - - - - - - - - - - - - - - - - - - - - - - - - - - - - - - - - - -


- - - - - - - - - - - - - - - - - - - - - - - - - - - - - - - - - - - - - -
 Random-effects Parameters |  Estimate  Std. Err. [ 95% Conf. Interval]
- - - - - - - - - - - - - - -+- - - - - - - - - - - - - - - - - - - - - - -
id: Identity               |
              var(_cons)   | .292878   .0408732      .22279   .3850151
- - - - - - - - - - - - - - -+- - - - - - - - - - - - - - - - - - - - - - -
            var(Residual)  | .2774438  .016191     .2474576   .3110638
- - - - - - - - - - - - - - - - - - - - - - - - - - - - - - - - - - - - - -
LR test vs. linear model: chibar2(01) = 257.78   Prob >= chibar2 = 0.0000
```

in the outputs of the linear mixed model analyses. However, for the indirect effect either the Sobel formula or bootstrap methods can be used. Unfortunately, both methods lead to much smaller confidence intervals than observed for the total effect and the direct effect. This is unusual, because the number of observations and the standard deviation of the variables used in the analyses are the same in all estimations. Therefore, the width of the confidence intervals for the three effects should be more or less the same.

Although fitness seems to mediate the relationship between cholesterol and the sum of skinfolds, it does not mean directly that there is a causal relationship between cholesterol, fitness and the sum of skinfolds. Looking at the example, it is also possible that the relationship is the other way round, i.e. the relationship between cholesterol and fitness is mediated by the sum of skinfolds. To illustrate this, the longitudinal mediation

models 1 and 2 were analysed the other way round. In the first mediation model, all relationships were assumed to be contemporaneous without a time lag, while in the second model the relationship between the sum of skinfolds and fitness is assumed to be contemporaneous, while the relationship between cholesterol and the sum of skinfolds and between cholesterol and fitness are assumed to have a time lag. Outputs 6.7a and 6.7b show the result of the longitudinal mediation analysis in which no time lags were modelled, while Outputs 6.8a and 6.8b show the result of the longitudinal mediation analysis in which a time lag is modelled for the relationship between cholesterol and the sum of skinfolds and between cholesterol and fitness, and no time lag for the relationship between the sum of skinfolds and fitness.

From the outputs it can be seen that the magnitude of the mediation by the sum of skinfolds regarding the relationship between cholesterol and

Output 6.4b Results of a linear mixed model mediation analysis to analyse the relationship between cholesterol, physical fitness and the sum of skinfolds (mediation model 2)

```
Mixed-effects ML regression              Number of obs     =      735
Group variable: id                       Number of groups  =      147

                                         Obs per group:
                                                        min =        5
                                                        avg =      5.0
                                                        max =        5

                                         Wald chi2(2)      =   175.82
Log likelihood = -696.17557              Prob > chi2       =   0.0000

- - - - - - - - - - - - - - - - - - - - - - - - - - - - - - - - - - - - - - - - -
         chol |     Coef.  Std. Err.      z  P>|z|  [ 95% Conf. Interval]
- - - - - - - -+- - - - - - - - - - - - - - - - - - - - - - - - - - - - - - - - -
     skinft_1 |  .1850714  .0273432    6.77  0.000   .1314797    .238663
   fitnesst_1 | -.2303257  .0486844   -4.73  0.000  -.3257453  -.1349061
        _cons |  5.042304  .3311341   15.23  0.000   4.393293   5.691315
- - - - - - - - - - - - - - - - - - - - - - - - - - - - - - - - - - - - - - - - -


- - - - - - - - - - - - - - - - - - - - - - - - - - - - - - - - - - - - - - - - -
Random-effects Parameters  | Estimate  Std. Err. [ 95% Conf. Interval]
- - - - - - - - - - - - - - -+- - - - - - - - - - - - - - - - - - - - - - - - - -
id: Identity               |
             var(_cons)    | .3212677  .0446304    .2446912   .4218088
- - - - - - - - - - - - - - -+- - - - - - - - - - - - - - - - - - - - - - - - - -
            var(Residual)| .2629499  .0154114    .2344145    .294959
- - - - - - - - - - - - - - - - - - - - - - - - - - - - - - - - - - - - - - - - -
LR test vs. linear model: chibar2(01) = 278.56    Prob >= chibar2 = 0.0000
```

Table 6.3 Data structure needed to perform mediation model 2

Id	Time	Outcome Y	Covariate X	Mediator M	X at t-1
1	1	3	3	10	Na
1	2	4	2	12	3
1	3	5	2	10	2
1	4	5	4	11	2
1	5	6	4	13	4
1	6	7	6	13	4

Na = not applicable; these lines are not used in the analysis.

fitness highly depends on the model used. When no time-lags are modelled the total effect of fitness on cholesterol equals –0.40 (Output 6.7a), while the direct effect equals –0.33 (Output 6.7b), which leads to an estimated indirect effect of –0.07. So,

the effect of fitness on cholesterol is for 17.5% mediated by the sum of skinfolds.

When a time lag is modelled between cholesterol and the sum of skinfolds and between cholesterol and fitness, the total effect of fitness on

Output 6.5a Results of a linear mixed model mediation analysis to analyse the relationship between cholesterol and the sum of skinfolds (mediation model 3)

```
Mixed-effects ML regression              Number of obs     =       735
Group variable: id                       Number of groups  =       147

                                         Obs per group:
                                                        min =         5
                                                        avg =       5.0
                                                        max =         5

                                         Wald chi2(1)      =    149.56
Log likelihood = -706.7596               Prob > chi2       =    0.0000

------------------------------------------------------------------------
       chol |    Coef.   Std. Err.      z   P>|z|   [95% Conf. Interval]
------------+-----------------------------------------------------------
    skinft_1 | .2638365  .0215735   12.23  0.000    .2215532   .3061198
       _cons | 3.544948  .0927765   38.21  0.000    3.363109   3.726786
------------------------------------------------------------------------


------------------------------------------------------------------------
Random-effects Parameters   | Estimate  Std. Err.  [95% Conf. Interval]
----------------------------+-------------------------------------------
id: Identity                |
              var(_cons)    |  .292878  .0408732     .22279   .3850151
----------------------------+-------------------------------------------
           var(Residual)    | .2774438  .016191    .2474576   .3110638
------------------------------------------------------------------------
LR test vs. linear model: chibar2(01) = 257.78    Prob >= chibar2 = 0.0000
```

cholesterol equals –0.44 (Output 6.8a), while the direct effect equals –0.23. This results in an indirect effect of –0.21, which leads to a mediation effect of around 48%.

So, it is obvious that the estimated mediation highly depends on the theoretical model used. Questions such as which variable is the covariate of interest, which variable is the potential mediator, and for which variables time-lags must be modelled are crucial for a proper interpretation of the result obtained.

6.2.2 Comments

Regarding the theoretical framework behind the research question of interest, the creation of a Directed Acyclic Graph (DAG) can be helpful. A DAG is a figure in which all possible relationships between the outcome and the covariate are shown. This includes the direct relationship, indirect relationships through possible mediators, and all other influencing variables, such as confounders and colliders. It is an acyclic framework, so it includes no cycles, and therefore no recursive processes. Although it is sometimes a simplification of the reality, it can be helpful in designing the analysis in order to estimate the causal relationship between the outcome and the covariate of interest (Krieger and Davey Smith, 2016).

In Section 6.2.1 the longitudinal mediation analysis was performed with linear mixed model analysis. There are more possibilities to estimate the different effects in a longitudinal mediation model. It is, for instance, possible to use structural equation modelling to estimate the different effects. When there are no latent variables (i.e. variables that are not observed) involved in the analysis, the

Output 6.5b Results of a linear mixed model mediation analysis to analyse the relationship between cholesterol, physical fitness and the sum of skinfolds (mediation model 3)

```
Mixed-effects ML regression              Number of obs    =       735
Group variable: id                       Number of groups =       147

                                         Obs per group:
                                                        min =         5
                                                        avg =       5.0
                                                        max =         5

                                         Wald chi2(2)     =    267.40
Log likelihood = -663.14831              Prob > chi2      =    0.0000


------------------------------------------------------------------------
       chol |      Coef.  Std. Err.     z   P>|z|    [ 95% Conf. Interval]
------------+-----------------------------------------------------------
   skinft_1 |   .1544256   .0236003   6.54  0.000     .1081699   .2006812
    fitness | -.3759705    .037702   -9.97  0.000    -.4498651  -.3020759
      _cons |  5.842352   .2494901  23.42  0.000     5.353361   6.331344
------------------------------------------------------------------------


------------------------------------------------------------------------
Random-effects Parameters |   Estimate  Std. Err.  [ 95% Conf. Interval]
--------------------------+---------------------------------------------
id: Identity              |
             var(_cons) |   .3576216  .0483208    .2744175   .4660534
--------------------------+---------------------------------------------
            var(Residual) |   .2305364  .0135237    .2054974   .2586264
------------------------------------------------------------------------
LR test vs. linear model: chibar2(01) = 334.12    Prob >= chibar2 = 0.0000
```

Table 6.4 Data structure needed to perform mediation model 3

Id	Time	Outcome Y	Covariate X	Mediator M	X at t-1	M at t-1
1	1	3	3	10	Na	Na
1	2	4	2	12	3	10
1	3	5	2	10	2	12
1	4	5	4	11	2	10
1	5	6	4	13	4	11
1	6	7	6	13	4	13

Na = not applicable; these lines are not used in the analysis.

result obtained from a structural equation model is the same as the result obtained from a linear mixed model analysis. When structural equation modelling is used for the analyses, the analyses performed in this chapter based on the models shown in Figure 6.3 are sometimes referred to as path analyses.

In recent years, potential outcome analysis has become popular to investigate mediation analysis. Within potential outcome analysis, the causal effect

Output 6.6a Results of a linear mixed model mediation analysis to analyse the relationship between cholesterol and the sum of skinfolds (mediation model 4)

```
Mixed-effects ML regression          Number of obs     =        588
Group variable: id                   Number of groups  =        147

                                     Obs per group:
                                                   min =          4
                                                   avg =        4.0
                                                   max =          4

                                     Wald chi2(1)      =      84.16
Log likelihood = -625.36416          Prob > chi2       =     0.0000


- - - - - - - - - - - - - - - - - - - - - - - - - - - - - - - - - - - - -
        chol |     Coef.  Std. Err.     z   P>|z|   [ 95% Conf. Interval]
- - - - - - -+- - - - - - - - - - - - - - - - - - - - - - - - - - - - - -
    skinft_2 | .2762735  .0301155   9.17  0.000   .2172481   .3352989
       _cons | 3.594035  .1167005  30.80  0.000   3.365306   3.822764
- - - - - - - - - - - - - - - - - - - - - - - - - - - - - - - - - - - - -


- - - - - - - - - - - - - - - - - - - - - - - - - - - - - - - - - - - - -
Random-effects Parameters  | Estimate Std. Err.  [ 95% Conf. Interval]
- - - - - - - - - - - - - - -+- - - - - - - - - - - - - - - - - - - - - -
id: Identity               |
              var(_cons)   |  .295427  .0449091   .2193085   .3979649
- - - - - - - - - - - - - - -+- - - - - - - - - - - - - - - - - - - - - -
            var(Residual)  | .3372098 .0227469   .2954481   .3848744
- - - - - - - - - - - - - - - - - - - - - - - - - - - - - - - - - - - - -
LR test vs. linear model: chibar2(01) = 147.18   Prob >= chibar2 = 0.0000
```

is defined as the difference between two potential outcomes, one outcome that has been observed and one outcome that would have been observed for a different exposure. Because a subject has only one possible exposure, the response to the other exposure values is simulated. Although the potential outcome method is relatively complex, when both the outcome and the mediator are continuous, the potential outcome analysis leads to exactly the same result as the linear mixed model analysis.

With longitudinal mediation analysis, an attempt is made to discover causal relationships in longitudinal observational studies. It should, however, be realised that with this kind of modelling real causation can only be determined when four non-confounding assumptions are met (VanderWeele, 2015):

1. No unmeasured confounding of the outcome-covariate relation.

2. No unmeasured confounding of the outcome-mediator relation.

3. No unmeasured confounding of the mediator-covariate relation.

4. No outcome-mediator confounders that are affected by the covariate.

Failing to adjust for confounding variables might result in bias, which means that the estimated effects will not have a real causal interpretation. Looking at these assumptions, it is obvious that the assumptions are never met in real-life observational longitudinal studies. This indicates that effect estimates derived from longitudinal mediation models cannot be interpreted directly as causal effects. Claims for proven causality based on the result of this kind of longitudinal data analysis must, therefore, be interpreted with great caution.

Output 6.6b Results of a linear mixed model mediation analysis to analyse the relationship between cholesterol, physical fitness and the sum of skinfolds (mediation model 4)

```
Mixed-effects ML regression          Number of obs    =        588
Group variable: id                   Number of groups =        147

                                     Obs per group:
                                                   min =          4
                                                   avg =        4.0
                                                   max =          4

                                     Wald chi2(2)     =     144.85
Log likelihood = -600.4941           Prob > chi2      =     0.0000

- - - - - - - - - - - - - - - - - - - - - - - - - - - - - - - - - - -
        chol |    Coef.   Std. Err.      z    P>|z|   [ 95% Conf. Interval]
- - - - - - -+- - - - - - - - - - - - - - - - - - - - - - - - - - - -
    skinft_2 |  .1672743  .0339376   4.93  0.000    .1007578   .2337908
   fitnesst_1 | -.382019   .0508198  -7.52  0.000   -.4816239   -.282414
        _cons |  5.95197   .3385552  17.58  0.000    5.288414   6.615526
- - - - - - - - - - - - - - - - - - - - - - - - - - - - - - - - - - -


- - - - - - - - - - - - - - - - - - - - - - - - - - - - - - - - - - -
Random-effects Parameters |  Estimate  Std. Err.   [ 95% Conf. Interval]
- - - - - - - - - - - - - -+- - - - - - - - - - - - - - - - - - - - - -
id: Identity              |
             var(_cons)|  .3600443  .0530431    .2697451   .4805717
- - - - - - - - - - - - - -+- - - - - - - - - - - - - - - - - - - - - -
           var(Residual)|  .2885277  .0197129    .2523662   .3298707
- - - - - - - - - - - - - - - - - - - - - - - - - - - - - - - - - - -
LR test vs. linear model: chibar2(01) = 188.20    Prob >= chibar2 = 0.0000
```

Table 6.5 Data structure needed to perform mediation model 4

Id	Time	Outcome Y	Covariate X	Mediator M	X at t-2	M at t-1
1	1	3	3	10	Na	Na
1	2	4	2	12	Na	10
1	3	5	2	10	3	12
1	4	5	4	11	2	10
1	5	6	4	13	2	11
1	6	7	6	13	4	13

Na = not applicable; these lines are not used in the analysis.

6.3 Other Methods that Claim to Estimate Causal Relationships

With the methods discussed so far, it was possible to estimate (quasi) causal relationships between time-dependent continuous outcomes and all kinds of time-dependent covariates. Other methods that claim to estimate causality are mostly limited to time-independent dichotomous outcomes or survival data (i.e. dichotomous outcomes including the time on which the dichotomous outcome occurs). Because of the time-independent outcome, these methods do not belong to the definition of longitudinal data used in this book (see Section 1.1), but because they are often seen as longitudinal methods, it is worthwhile to include a short explanation of these methods to this chapter.

Table 6.6 Overview of the results of the four longitudinal mediation models

Mediation model	Total effect	Direct effect	Indirect effect
1	0.19	0.07	0.12
2	0.26	0.19	0.07
3	0.26	0.15	0.11
4	0.28	0.17	0.11

6.3.1 G-methods

G-methods are developed to deal with time-varying confounding. Dealing with time-varying confounding is not very special, because standard mixed model analysis can also deal with time-varying confounding. In research situations when the outcome variable is repeatedly measured over time and when both the covariate and the possible confounder are repeatedly measured over time, a standard mixed model analysis can be used to adjust for the time-varying confounder. This is done by simply adding the potential confounder to the mixed model analysis. The main advantage of using G-methods is that it can model the fact that the covariate at a certain time-point influences the possible confounder at one (or more) time-points later. This particular situation cannot be analysed by standard mixed model analysis.

Output 6.7a Results of a linear mixed model mediation analysis to analyse the relationship between cholesterol and physical fitness (mediation model 1)

```
Mixed-effects ML regression            Number of obs     =       882
Group variable: id                     Number of groups  =       147

                                       Obs per group:
                                                     min =         6
                                                     avg =       6.0
                                                     max =         6

                                       Wald chi2(1)      =    175.81
Log likelihood = -796.92205            Prob > chi2       =    0.0000

------------------------------------------------------------------------------
      chol |      Coef.  Std. Err.       z   P>|z|    [95% Conf. Interval]
-----------+------------------------------------------------------------------
   fitness | -.3998117  .0301532  -13.26   0.000    -.458911    -.3407125
     _cons |  6.548087  .1631421   40.14   0.000    6.228335     6.86784
------------------------------------------------------------------------------


------------------------------------------------------------------------------
Random-effects Parameters  | Estimate Std. Err.   [95% Conf. Interval]
---------------------------+--------------------------------------------------
id: Identity               |
             var(_cons)    | .3581673  .0468052    .277237     .4627225
---------------------------+--------------------------------------------------
           var(Residual)   | .2437897  .0127297    .2200742    .2700608
------------------------------------------------------------------------------
LR test vs. linear model: chibar2(01) = 451.40    Prob >= chibar2 = 0.0000
```

Output 6.7b Results of a linear mixed model mediation analysis to analyse the relationship between cholesterol, the sum of skinfolds and physical fitness (mediation model 1)

```
Mixed-effects ML regression              Number of obs     =      882
Group variable: id                       Number of groups  =      147

                                         Obs per group:
                                                       min =        6
                                                       avg =      6.0
                                                       max =        6

                                         Wald chi2(2)      =   187.01
Log likelihood = -791.79549              Prob > chi2       =   0.0000


- - - - - - - - - - - - - - - - - - - - - - - - - - - - - - - - - - - - - - -
      chol |     Coef.  Std. Err.     z    P>|z|    [ 95% Conf. Interval]
- - - - - -+- - - - - - - - - - - - - - - - - - - - - - - - - - - - - - - - -
   fitness | -.3271325  .0372392  -8.78  0.000    -.40012     -.2541449
     skinf |  .0710136  .021954    3.23  0.001    .0279845      .1140427
     _cons |  5.909606  .2537431  23.29  0.000    5.412279      6.406934
- - - - - - - - - - - - - - - - - - - - - - - - - - - - - - - - - - - - - - -


- - - - - - - - - - - - - - - - - - - - - - - - - - - - - - - - - - - - - - -
Random-effects Parameters | Estimate  Std. Err.  [ 95% Conf. Interval]
- - - - - - - - - - - - - -+- - - - - - - - - - - - - - - - - - - - - - - - -
id: Identity              |
              var(_cons)  | .3378504  .0448049   .2605195     .4381356
- - - - - - - - - - - - - -+- - - - - - - - - - - - - - - - - - - - - - - - -
           var(Residual)  | .2429576  .0127082   .2192842     .2691868
- - - - - - - - - - - - - - - - - - - - - - - - - - - - - - - - - - - - - - -
LR test vs. linear model: chibar2(01) = 410.84    Prob >= chibar2 = 0.0000
```

One of the problems with G-methods is that they are suitable for the analysis of time-independent dichotomous outcomes (measured at the end of the study) or for the analysis of survival outcomes and that the methods are specifically developed for situations in which the covariate of interest is dichotomous (i.e. exposure versus non-exposure).

The classical example always used to explain G-methods is a longitudinal observational study of the effect of antiretroviral therapy (ART) in HIV patients. The covariate of interest in this study is whether a patient is prescribed ART at a certain time-point. This is a dichotomous time-dependent variable. The time-varying confounder is the CD4 count at a certain time-point. The outcome variable in this study is whether the patient develops AIDS in a certain time-interval (which makes it a survival outcome). The specific feature of this observational study example is the fact that the decision to treat a patient with ART at a certain time-point depends on the CD4 count at the same time-point, but treatment with ART at a certain time-point leads to an increase of the CD4 count one time-point later. So, the possible time-varying confounder (i.e. CD4 count) is influenced by the covariate (i.e. ART). It is, however, questionable whether in this particular situation CD4 count can be seen as a time-varying confounder, because when ART leads to an increase in CD4 count and, therefore, in a lower probability to develop AIDS, CD4 count also acts as a mediator in the relationship between ART and the development of AIDS. So, basically, the time-varying confounder partly acts as a confounder, but also partly acts as a mediator.

Basically G-methods can be divided into G-estimation and marginal structural models. The

Output 6.8a Results of a linear mixed model mediation analysis to analyse the relationship between cholesterol and physical fitness (mediation model 2)

```
Mixed-effects ML regression                Number of obs     =        735
Group variable: id                         Number of groups  =        147

                                           Obs per group:
                                                         min =          5
                                                         avg =        5.0
                                                         max =          5

                                           Wald chi2(1)      =     123.68
Log likelihood = -718.27422                Prob > chi2       =     0.0000

-----------------------------------------------------------------------------
       chol |    Coef.   Std. Err.      z    P>|z|    [ 95% Conf. Interval]
------------+----------------------------------------------------------------
  fitnesst_1 | -.438006  .0393857  -11.12   0.000   -.5152005  -.3608115
       _cons |  6.80997  .2135079   31.90   0.000    6.391502   7.228437
-----------------------------------------------------------------------------


-----------------------------------------------------------------------------
Random-effects Parameters | Estimate  Std. Err.   [ 95% Conf. Interval]
--------------------------+--------------------------------------------------
id: Identity              |
            var(_cons)    | .3629983  .0493559    .2780796   .4738491
--------------------------+--------------------------------------------------
          var(Residual)   | .275655   .0161137    .2458148   .3091176
-----------------------------------------------------------------------------
LR test vs. linear model: chibar2(01) = 310.21    Prob >= chibar2 = 0.0000
```

difference between the two is the estimation method. With G-estimation, a two-step method is used to estimate the effect of a particular covariate (i.e. exposure) on the outcome. The first step is a casual model that includes the covariate and links the outcome under no exposure during follow-up (i.e. the outcome that would have been observed under no exposure during the follow-up) to the weighted sum of time spent in a given exposure status. The second step is a logistic regression analysis for predicting exposure at each time-point based on the previous exposure, confounding history and the outcome. G-estimation succeeds in adjusting for time-varying confounders that are affected by previous exposure by separately analysing the association between outcome and exposure at each time-point and adjusting only for the time-varying confounder at the previous time-points.

Marginal structural models on the other hand use inverse probability weighting for the estimation. Inverse probability weighting is a complicated method in which an artificial population is generated in which exposures are independent of (time-varying) confounders. An analysis on this artificial population, therefore, is adjusted for the (time-varying) confounding.

It has been mentioned before that the outcome variable used in G-methods is either a dichotomous variable measured at the end of the study or a survival outcome. For both there is no need to take into account the correlated observations within the subject in the outcome variable, so there is no need to use for instance mixed model analysis. However, because the covariate and potential confounders are (or can be) time-dependent, an alternative way is used to take into account the dependency of the observations within the subjects in the

Output 6.8b Results of a linear mixed model mediation analysis to analyse the relationship between cholesterol, the sum of skinfolds and physical fitness (mediation model 2)

```
Mixed-effects ML regression                    Number of obs     =       735
Group variable: id                             Number of groups  =       147

                                               Obs per group:
                                                            min =         5
                                                            avg =       5.0
                                                            max =         5

                                               Wald chi2(2)      =    175.82
Log likelihood = -696.17557                    Prob > chi2       =    0.0000
```

chol	Coef.	Std. Err.	z	P>|z|	[95% Conf. Interval]	
fitnesst_1	-.2303257	.0486844	-4.73	0.000	-.3257453	-.1349061
skinft_1	.1850714	.0273432	6.77	0.000	.1314797	.238663
_cons	5.042304	.3311341	15.23	0.000	4.393293	5.691315

Random-effects Parameters	Estimate	Std. Err.	[95% Conf. Interval]	
id: Identity				
var(_cons)	.3212677	.0446304	.2446912	.4218088
var(Residual)	.2629499	.0154114	.2344145	.294959

```
LR test vs. linear model: chibar2(01) = 278.56    Prob >= chibar2 = 0.0000
```

time-dependent covariate and potential confounders. Within G-methods this is done by adding lagged variables to the statistical models. With lagged variables, for instance, the covariate or possible confounder at a certain time-point is adjusted for the same variable one time-point earlier. Figure 6.4 shows the theoretical framework behind G-methods.

Although the use of G-methods makes some sense it should be realised that data which is suitable for using G-methods on is rare and does not often occur in real life. Furthermore, G-methods are not much used in medical studies because both the conceptual and technical details of the methods are very complicated. Therefore, the application of G-methods in real-life medical studies is rather limited. For further details about G-methods one is referred to Robins et al. (2000),

Rhian et al. (2011), Mansournia et al. (2017) and Naimi et al. (2017).

6.3.2 Joint Models

Joint models were introduced to combine longitudinal data of a particular covariate with a survival analysis. When longitudinal information of the covariate is available in combination of survival data, usually time-varying Cox regression analysis is used to estimate the effect of the covariate on the survival outcome. An alternative to the time-varying Cox regression analysis is to perform two separate analyses. In the first analysis, the longitudinal development of the covariate over time is estimated with a longitudinal regression analysis, such as a mixed model analysis. In the second analysis, the predicted linear

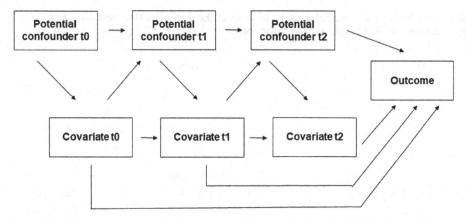

Figure 6.4 Illustration of a causal diagram with a covariate and a time-varying confounder both measured three times and an outcome measured at the end of follow-up. In the framework other measured and unmeasured possible confounders are omitted.

development over time (or another parameter derived from the longitudinal regression analysis) is used as covariate in a Cox regression analysis. The general idea behind joint models is that the two analyses (i.e. the longitudinal regression analysis and the survival analysis) are combined into one analysis.

So, because the outcome of a joint model analysis is a survival outcome, joint models do not belong to the definition of longitudinal data used in this book (see Section 1.1). However, because the first step in the joint model analysis is a longitudinal regression analysis, it is worthwhile to include a short description of this method including a corresponding example into this chapter.

6.3.2.1 Example

The example dataset is taken from a hypothetical study in which the first occurrence of hypercholesterolemia is related to the development of physical fitness. In this observational study, at most, six repeated measurements were performed. From the 147 subjects who started the study, 13 were diagnosed with hypercholesterolemia at time-point 4, 29 were diagnosed at time-point 5 and 33 were diagnosed at time-point 6. The data were analysed with a joint model analysis as well as with a two-step method in which first the linear development over time in physical fitness was estimated with a linear mixed model analysis including a random intercept and a random slope for time. In the second step of the two-step method, the individual predicted slope (using both the fixed and random components of the mixed model analysis) was used as covariate in a

Cox regression analysis with the (time to) occurrence of hypercholesterolemia as outcome. Output 6.9 shows the result of the linear mixed model analysis to estimate the individual development over time. The model included a random intercept and a random slope for time.

From Output 6.9 it can be seen that there is a decrease in fitness over time. The regression coefficient for time (i.e. −2.108964) indicates that there is a decrease of 2.11 units in fitness for each year of measurement. Based on the results of the mixed model analysis (including the regression coefficient for time, the random intercept and the random slope for time) the slope in physical fitness for each subject can be predicted. This predicted slope can then be used in a Cox regression analysis to analyse the relationship with the first occurrence of hypercholesterolemia. Output 6.10 shows the result of this analysis

From Output 6.10, it can be seen that the hazard ratio for the predicted slope equals 0.9560501, which means that for each unit difference in the predicted slope the hazard for hypercholesterolemia is 0.956 times as high. So an increase in fitness, or a lesser decrease in fitness, is preventive against the occurrence of hypercholesterolemia.

In the two-step method, a Cox regression analysis was used for the survival analysis. One of the reasons why Cox regression analysis is mostly used for survival analysis is that there are no assumptions about the shape of the baseline hazard function. Cox regression analysis is, therefore, known as a semi-parametric survival analysis. When a joint model analysis is used it is not possible to use a Cox regression analysis for the

Output 6.9 Results of a linear mixed model analysis to analyse the linear development over time in fitness (including a random intercept and random slope for time)

```
Mixed-effects ML regression                    Number of obs      =        827
Group variable: id                             Number of groups   =        147

                                               Obs per group:
                                                            min =          4
                                                            avg =        5.6
                                                            max =          6

                                               Wald chi2(1)       =     408.22
Log likelihood = -2495.5976                    Prob > chi2        =     0.0000


- - - - - - - - - - - - - - - - - - - - - - - - - - - - - - - - - - - - - - - -
   fitness |     Coef.   Std. Err.      z     P>|z|    [ 95% Conf. Interval]
- - - - - - + - - - - - - - - - - - - - - - - - - - - - - - - - - - - - - - - -
      time | -2.108964   .1043808   -20.20   0.000    -2.313546  -1.904381
      _cons |  56.57512   .5925217    95.48   0.000     55.4138    57.73644
- - - - - - - - - - - - - - - - - - - - - - - - - - - - - - - - - - - - - - - -


- - - - - - - - - - - - - - - - - - - - - - - - - - - - - - - - - - - - - - - -
Random-effects Parameters | Estimate  Std. Err.   [ 95% Conf. Interval]
- - - - - - - - - - - - - - - + - - - - - - - - - - - - - - - - - - - - - - - -
id: Unstructured          |
             var(start) |  .6795149  .1951595    .3870172   1.193075
             var(_cons) |  44.43301  6.033639    34.05019   57.98184
      cov(start,_cons) | -1.552841  .8150746   -3.150358    .0446759
- - - - - - - - - - - - - + - - - - - - - - - - - - - - - - - - - - - - - - - -
          var(Residual) |  13.20972  .8096939    11.71437   14.89595
- - - - - - - - - - - - - - - - - - - - - - - - - - - - - - - - - - - - - - - -
LR test vs. linear model: chi2(3) = 680.62              Prob > chi2 = 0.0000
```

Output 6.10 Results of a Cox regression analysis to analyse the relationship between the (time to) first occurrence of hypercholesterolemia and the predicted linear development over time in fitness

```
Cox regression - Breslow method for ties

No. of subjects =           147          Number of obs      =        827
No. of failures =            75
Time at risk    =           827
                                         LR chi2(1)         =       5.90
Log likelihood = -357.54393              Prob > chi2        =     0.0151


- - - - - - - - - - - - - - - - - - - - - - - - - - - - - - - - - - - - - - -
      _t | Haz. Ratio  Std. Err.        z     P>|z|   [95% Conf. Interval]
- - - - - - + - - - - - - - - - - - - - - - - - - - - - - - - - - - - - - - - -
    slope |  .9560501   .0178397     -2.41   0.016    .9217166   .9916625
- - - - - - - - - - - - - - - - - - - - - - - - - - - - - - - - - - - - - - -
```

Output 6.11 Results of a joint model analysis to analyse the relationship between the (time to) first occurrence of hypercholesterolemia and the development of fitness using a Weibull distribution for the baseline hazard

```
Joint model estimates                    Number of obs.     =    827
Panel variable: id                       Number of panels   =    147
                                         Number of failures =     75


Log-likelihood = -2649.4308


- - - - - - - - - - - - - - - - - - - - - - - - - - - - - - - - - - - - - - - -
               |    Coef.   Std. Err.     z   P>|z|   [ 95% Conf. Interval]
- - - - - - - -+- - - - - - - - - - - - - - - - - - - - - - - - - - - - - - - -
Longitudinal  |
     _time_1  | -2.125825 .1044802  -20.35  0.000   -2.330602 -1.921048
       _cons  | 56.59577  .5923011   95.55  0.000   55.43488  57.75665
- - - - - - - - - - - - - - - - - - - - - - - - - - - - - - - - - - - - - - - -

    Survival  |
 assoc:value  |
       _cons  | -.0504124  .018881   -2.67  0.008   -.0874185 -.0134062
   ln_lambda  |
       _cons  | -11.46199 1.857622   -6.17  0.000   -15.10286  -7.82112
    ln_gamma  |
       _cons  |  2.005993 .114317    17.55  0.000    1.781935  2.23005
- - - - - - - - - - - - - - - - - - - - - - - - - - - - - - - - - - - - - - - -


- - - - - - - - - - - - - - - - - - - - - - - - - - - - - - - - - - - - - - - -
Random effects Parameters  | Estimate Std. Err.  [ 95% Conf. Interval]
- - - - - - - - - - - - - - -+- - - - - - - - - - - - - - - - - - - - - - - - -
   id: Unstructured         |
           sd(_time_1)  |  .8212008  .1176223   .6201975  1.087348
            sd(_cons)   | 6.661769  .4522539   5.831808  7.609847
     corr(_time_1,_cons)| -.2775905  .1222785  -.4965678 -.0253933
- - - - - - - - - - - - - - -+- - - - - - - - - - - - - - - - - - - - - - - - -
             sd(Residual)|  3.635472  .1112869   3.423769  3.860267
- - - - - - - - - - - - - - - - - - - - - - - - - - - - - - - - - - - - - - - -
```

survival part of the analysis; it is only possible to use a parametric survival analysis. With a parametric survival analysis it is assumed that the baseline hazard function has a particular shape. The most commonly used parametric survival analyses are the one assuming an exponential baseline hazard function and the one assuming a Weibull baseline hazard function. With the exponential hazard function, the baseline hazard is assumed to be constant over time, while with the Weibull hazard function, the baseline hazard is assumed to increase or decrease over time. A slightly more flexible option is the use of the flexible parameter method.

This method uses restricted cubic spline functions to model the baseline hazard. A detailed description of the different parametric survival analysis goes beyond the scope of this book; see for further details, for instance, Lambert and Royston, 2009; Cleves et al., 2010; Royston et al., 2011. In the present example both the Weibull survival model and the flexible parameter model were used to analyse the relationship between the first occurrence of hypercholesterolemia and (the linear development of) physical fitness. Output 6.11 shows the result of the joint model analysis using a Weibull distribution for the baseline hazard

Output 6.12   Results of a joint model analysis to analyse the relationship between the (time to) first occurrence of hypercholesterolemia and the development of fitness using a flexible parameter approach

```
Joint model estimates                     Number of obs.     =        827
Panel variable: id                        Number of panels   =        147
                                          Number of failures =         75

                                          Log-likelihood     = -2649.4653


-------------------------------------------------------------------------
             |    Coef.   Std. Err.     z    P>|z|   [ 95% Conf. Interval]
-------------+-----------------------------------------------------------
Longitudinal |
     _time_1 | -2.127614  .1043759  -20.38  0.000  -2.332187  -1.923041
       _cons |  56.59798  .5921285   95.58  0.000   55.43743   57.75853
-------------+-----------------------------------------------------------
    Survival |
 assoc:value |
       _cons | -.0495594  .0187288   -2.65  0.008  -.0862671   -.0128516
          xb |
       _rcs1 |  4.425586  .515262     8.59  0.000   3.415691    5.435481
       _cons | -3.705836  1.1078     -3.35  0.001  -5.877083   -1.534588
-------------------------------------------------------------------------


-------------------------------------------------------------------------
Random effects Parameters | Estimate  Std. Err.   [ 95% Conf. Interval]
--------------------------+----------------------------------------------
id: Unstructured          |
          sd(_time_1) |  .818273   .1175346   .6174956   1.084333
           sd(_cons) |  6.65904   .4520523   5.829447   7.606692
   corr(_time_1,_cons) | -.2758098  .1225533  -.4953445  -.0231603
--------------------------+----------------------------------------------
          sd(Residual) |  3.636692  .1113438   3.424881   3.861602
-------------------------------------------------------------------------
```

function, while Output 6.12 shows the result of the joint model analysis using the flexible parameter method.

In both joint model outputs, the first part of the output shows the result of the linear mixed model analysis in order to analyse the linear development over time in fitness. The regression coefficients for the development over time are slightly different for both joint models and are also slightly different from the result obtained from the mixed model analysis shown in Output 6.9. However, the differences between the estimates are very small. In the second part of the output of the joint model analysis, the result of the survival analysis is shown. The most important coefficient of this part of the output

is the value given by _cons. This is the regression coefficient for the relationship between the first occurrence of hypercholesterolemia and the development of fitness. This regression coefficient should be transformed into a hazard ratio by taking the e-power. For both joint models, the hazard ratio equals EXP[−0.05] = 0.95, with a 95% confidence interval ranging from EXP[−0.09] = 0.92 to EXP[−0.013] = 0.99. The hazard ratio and the 95% confidence interval are more or less the same as the hazard ratio and the 95% confidence interval derived from the Cox regression analysis with predicted slope of fitness as covariate. Besides the regression coefficient for the development of fitness, the output of the joint model analysis also provides some information about the baseline hazard function used in the particular survival analysis. This information is not really important in light of the scope of this book (see for specific details for instance Royston, 2001 and Cleves et al., 2010). In the last part of the output of the joint model analysis, the random intercept and slope variances are given. It should be realised that in the output of the joint model analysis, standard deviations are given instead of variances. When the standard deviations are squared it can be seen that the variances estimated by the joint model analysis are more or less the same as the variances estimated with the linear mixed model analysis (see Output 6.9).

In general, it seems that the result obtained from a joined model analysis is not that different from the result obtained from the two-step method. And although it is argued that joint modelling reduces bias and improves precision (see for details Rizopoulos, 2011, Crowther et al., 2013 and Mchunu et al., 2020), based on the result of the example, it is questionable what the added value of the use of joint models really is. One of the limitations of a joint model analysis is that only the slope of the longitudinally measured covariate is used in the survival analysis. It is, however, highly possible that also the average value or the heterogeneity of the longitudinally measured covariate are related to survival as well. With the two-step method these additional indicators can be estimated in a relatively simple way and used in the survival analysis. This makes the two-step method slightly more flexible than the joint model method.

Dichotomous Outcome Variables

7.1 Two Measurements

When a dichotomous outcome variable is measured twice over time in the same subjects, a 2×2 table can be constructed as shown below (where n stands for the number of subjects and p stands for the proportion of the total number of subjects N).

	t_2		
	1	2	Total
t_1 1	n_{11}/p_{11}	n_{12}/p_{12}	$n_{1(t1)}/p_{1(t1)}$
2	n_{21}/p_{21}	n_{22}/p_{22}	$n_{2(t1)}/p_{2(t1)}$
Total	$n_{1(t2)}/p_{1(t2)}$	$n_{2(t2)}/p_{2(t2)}$	N

The simplest way to estimate the development over time is to compare the proportion of subjects in group 1 at $t = 1$ with the proportion of subjects in group 1 at $t = 2$. Equation 7.1 shows how to calculate the standard error of the difference in proportions:

$$se\left(p_{1(t2)} - p_{1(t1)}\right) = \frac{\sqrt{\left(n_{1(t2)} - n_{1(t1)}\right)}}{N} \qquad (7.1)$$

where $p_{1(t2)}$ is the proportion of subjects in group 1 at $t = 2$, $p_{1(t1)}$ is the proportion of subjects in group 1 at $t = 1$, $n_{1(t2)}$ is the number of subjects in group 1 at $t = 2$, $n_{1(t1)}$ is the number of subjects in group 1 at $t = 1$, and N is the total number of subjects.

The standard error can be used to calculate the 95% confidence interval for the difference (difference ± 1.96 times the standard error) which can be used to answer the question of whether there is a significant change over time. The problem with the difference in proportions is that it basically provides an indication of the difference between the change in opposite directions. If all subjects from group 1 at $t = 1$ move to group 2 at $t = 2$, and all subjects from group 2 at $t = 1$ move to

group 1 at $t = 2$, the difference in proportions reveals no change over time.

A widely used method to determine whether there is a change over time in a dichotomous outcome variable is the McNemar test. This is an alternative Chi-square test, which takes into account the fact that the observed proportions in the 2×2 table are not independent. The McNemar test is, in principle, based on the difference between the number of subjects moving from group 1 to group 2 and the number of subjects moving from group 2 to group 1, and the test statistic follows a Chi-square distribution with one degree of freedom (Equation 7.2):

$$\chi^2 = \frac{\left(n_{12} - n_{21} - 1\right)^2}{n_{12} + n_{21}} \qquad (7.2)$$

where n_{12} is the number of subjects in group 1 at $t = 1$ and in group 2 at $t = 2$, and n_{21} is the number of subjects in group 2 at $t = 1$ and in group 1 at $t = 2$.

The McNemar test determines whether the change in one direction is equal to the change in another direction. So, the McNemar test has the same disadvantage as has been mentioned above for the difference in proportions. It tests the difference between the change in opposite directions.

A possible way in which to estimate the total change over time is to calculate the proportion of subjects who change from one group to another. The standard error of this proportion is calculated as:

$$se\left(p_{change}\right) = \sqrt{\frac{p_{change} - \left(1 - p_{change}\right)}{N}} \qquad (7.3)$$

where se is the standard error, p_{change} is the proportion of change equal to $p_{12} + p_{21}$, and N is the total number of subjects.

If one is only interested in the proportion of subjects who change in a certain direction (i.e. only a decrease or increase over time) the same method can be followed for separate changes. In this respect, a proportion of increase or a proportion of decrease can be calculated and a 95% confidence interval can be constructed, based on the standard error calculated with Equation 7.3.

It should be noted that when all individuals belong to the same group at $t = 1$, the estimate of the change in opposite directions is equal to the estimate of the total change over time. In that situation, which often occurs in intervention studies (see Chapter 10), all methods discussed so far can be used to estimate the change over time in a dichotomous outcome variable.

7.2 More than Two Measurements

When more than two measurements are performed on the same subjects, the multivariate extension of the McNemar test can be used. This multivariate extension is known as Cochran's Q, and it has the same disadvantage as the McNemar test. It is a test for the difference between the change in opposite directions, while in longitudinal studies one is generally interested in the total change over time. To analyse the total change over time, the proportion of change can be calculated in the same way as in the situation with two measurements. To do this, $(T - 1)$ 2×2 tables must first be constructed (for $t = 1$ and $t = 2$, for $t = 2$ and $t = 3$, and so on). The next step is to calculate the proportion of change for each 2×2 table. To calculate the total proportion of change, Equation 7.4 can be applied:

$$\bar{p} = \frac{1}{N(T-1)} \sum_{i=1}^{N} c_i \qquad (7.4)$$

where $\bar{p}$ is the total proportion of change, N is the number of subjects, T is the number of measurements, and c_i is the number of changes for individual i over time.

7.3 Comparing Groups

To compare the development over time between two groups, for a dichotomous outcome variable the proportion of change in the two groups can be compared. This can be done by applying the test for two independent proportions. The standard error of this difference (needed to create a 95% confidence interval and for testing whether there is a significant difference between the two groups) is calculated by Equation 7.5:

$$se\left(p_{g1} - p_{g2}\right) = \sqrt{\left[\frac{p_{g1}\left(1 - p_{g1}\right)}{N_{g1}}\right] + \left[\frac{p_{g2}\left(1 - p_{g2}\right)}{N_{g2}}\right]}$$

$$(7.5)$$

where se is the standard error, p_{g1} is the proportion of change in group 1, p_{g2} is the proportion of change in group 2, N_{g1} is the number of subjects in group 1, and N_{g2} is the number of subjects in group 2.

Of course, this method can also be carried out to determine the proportion of change in a certain direction (i.e. the proportion of increase or the proportion of decrease). It should be realised that the calculation of the proportion of change over a particular time period is primarily useful for the longitudinal analysis of datasets with only two repeated measurements. For more information on the analysis of proportions and differences in proportions, reference is made to the classical work of Fleiss (1981).

7.4 Example

7.4.1 Introduction

The dataset used to illustrate longitudinal analyses with a dichotomous outcome variable is the same as that used to illustrate longitudinal analyses with a continuous outcome variable. The only difference is that the outcome variable cholesterol is dichotomised into hypercholesterolemia. This is done by taking the 66th percentile. At each of the repeated measurements the upper 33% are coded as 1, and the lower 66% are coded as 0.

7.4.2 Development over Time

To analyse the development of hypercholesterolemia over time, the situation with two measurements will first be illustrated. From the example dataset the first $(t = 1)$ and the last $(t = 6)$ measurements will be considered. Table 7.1 shows the corresponding 2×2 table.

Because the dichotomisation of hypercholesterolemia was based on a fixed value (the 66th percentile) at each of the repeated measurements, by definition, there is no difference between the change over time in opposite directions. The proportion of subjects in group 1 at $t = 1$ (33.3%) is almost equal to the proportion of subjects in group 1 at $t = 6$ (34.0%). Therefore, the McNemar test is not very informative in this particular situation. However, just as an example, Output 7.1 shows the result of the McNemar test.

As expected, the McNemar test statistic Chi-square = 0.0000 and the corresponding p-value = 1.0000, which indicates that there is no change over time for hypercholesterolemia. The output of the McNemar test illustrates perfectly the limitation of the method, i.e. only the difference between the change over time in opposite directions is taken into account.

From the 2 × 2 table, the total proportion of change and the corresponding 95% confidence interval can also be calculated. The proportion of change is (18 + 17)/147 = 0.24. The standard error of this proportion, which is calculated with Equation 7.3, is 0.035. With these two components the 95% confidence interval can be calculated, which leads to an interval that ranges from 0.17

to 0.31, indicating a highly significant change over time. Note that this calculation deals with the change over time in both directions, which is different from the McNemar test, which deals with the difference in change in opposite directions.

When the development over time of hypercholesterolemia is analysed using all six measurements, the multivariate extension of the McNemar test (Cochran's Q) can be used. However, Cochran's Q has the same limitations as the McNemar test. So again, it is not very informative in this particular situation, in which the groups are defined according to the same (fixed) percentile at each measurement. However, Output 7.2 shows the result of Cochran's Q test. As expected, the significance level of Cochran's Q (0.9945) is close to one, indicating no difference between the change over time in opposite directions.

To evaluate the total change over time, Equation 7.4 can be used. First of all, the $(T − 1)$ 2 × 2 tables must be constructed (see Table 7.2). From these tables, the total proportion of change can be calculated.

The sum of the changes is 143, so the proportion of change is $143/(147 \times 5) = 0.19$. The corresponding 95% confidence interval (based on the standard error calculated with Equation 7.3) ranges from 0.16 to 0.22, indicating a highly significant change over time. Again, this change over time deals with the total change over time in both directions.

Table 7.1 2 × 2 table with the number of subjects with hypercholesterolemia at $t = 1$ and $t = 6$

Hypercholesterolemia at $t = 1$	Hypercholesterolemia at $t = 6$		
	0	1	Total
0	80	17	97
1	18	32	50
Total	98	49	147

Output 7.1 Results of a McNemar test to analyse the development over time of hypercholesterolemia between $t = 1$ and $t = 6$

```
- - - - - - - - - - - - - - - - - - - - - - - - - - - - - -
hypercholesterolemia | hypercholesterolemia
at t=1               | at t=6
                     |   0        1      Total
- - - - - - - - - - -+- - - - - - - - - - - - - -
                 0 | 80        17       97
                 1 | 18        32       50
                   |
             Total | 98        49      147
- - - - - - - - - - - - - - - - - - - - - - - - - - -

                              chi2      df     Prob>chi2
- - - - - - - - - - - - - - - - - - - - - - - - - - - - - -
           McNemar Test |    0.00       2       1.0000
- - - - - - - - - - - - - - - - - - - - - - - - - - - - - -
```

Output 7.2 Results of a Cochran's Q test to analyse the development over time of hypercholesterolemia from $t = 1$ to $t = 6$, using data from all repeated measurements

Cochran Q Test

Cases

	=0	=1	Variable	
	97	50	hypercholt1	hypercholesterolemia at t=1
	99	48	hypercholt2	hypercholesterolemia at t=2
	96	51	hypercholt3	hypercholesterolemia at t=3
	98	49	hypercholt4	hypercholesterolemia at t=4
	99	48	hypercholt5	hypercholesterolemia at t=5
	98	49	hypercholt6	hypercholesterolemia at t=6

Cases		Cochran Q	DF	Significance
147		0.4298	5	0.9945

7.4.3 Comparing Groups

When the aim of the study is to investigate whether there is a difference in development over time between several groups, the proportion of change in the groups can be compared. In the example dataset, the population can be divided into two groups, according to sex (i.e. males and females). For both groups, first a 2×2 table can be constructed (see Table 7.3), indicating the changes in hypercholesterolemia between $t = 1$ and $t = 6$.

The next step is to calculate the proportion of change for both groups. For males the proportion of change = 13/69 = 0.19; while for females, the proportion of change = 0.28. From these two proportions the difference and the 95% confidence interval can be calculated. The latter is based on the standard error calculated with Equation 7.5. The difference in proportion of change between the two groups is 0.09, with a 95% confidence interval ranging between –0.05 and 0.23. So, there is a difference between the two groups (i.e. females have a 9% greater change over time), but this difference is not statistically significant.

When there are more than two measurements, Equation 7.4 can be used to calculate the proportion of change in both groups. After creating $(T - 1)$ separate 2×2 tables, for males this proportion equals 0.18, and for females, this proportion equals 0.21. So, the difference in proportion of change between the two groups equals 0.03. The

95% confidence interval can be calculated with the standard error, which is calculated with Equation 7.5. This interval ranges between –0.03 and 0.09, so the (small) difference observed between the two groups is not statistically significant.

7.5 Longitudinal Regression Methods

7.5.1 Introduction

In general, when a dichotomous outcome variable is used in a longitudinal study, and the objective of the study is to analyse the longitudinal relationship between such a variable and one or more covariates, it is possible to use generalised estimating equations (GEE) analysis and mixed model analysis. In Chapter 3, it was extensively explained that for continuous outcome variables in longitudinal studies these methods can be considered as longitudinal linear regression analysis. Analogous to this, GEE analysis and mixed model analysis with a dichotomous outcome variable in longitudinal studies can be considered as longitudinal logistic regression analysis. So, comparable to Equation 3.1, the longitudinal logistic model can be formulated as in Equation 7.6.

$$ln\left(\frac{pr(Y_{it} = 1)}{1 - pr(Y_{it} = 1)}\right) = \beta_0 + \beta_1 X_{it} \qquad (7.6a)$$

119

Table 7.2 Five 2 × 2 tables with the number of subjects with hypercholesterolemia at $t = 1$ till $t = 6$

Hypercholesterolemia at $t = 1$	Hypercholesterolemia at $t = 2$		
	0	1	Total
0	83	14	97
1	16	34	50
Total	99	48	147

Hypercholesterolemia at $t = 2$	Hypercholesterolemia at $t = 3$		
	0	1	Total
0	83	16	99
1	13	35	48
Total	96	51	147

Hypercholesterolemia at $t = 3$	Hypercholesterolemia at $t = 4$		
	0	1	Total
0	84	12	96
1	14	37	51
Total	98	49	147

Hypercholesterolemia at $t = 4$	Hypercholesterolemia at $t = 5$		
	0	1	Total
0	86	12	98
1	13	36	49
Total	99	48	147

Hypercholesterolemia at $t = 5$	Hypercholesterolemia at $t = 6$		
	0	1	Total
0	82	17	99
1	16	32	48
Total	98	49	147

Table 7.3 2 × 2 tables with the number of subjects with hypercholesterolemia at $t = 1$ and $t = 6$ for two groups divided by sex (males versus females)

Males	Hypercholesterolemia at $t = 6$		
Hypercholesterolemia at $t = 1$	0	1	Total
0	40	5	45
1	8	16	24
Total	48	21	69
Females	Hypercholesterolemia at $t = 6$		
Hypercholesterolemia at $t = 1$	0	1	Total
0	40	12	52
1	10	16	26
Total	50	28	78

In a different notation:

$$pr(Y_{it} = 1) = \frac{1}{1 + exp\left[-(\beta_0 + \beta_1 X_{it})\right]} \quad (7.6b)$$

where $pr(Y_{it} = 1)$ is the probability that the observations of the outcome for subject i at time t equal 1 (where 1 means that subject i belongs to the group of interest), β_0 is the intercept, X_{it} are observations of the covariate of subject i at time t and β_1 is the regression coefficient for the covariate.

Although the model looks quite complicated, it is in fact nothing more than an extension of a cross-sectional logistic regression model. The extension is presented in the subscript t, which indicates that the same subject is repeatedly measured over time. Like in cross-sectional logistic regression analysis, the covariate(s) can be continuous, dichotomous or categorical, although in the latter situation dummy coding can or must be used. The coefficient of interest is β_1, because this coefficient reflects the longitudinal relationship between belonging to the group of interest over time and a particular covariate. Like in cross-sectional logistic regression, this coefficient (β_1) can be transformed into an odds ratio (EXP$[\beta_1]$). The interpretation of the regression coefficient (i.e. odds ratio) is equivalent to the pooled interpretation of the regression coefficient derived from a longitudinal regression analysis with a continuous outcome variable, i.e. partly between-subjects and partly within-subjects. (See the example in Section 7.2.2 for a detailed explanation.)

Analogous to the situation with continuous outcome variables, with GEE analysis an adjustment is made for the within-subjects correlations between the repeated measurements by assuming a (working) correlation structure, while with mixed model analysis this adjustment is made by allowing different regression coefficients to vary between subjects, by adding a random intercept and (if necessary) random slopes to the model.

7.5.2 Generalised Estimating Equations

Also for dichotomous outcome variables, GEE analysis requires an a priori choice of a correlation structure. Although there are the same possibilities as has been discussed for continuous outcome variables (see Section 3.4.2), it is not really possible to use the correlation structure of the observed data as a guide for the choice of the correlation structure. This is because a correlation coefficient is basically only defined for continuous variables. In this example, an exchangeable correlation structure (which is the default option in many software packages) will be used. Output 7.3 presents the result of the logistic GEE analysis to analyse the relationship between hypercholesterolemia and the sum of skinfolds.

The output of the logistic GEE analysis is comparable to the output of a linear GEE analysis, which was discussed in Section 3.4.3. The outcome variable is hypercholesterolemia which is the dichotomised version of cholesterol, and the correlation structure used is exchangeable. The difference between the outputs is found in the link function and the family. In a logistic regression analysis, the link function is the logit and the family is binomial, while with a continuous outcome the link function is identity and the family Gaussian.

The second part of the output shows the regression coefficients. For the sum of skinfolds the regression coefficient, the standard error, the z-value (obtained from dividing the regression coefficient by its standard error), the corresponding p-value, and the 95% confidence interval around the regression coefficient are presented. The latter is calculated in the regular way, i.e. by the regression coefficient $\pm$ 1.96 times the standard error.

It can be seen that hypercholesterolemia is significantly related to the sum of skinfolds. The regression coefficient is 0.2789969, and the odds ratio is therefore EXP[0.2789969] = 1.32. The 95% confidence interval around the odds ratio ranges between EXP[0.1729089] = 1.19 and EXP[0.3850849] = 1.47. The interpretation of this odds ratio is somewhat complicated, because, as for continuous outcome variables, the odds ratio pools two interpretations. (1) The between-subjects interpretation: a subject with a one-unit higher score for the sum of skinfolds, compared to another subject, has 1.32 times higher odds of being in the hypercholesterolemia group compared to the odds of being in the non-hypercholesterolemia group. (2) The within-subjects interpretation: an increase of one unit in the sum of skinfolds within a subject is associated with 1.32 times higher odds of moving to the hypercholesterolemia group compared to the odds of staying in the non-hypercholesterolemia group. The magnitude of the regression coefficient (i.e. the magnitude of the odds ratio) is a weighted average of both relationships.

Output 7.3 Results of a logistic GEE analysis to analyse the relationship between hypercholesterolemia and the sum of skinfolds

```
GEE population-averaged model          Number of obs      =      882
Group variable:                  id    Number of groups   =      147
Link:                         logit    Obs per group:
Family:                    binomial                  min  =        6
Correlation:           exchangeable                  avg  =      6.0
                                                      max  =        6
                                       Wald chi2(1)       =    26.57
Scale parameter:                   1   Prob > chi2        =   0.0000

                                (Std. Err. adjusted for clustering on id)
- - - - - - - - - - - - - - - - - - - - - - - - - - - - - - - - - - - - - - -
            |              Robust
  hyperchol |    Coef.   Std. Err.     z  P>|z|   [ 95% Conf. Interval]
- - - - - - +- - - - - - - - - - - - - - - - - - - - - - - - - - - - - - - - -
      skinf |  .2789969   .0541275   5.15  0.000   .1729089   .3850849
      _cons | -1.777271   .2688893  -6.61  0.000  -2.304285  -1.250258
- - - - - - - - - - - - - - - - - - - - - - - - - - - - - - - - - - - - - - -
```

It should be realised that the scale parameter which is given in the output of a logistic GEE analysis has a slightly different interpretation than the scale parameter given in the output of a linear GEE analysis. This has to do with the characteristics of the binomial distribution on which the logistic GEE analysis is based. In the binomial distribution the variance is directly linked to the mean value (Equation 7.7). So, for the logistic GEE analysis, the scale parameter has to be one (i.e. a direct connection between the variance and the mean).

$$\sigma^2(\bar{p}) = \bar{p}(1 - \bar{p}) \qquad (7.7)$$

where σ^2 is the variance, and $\bar{p}$ is the average probability.

Comparable to the situation already described for continuous outcome variables, GEE analysis requires the choice of a particular correlation structure. It has already been mentioned that for a dichotomous outcome variable it is not really possible to base that choice on the correlation structure of the observed data. It is therefore interesting to investigate the difference in estimated regression coefficients when different correlation structures are chosen. Output 7.4 shows the results of several GEE analyses with different correlation structures. and Table 7.4 summarises the results of the different GEE analyses.

The most important conclusion which can be drawn from Table 7.4 is that the results of the GEE analyses with different dependent correlation structures are comparable. Only the analysis with an autoregressive correlation structure leads to a slightly higher regression coefficient. This finding is different from that observed in the analysis of a continuous outcome variable (see Table 3.7), for which a remarkable difference was found between the results of the analyses with different correlation structures. So, (probably) the statement in the literature that GEE analysis is robust against the wrong choice of a correlation structure is particularly true for dichotomous outcome variables (see for instance also Liang and Zeger, 1993).

Furthermore, from Table 7.4 it can be seen that there are remarkable differences between the results obtained from the analysis with an independent correlation structure and the results obtained from the analyses with the four dependent correlation structures. It should further be noted that comparable to the situation with a continuous outcome variable, the standard errors obtained from the analysis with an independent correlation structure are higher than those obtained from the analysis with any of the dependent correlation structures.

To put the results of the GEE analysis in a somewhat broader perspective, they can be

Output 7.4 Results of logistic GEE analyses with different correlation structures to analyse the relationship between hypercholesterolemia and the sum of skinfolds

```
GEE population-averaged model        Number of obs     =      882
Group variable:                id    Number of groups =      147
Link:                       logit    Obs per group:
Family:                  binomial                 min =        6
Correlation:          independent                 avg =      6.0
                                                  max =        6
                                     Wald chi2(1)      =    31.81
Scale parameter:               1     Prob > chi2       =   0.0000


Pearson chi2(882):        876.96     Deviance          =  1052.33
Dispersion (Pearson):   .9942859     Dispersion        = 1.193114


                              (Std. Err. adjusted for clustering on id)
- - - - - - - - - - - - - - - - - - - - - - - - - - - - - - - - - -
           |            Robust
 hyperchol |    Coef. Std. Err.      z    P>|z|   [ 95% Conf. Interval]
- - - - - -+- - - - - - - - - - - - - - - - - - - - - - - - - - - -
     skinf | .4036003 .0715571    5.64   0.000    .2633509  .5438497
     _cons | -2.243682 .3319424  -6.76   0.000   -2.894277 -1.593086
- - - - - - - - - - - - - - - - - - - - - - - - - - - - - - - - - -


GEE population-averaged model        Number of obs     =      882
Group and time vars:      id time    Number of groups =      147
Link:                       logit    Obs per group:
Family:                  binomial                 min =        6
Correlation:        stationary(5)                 avg =      6.0
                                                  max =        6
                                     Wald chi2(1)      =    29.88
Scale parameter:               1     Prob > chi2       =   0.0000


                              (Std. Err. adjusted for clustering on id)
- - - - - - - - - - - - - - - - - - - - - - - - - - - - - - - - - -
           |            Robust
 hyperchol |    Coef. Std. Err.      z   P>|z|    [ 95% Conf. Interval]
- - - - - -+- - - - - - - - - - - - - - - - - - - - - - - - - - - -
     skinf | .2842957 .0520134    5.47   0.000    .1823512  .3862402
     _cons | -1.791111 .2617465  -6.84   0.000   -2.304125 -1.278097
- - - - - - - - - - - - - - - - - - - - - - - - - - - - - - - - - -


GEE population-averaged model        Number of obs     =      882
Group and time vars:      id time    Number of groups =      147
Link:                       logit    Obs per group:
Family:                  binomial                 min =        6
Correlation:              AR(1)                    avg =      6.0
                                                  max =        6
                                     Wald chi2(1)      =    37.72
Scale parameter:               1     Prob > chi2       =   0.0000


                              (Std. Err. adjusted for clustering on id)
- - - - - - - - - - - - - - - - - - - - - - - - - - - - - - - - - -
```

Output 7.4 (*cont.*)

```
            |                  Robust
  hyperchol |      Coef.     Std. Err.       z    P>|z|  [ 95% Conf. Interval]
------------+----------------------------------------------------------------
      skinf |    .3278797    .0533889     6.14   0.000    .2232394    .4325199
      _cons |    -1.94179    .2685998    -7.23   0.000   -2.468236   -1.415344
------------+----------------------------------------------------------------
```

```
GEE population-averaged model              Number of obs     =      882
Group and time vars:           id time     Number of groups  =      147
Link:                            logit     Obs per group:
Family:                       binomial                    min =        6
Correlation:              unstructured                    avg =      6.0
                                                          max =        6
                                           Wald chi2(1)      =    29.66
Scale parameter:                    1      Prob > chi2       =   0.0000
```

```
                               (Std. Err. adjusted for clustering on id)
-----------------------------------------------------------------------------
            |                  Robust
  hyperchol |      Coef.     Std. Err.      z    P>|z|   [ 95% Conf. Interval]
------------+----------------------------------------------------------------
      skinf |   .2801254    .0514332     5.45   0.000     .1793181    .3809327
      _cons |  -1.797615    .2634358    -6.82   0.000    -2.31394    -1.28129
------------------------------------------------------------------------------
```

Table 7.4 Regression coefficients and standard errors for the sum of skinfolds estimated by GEE analysis with different correlation structures

Correlation structure	Regression coefficient (se)
Exchangeable	0.279 (0.054)
Independent	0.404 (0.071)
Stationary five-dependent	0.284 (0.052)
Autoregressive	0.328 (0.053)
Unstructured	0.280 (0.051)

compared with the results of a naive logistic regression analysis, in which the dependency of observations is ignored. Output 7.5 presents the result of this naive logistic regression analysis.

The comparison between the results of the naive logistic regression analysis and the results of the GEE analysis with an independent correlation structure are comparable to what has been observed for continuous outcome variables. The regression coefficients of both analyses are exactly the same, while the standard errors obtained from the GEE analysis are higher than those obtained for the naive logistic regression analysis.

7.5.3 Mixed Model Analysis

Comparable to the situation with continuous outcome variables, in the case of dichotomous outcome variables it is also possible to analyse the relationship between a dichotomous outcome variable and covariate(s) with a mixed model analysis. The first step is to perform an analysis with only a random intercept. Output 7.6 shows the result of the logistic mixed model analysis with only a random intercept to analyse the relationship between hypercholesterolemia and the sum of skinfolds.

The output of a logistic mixed model analysis is comparable to the output observed for a linear mixed model analysis. The first part provides some general information about the model. It shows that a logistic mixed model analysis was performed, that there are 882 observations within

Output 7.5 Results of a naive logistic regression analysis to analyse the relationship between hypercholesterolemia and the sum of skinfolds

```
Logistic regression                          Number of obs    =        882
                                             LR chi2(1)       =      71.87
                                             Prob > chi2      =     0.0000
Log likelihood = -526.1634                   Pseudo R2        =     0.0639

--------------------------------------------------------------------------
  hyperchol |     Coef.   Std. Err.      z    P>|z|    [ 95% Conf. Interval]
----------+---------------------------------------------------------------
     skinf |  .4036002   .0499853    8.07   0.000     .3056308    .5015697
     _cons | -2.243681   .2097814  -10.70   0.000    -2.654845   -1.832517
--------------------------------------------------------------------------
```

Output 7.6 Results of a logistic mixed model analysis with only a random intercept to analyse the relationship between hypercholesterolemia and the sum of skinfolds

```
Mixed-effects logistic regression            Number of obs    =        882
Group variable:              id              Number of groups =        147

                                             Obs per group:
                                                       min =           6
                                                       avg =         6.0
                                                       max =           6

Integration method: mvaghermite              Integration pts. =         7

                                             Wald chi2(1)     =      28.19
Log likelihood = -403.09316                  Prob > chi2      =     0.0000
--------------------------------------------------------------------------
  hyperchol |     Coef.   Std. Err.      z    P>|z|    [ 95% Conf. Interval]
----------+---------------------------------------------------------------
     skinf |  .5610047   .1056666    5.31   0.000     .3539019    .7681075
     _cons | -3.641963   .4951684   -7.35   0.000    -4.612475   -2.671451
----------+---------------------------------------------------------------
id          |
  var(_cons)|  7.180246   1.688216                     4.529031   11.38344
--------------------------------------------------------------------------
LR test vs. logistic model: chibar2(01) = 246.14   Prob >= chibar2 = 0.0000
```

147 subjects. Again, there is no missing data; the minimum, maximum and average number of observations within a subject are all equal to six.

Furthermore, the log likelihood of the model (i.e. −403.09316) and the result of a Wald test (Wald chi2(4) = 28.19), and the corresponding p-value (prob > chi2 = 0.000) are presented. This Wald test is a generalised Wald test for all covariates in the model, which is not interesting. As for a linear mixed model analysis, the log

likelihood can be used for the likelihood ratio test, which, for instance, can be used to evaluate whether a random slope should be added to the model.

The output also shows the integration method (mvaghermite). The latter stands for mean variance adaptive Gauss–Hermite quadrature. It is a complicated method that has been used for the logistic mixed model analysis. See for mathematical details, for instance, Liu and Pierce (1994),

Lesaffre and Spiessens (2001), Rabe-Hesketh et al. (2002), Skrondal and Rabe-Hesketh (2004) or Rabe-Hesketh et al. (2005). It should be noted that there are more estimation methods available to estimate the parameters of a logistic mixed model analysis (Stroup and Claassen, 2002) and that different software programmes can use a different estimation method. In Section 13.5 this will be further discussed.

The second part of the output shows the most important information obtained from the analysis, i.e. the (fixed) regression coefficients. This information is exactly the same as has been discussed for continuous outcome variables, although the regression coefficients can be transformed into odds ratios by taking EXP[regression coefficient]. Again, the interpretation of the regression coefficient is the same as has been discussed for the logistic GEE analysis, i.e. a pooled between-subjects and within-subjects interpretation. (1) The between-subjects interpretation: a subject with a one-unit higher score for the sum of skinfolds, compared to another subject, has a EXP (0.5610047) = 1.75 times higher odds of being in the hypercholesterolemia group compared to the odds of being in the non-hypercholesterolemia group. (2) The within-subjects interpretation: an increase of one unit in the sum of skinfolds within a subject is associated with 1.75 times higher odds of moving to the hypercholesterolemia group compared to the odds of staying in the non-hypercholesterolemia group.

The last part of the output shows information about the random part of the model. In this situation only the random intercept variance is given, i.e. 7.180246. Also, for the logistic mixed model analysis, the assumption is that the intercepts are normally distributed. From this normal distribution, the variance is calculated. It should be noted that in the output of the logistic mixed model analysis no error variance is given. This has to do with the fact that in a logistic regression analysis the probability of belonging to a certain group is estimated without error. The error in the analysis is outside the model, i.e. in the difference between the calculated probability and the observed dichotomous value (which is either 0 or 1).

Because there is no error variance in the logistic mixed model analysis, the ICC cannot be calculated in the same way as has been discussed for continuous outcome variables. For logistic mixed model analysis, the ICC can be calculated by Equation 7.8 (Twisk, 2006; Twisk, 2019) . In the example, the ICC is therefore equal to 7.18 / (7.18 + $(3.14)^2$ / 3) = 69%.

$$ICC = \sigma_b^2 \bigg/ \left(\sigma_b^2 + \frac{\pi^2}{3} \right) \qquad (7.8)$$

where σ_b^2 = between group variance, and $\pi = 3.14$

The last line of the output gives the result of the likelihood ratio test comparing the model with a random intercept with a model without a random intercept, i.e. a naive logistic regression analysis. Apparently, this difference is 246.14, which follows a Chi-square distribution with one degree of freedom (i.e. the random intercept), and which is highly significant. In other words, the results of the likelihood ratio test suggest that it is necessary to add a random intercept to the model. As previously mentioned in Chapter 3, where a linear mixed model analysis was discussed, this likelihood ratio test is not very interesting, because theoretically, there must be an adjustment for the dependency of the observations within a subject, so there must be a random intercept.

The results of this likelihood ratio test can be verified by comparing the –2 log likelihood of the naive logistic regression analysis presented in Output 7.5 with the –2 log likelihood of the logistic mixed model analysis with only a random intercept presented in Output 7.6. This difference is indeed equal to 246.14.

The next step in this logistic mixed model analysis is to evaluate the necessity of a random slope for sum of skinfolds. As has been mentioned before, a random slope is only possible for time-dependent covariates, so a random slope for the sum of skinfolds can be added to the model. When a random slope for the sum of skinfolds is added to the model (depending on the software package used) it is possible that the model will not converge. This happens quite often when random slopes are added to a logistic mixed model analysis. The reason for this is that the mathematics behind logistic mixed model analysis is complicated and therefore, it is sometimes not possible to add random slopes to the model. Output 7.7 shows the results of the logistic mixed model analysis with a random slope for the sum of skinfolds.

From the random part of Output 7.7, it can be seen that the random slope variance for the sum of skinfolds (var(skinf)) as well as the covariance

Output 7.7 Results of a logistic mixed model analysis with a random intercept and a random slope for the sum of skinfolds to analyse the relationship between hypercholesterolemia and the sum of skinfolds

```
Mixed-effects logistic regression        Number of obs      =      882
Group variable:              id          Number of groups   =      147

                                         Obs per group:
                                                       min =        6
                                                       avg =      6.0
                                                       max =        6

Integration method: mvaghermite          Integration pts.   =        7

                                         Wald chi2(1)       =    28.17
Log likelihood = -403.09316              Prob > chi2        =   0.0000
-----------------------------------------------------------------------
   hyperchol |    Coef.  Std. Err.     z    P>|z|   [ 95% Conf. Interval]
-------------+---------------------------------------------------------
       skinf |  .5607602  .1056562   5.31  0.000    .3536778   .7678426
       _cons | -3.640467  .4950777  -7.35  0.000   -4.610801  -2.670132
-------------+---------------------------------------------------------
id           |
  var(skinf) |  1.11e-13  6.95e-09                      .          .
  var(_cons) |  7.179823  1.688199                  4.528662  11.38302
-------------+---------------------------------------------------------
id           |
  cov(_cons, |
      skinf) |  1.32e-11  6.40e-07   0.00  1.000   -1.25e-06  1.25e-06
-----------------------------------------------------------------------
LR test vs. logistic model: chi2(3) = 246.14        Prob > chi2 = 0.0000
```

between the random intercept and the random slope (cov(_cons,skinf)) are extremely low, so it is obvious that a random slope for the sum of skinfolds should not be added to the model. This is also reflected in the –2 log likelihood of the model, which is exactly the same as the –2 log likelihood obtained from a model with only a random intercept (see Output 7.6).

7.5.4 Comparison between GEE Analysis and Mixed Model Analysis

For continuous outcome variables it was seen that GEE analysis with an exchangeable correlation structure and a mixed model analysis with only a random intercept provided identical regression coefficients in the analysis of a longitudinal dataset. For dichotomous outcome variables, however, the situation is more complex. Logistic GEE analysis with an exchangeable correlation structure and

the logistic mixed model analysis with only a random intercept give a totally different result. In Output 7.3 it was shown that the regression coefficient for the sum of skinfolds derived from a logistic GEE analysis with an exchangeable correlation structure was 0.2789969 with a standard error of 0.0541275, while the regression coefficient for the sum of skinfolds derived from a logistic mixed model analysis with only a random intercept was 0.5610047 with a standard error of 0.1056666 (see Output 7.6). The regression coefficient and standard error obtained from the logistic GEE analysis are much lower than those obtained from a logistic mixed model analysis. This is always the case and it also holds for the estimated standard errors.

In Chapter 3 it was explained that the difference between mixed model analysis and GEE analysis is that within mixed model analysis the adjustment for the dependency of the observations within the subject is performed by estimating the difference between the subjects with a random intercept variance. Within GEE analysis the adjustment is performed by directly estimating the correlation between the repeated measurements. However, there is also another difference between the two methods. GEE analysis is known as a population average method, while mixed model analysis is known as a subject specific method (Hu et al., 1998). This does not influence the values of the estimated regression coefficients obtained from a linear GEE analysis and a linear mixed model analysis, but it does influence the values of the estimated regression coefficients obtained from a logistic GEE analysis and a logistic mixed model analysis. The difference in regression coefficients is a theoretical one, which is always in favour of a mixed model analysis, meaning that the regression coefficients obtained from a logistic mixed model analysis will always be higher (i.e. further away from zero) compared to the regression coefficients obtained from a logistic GEE analysis. This difference is based on a mathematical relationship and depends on the magnitude of the between-subject variance (see Equation 7.9) (Hu et al., 1998). When there is more between-subject variance, the difference between the regression coefficients will be larger:

$$\beta^{(pa)} = \left[\left(\frac{16\sqrt{3}}{15\pi} \right)^2 \sigma_b^2 + 1 \right]^{-1/2} \beta^{(ss)} \qquad (7.9a)$$

$$\frac{16\sqrt{3}}{15\pi} = 0.588 \qquad (7.9b)$$

where $\beta^{(pa)}$ is the population average regression coefficient obtained from a logistic GEE analysis, σ_b^2 is the between-subject variance and $\beta^{(ss)}$ is the subject-specific regression coefficient obtained from a logistic mixed model analysis.

In Figure 7.1, the difference between the population average method and the subject-specific method is illustrated for both the linear model (i.e. with a continuous outcome variable) and the logistic model (i.e. with a dichotomous outcome variable). For the linear longitudinal regression analysis, both GEE analysis and mixed model analysis produce exactly the same result, i.e. the population average method is equal to the subject-specific method. For the logistic longitudinal regression analysis, however, the two methods produce a different result. From Figure 7.1 it can

be seen that the regression coefficients calculated with a logistic GEE analysis will always be lower than the coefficients calculated with a logistic mixed model analysis. (See also, for instance, Neuhaus et al., 1991; Hu et al., 1998; Twisk et al., 2017.)

Because of the remarkable difference in regression coefficients, it is important to get an answer to the question of which method should be used. To answer that question, data from a randomised controlled trial (RCT) is used in which the effectiveness of a classification-based treatment was compared to usual physical therapy care in patients with subacute or chronic lower back pain (Apeldoorn et al., 2012). The outcome variable of interest was good or bad functional status, in which bad functional status was the event of interest. For this particular example, the outcome variable was assessed at 8 and 26 weeks after the start of treatment. For the illustration, two analyses were performed with both logistic mixed model analysis and logistic GEE analysis. One analysis was performed on a complete dataset and one analysis on the real dataset with around 10% missing data. In Chapter 3 it was mentioned that mixed model analysis deals better with missing data than GEE analysis and that this is the most important reason why mixed model analysis is preferred above GEE analysis when a continuous outcome variable is analysed in a longitudinal study. Therefore, it is interesting to evaluate whether this is also the case when a dichotomous outcome variable is analysed in a longitudinal study.

To evaluate the performance of the different methods, the estimated probabilities of the outcome variable obtained from the analyses were compared to the observed percentages at the two time points. Table 7.5 shows the results of the two analyses on the complete dataset. As expected, the regression coefficients obtained from the logistic GEE analysis were much lower (closer to zero) than the coefficients obtained from the logistic mixed model analysis. Table 7.6 shows the predicted probabilities and the observed percentages of bad functional status in the intervention and usual care group at the two follow-up measurements. From Table 7.6 it can be seen that the predicted probabilities derived from the logistic GEE analysis are exactly the same as the observed percentages. The predicted probabilities derived from the logistic mixed model analysis are highly overestimated, i.e. higher probabilities when the

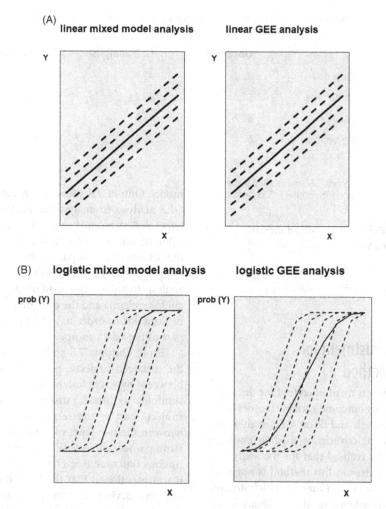

(A)
linear mixed model analysis   **linear GEE analysis**

(B)   **logistic mixed model analysis**   **logistic GEE analysis**

Figure 7.1 Illustration of the population average method of GEE analysis and the subject-specific method of mixed model analysis, illustrating both the situation with (A) a continuous outcome variable and (B) the situation with a dichotomous outcome variable.

Table 7.5 Results of a logistic GEE analysis and a logistic mixed model analysis performed on the complete RCT dataset

	GEE analysis	Mixed model analysis
8 weeks	−0.44 (0.36)	−0.80 (0.66)
26 weeks	−0.57 (0.37)	−0.97 (0.68

observed percentages are higher than 50% and lower probabilities when the observed percentages are lower than 50%.

When the real dataset (with around 10% missing data) is analysed, the result of the comparison is almost the same as has been observed in the analysis on the complete dataset. Again, the regression coefficients of the logistic GEE analysis are lower (closer to zero) than the regression coefficients of the logistic mixed model analysis (see Table 7.7). The differences between the observed percentages and predicted probabilities are less pronounced than for the complete dataset, but the differences are still in favour of the logistic GEE analysis (see Table 7.8). So, in conclusion, the results of the analysis on this example dataset indicate the lower regression coefficients obtained from the logistic GEE analysis are more valid than the regression coefficients obtained from the logistic mixed model analysis, even in situations where there is missing data. Therefore, it is advised to use logistic GEE analysis for the longitudinal analysis of a dichotomous outcome.

Table 7.6 Observed percentages of bad functional status and predicted probabilities derived from the logistic GEE analysis and logistic mixed model analysis on the complete RCT dataset

		Observed	GEE analysis	Mixed model analysis
8 weeks	Usual care	42.2	42.2	35.7
	Intervention	53.2	53.2	55.2
26 weeks	Usual care	56.2	56.2	61.6
	Intervention	69.4	69.4	80.8

Table 7.7 Results of a logistic GEE analysis and a logistic mixed model analysis performed on the RCT dataset with missing data

	GEE analysis	Mixed model analysis
8 weeks	−0.29 (0.34)	−0.51 (0.60)
26 weeks	−0.51 (0.35)	−0.86 (0.62)

7.5.5 The Adjustment for Covariance Method

In Section 3.6, it was mentioned that for the analysis of a continuous outcome variable besides linear mixed model analysis and linear GEE analysis also the adjustment for covariance method could be used. It should be realised that for the analysis of a dichotomous outcome, this method is not available. This is due to the fact that for a dichotomous outcome, the covariance of the residuals is not defined. So, for the analysis of a dichotomous outcome, only logistic GEE analysis or logistic mixed model analysis can be used.

7.5.6 Models to Disentangle the Between- and Within-subjects Relationship

In Chapter 5, hybrid models were introduced as a possibility to disentangle the between- and within-subjects relationship. A model of changes and an autoregressive model were used in order to estimate only the within-subjects part of the relationship. All these models can also be used for dichotomous outcomes. Regarding the overall example used throughout the book, for instance, the relationship between hypercholesterolemia and the sum of skinfolds can be analysed with a hybrid

model. Output 7.8 shows the result of the logistic GEE analysis to analyse the relationship between hypercholesterolemia and the individual mean value of the sum of skinfolds in order to obtain the between-subjects part of the relationship, while Output 7.9 shows the result of the logistic GEE analysis to analyse the relationship between hypercholesterolemia and the deviation score of the sum of skinfolds in order to obtain the within-subjects part of the relationship.

From Outputs 7.8 and 7.9 it can be seen that the between-subjects part of the relationship between hypercholesterolemia and the sum of skinfolds is much stronger that the within-subjects part of the relationship. The difference between the two parts of the relationship was less strong when cholesterol was analysed as a continuous outcome (see Output 5.3). In Section 5.2 it was mentioned that the individual mean value and the deviation score are uncorrelated and, therefore, the two variables could be analysed in the same model leading to exactly the same regression coefficients. For illustration, Output 7.10 shows the results of the logistic GEE analysis to analyse the relationship between hypercholesterolemia and both the individual mean value and the deviation score of the sum of skinfolds.

Surprisingly, the two regression coefficients obtained from the combined model are slightly different from the ones obtained from the two separate models. This is not really expected, because the correlation between the individual mean value and the deviation score of the sum of skinfolds are equal to zero and therefore, they should not influence each other in a multiple regression model. However, in a logistic model the situation is slightly different. This has to do with the non-collapsibility phenomenon. Theoretically, this non-collapsibility phenomenon arises from the difference in the total variance

Table 7.8 Observed percentages of bad functional status and predicted probabilities derived from the logistic GEE analysis and logistic mixed model analysis on the RCT dataset with missing data

		Observed	GEE analysis	Mixed model analysis
8 weeks	Usual care	43.7	44.0	39.0
	Intervention	51.5	51.2	51.5
26 weeks	Usual care	56.2	56.2	61.1
	Intervention	68.7	68.0	78.8

Output 7.8 **Results of a logistic GEE analysis to analyse the relationship between hypercholesterolemia and the individual mean value of the sum of skinfolds**

```
GEE population-averaged model          Number of obs    =       882
Group variable:                 id     Number of groups =       147
Link:                        logit     Obs per group:
Family:                   binomial                        min =       6
Correlation:          exchangeable                        avg =     6.0
                                                           max =       6
                                       Wald chi2(1)     =     22.26
Scale parameter:                 1     Prob > chi2      =    0.0000


                                     (Std. Err. adjusted for clustering on id)
-----------------------------------------------------------------------
             |            Robust
     chol01 |     Coef.  Std. Err.     z   P>|z|   [95% Conf. Interval]
-----------+-----------------------------------------------------------
 mean_skinf |  .4823638  .1022276   4.72  0.000   .2820015   .6827261
      _cons | -2.542548  .4395854  -5.78  0.000   -3.40412  -1.680977
-----------------------------------------------------------------------
```

between a logistic regression analysis with one covariate and a logistic regression analysis with more than one covariate. In a linear model, the total variance is the summation of explained and unexplained variance. When a covariate is added to a linear regression model, the unexplained variance decreases while the explained variance increases with the same amount. However, in a logistic model, the unexplained variance is a fixed number. So, when a covariate that is related to the outcome is added to a logistic model which already contains another covariate, the total variance will increase. Because of this increased variance it is often said that adding a covariate to the logistic model that is related to the outcome changes the scale on which the regression coefficients must be interpreted. Because of this, the regression coefficient will change,

even though the correlation between the two variables equals zero. However, although the noncollapsibility phenomenon can lead to biased effect estimates, it should be realised that the influence is not extremely high. This was illustrated in the hybrid model analysis in which both variables (the individual mean value and the deviation score for the sum of skinfolds) are highly related to hypercholesterolemia, but the regression coefficients obtained from the combined model are only slightly different from the ones obtained from the separate models.

When the model of changes between subsequent measurements is used to obtain an estimate for the within-subjects part of the relationship with a dichotomous outcome, another problem arises. This has to do with the fact that changes in a dichotomous outcome variable result in a

Output 7.9 Results of a logistic GEE analysis to analyse the relationship between hypercholesterolemia and the deviation score of the sum of skinfolds

```
GEE population-averaged model          Number of obs    =      882
Group variable:                   id   Number of groups =      147
Link:                          logit   Obs per group:
Family:                     binomial                 min =        6
Correlation:            exchangeable                 avg =      6.0
                                                     max =        6
                                       Wald chi2(1)     =    10.38
Scale parameter:                   1   Prob > chi2      =   0.0013

                                (Std. Err. adjusted for clustering on id)
-----------------------------------------------------------------------
             |               Robust
    chol01   |     Coef.   Std. Err.      z    P>|z|    [ 95% Conf. Interval]
-------------+---------------------------------------------------------
  dev_skinf  |  .2126421   .0660035    3.22   0.001    .0832776   .3420066
      _cons  | -.6944896   .1367522   -5.08   0.000   -.9625191  -.4264602
-----------------------------------------------------------------------
```

Output 7.10 Results of a logistic GEE analysis to analyse the relationship between hypercholesterolemia and both the individual mean value and the deviation score of the sum of skinfolds

```
GEE population-averaged model          Number of obs    =      882
Group variable:                   id   Number of groups =      147
Link:                          logit   Obs per group:
Family:                     binomial                 min =        6
Correlation:            exchangeable                 avg =      6.0
                                                     max =        6
                                       Wald chi2(2)     =    33.28
Scale parameter:                   1   Prob > chi2      =   0.0000

                                (Std. Err. adjusted for clustering on id)
-----------------------------------------------------------------------
             |               Robust
    chol01   |     Coef.   Std. Err.      z    P>|z|    [ 95% Conf. Interval]
-------------+---------------------------------------------------------
 mean_skinf  |  .4671199   .1046545    4.46   0.000    .2620009   .6722389
  dev_skinf  |  .2210443   .0670186    3.30   0.001    .0896903   .3523983
      _cons  |  -2.50239   .4455472   -5.62   0.000   -3.375646  -1.629133
-----------------------------------------------------------------------
```

categorical variable with four groups (i.e. subjects who stay in one group, subjects who stay in another group and two groups in which subjects move from one group to another (see Figure 7.2)). So, changes between subsequent measurements in a dichotomous outcome variable result in a categorical outcome, which longitudinal analysis is even more complicated than the longitudinal analysis of a dichotomous outcome (see Chapter 8).

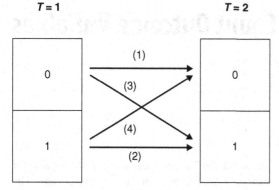

$T = 1$ $T = 2$

Figure 7.2 Changes in a dichotomous variable between two time-points lead to a categorical variable with four groups.

7.5.7 Comments

In Chapter 6, different methods were introduced which aim to estimate causality in observed longitudinal studies. These models can also be applied to dichotomous outcomes. However, for the longitudinal mediation models, the problem of non-collapsibility also occurs, so these models should be interpreted with some caution.

In this chapter, the longitudinal analysis of a dichotomous outcome variable is explained in a rather simple way. It should be realised that the mathematical details of these analyses are very complicated, and therefore, a detailed explanation goes beyond the scope of this book. For further details, reference is made to other publications, with regard to GEE analysis, for instance Liang and Zeger, 1986; Prentice, 1988; Lipsitz et al., 1991; Carey et al., 1993; Lipsitz et al., 1994b; Wiliamson et al., 1995; Lipsitz and Fitzmaurice, 1996; and with regard to mixed model analysis for instance Conway, 1990; Goldstein, 1995; Rodriguez and Goldman, 1995; Goldstein and Rasbash, 1996; Gibbons and Hedeker, 1997; Barbosa and Goldstein, 2000; Yang and Goldstein, 2000; Rodriguez and Goldman, 2001).

Chapter 8

Categorical and Count Outcome Variables

8.1 Categorical Outcome Variables

8.1.1 Two Measurements

Longitudinal analysis with a categorical outcome variable is more problematic than the longitudinal analysis with a continuous or dichotomous outcome variable. Until recently only simple methods were available to analyse such outcome variables. Therefore, categorical variables are sometimes treated as continuous, especially when they are ordinal and have a sufficient number (usually five or more) of categories. Another method is to reduce the categorical outcome variable into a dichotomous one by combining two or more categories. However, this results in a loss of information, and is only recommended when there are only a few subjects in one or more categories of the categorical variable.

The simplest form of longitudinal study with a categorical outcome variable is one where the categorical outcome variable is measured twice in time. This situation (when the categorical variable consists of three groups) is illustrated in the 3×3 table presented below (where n stands for number of subjects and p stands for the proportion of the total number of subjects N).

To determine whether there is a change over time in a categorical outcome variable, an extension of the McNemar test (which has been discussed for dichotomous outcome variables, see Section 7.1) can be used. This extension is known

as the Stuart–Maxwell test, and is only suitable for outcome variables with three categories. The Stuart–Maxwell test statistic follows a Chi-square distribution with one degree of freedom, and is defined as shown in Equation 8.1:

$$\chi^2 = \frac{\bar{n}_{23}d_1^2 + \bar{n}_{13}d_2^2 + \bar{n}_{12}d_3^2}{2(\bar{n}_{12}\bar{n}_{13} + \bar{n}_{12}\bar{n}_{23} + \bar{n}_{13}\bar{n}_{23})} \quad (8.1a)$$

$$\bar{n}_{ij} = \frac{n_{ij} + n_{ji}}{2} \quad (8.1b)$$

$$d_i = n_{it1} - n_{it2} \quad (8.1c)$$

where n_{ij} is the number of subjects in group i at $t = 1$ and in group j at $t = 2$, and n_{ji} is the number of subjects in group j at $t = 1$ and in group i at $t = 2$.

Like the McNemar test, the Stuart–Maxwell test gives an indication of the differences between the change over time in opposite directions, while the main interest is usually the total change over time. Therefore, the proportion of change can be calculated. This proportion of change is a summation of all the off-diagonal proportions of the categorical 3×3 table. Around this proportion a 95% confidence interval can be calculated in the usual way. For calculation of the standard error of the proportion of change, Equation 8.2 can be used:

$$se\left(p_{change}\right) = \sqrt{\frac{p_{change} - \left(1 - p_{change}\right)}{N}} \quad (8.2)$$

		t_2			
		1	2	3	Total
t_1	1	n_{11}/p_{11}	n_{12}/p_{12}	n_{13}/p_{13}	$n_{1(t1)}/p_{1(t1)}$
	2	n_{21}/p_{21}	n_{22}/p_{22}	n_{23}/p_{23}	$n_{2(t1)}/p_{2(t1)}$
	3	n_{31}/p_{31}	n_{32}/p_{32}	n_{33}/p_{33}	$n_{3(t1)}/p_{3(t1)}$
	total	$n_{1(t2)}/p_{1(t2)}$	$n_{2(t2)}/p_{2(t2)}$	$n_{3(t2)}/p_{3(t2)}$	N

where *se* is the standard error, p_{change} is the proportion of change equal to $1 - (p_{11} + p_{22} + p_{33})$ when there are three categories, and N is the total number of subjects.

As for the dichotomous outcome variables, this method can be carried out for the proportion of subjects that increases over time or the proportion of subjects that decreases over time. It is obvious that the calculation of the proportion of change is not limited to categorical variables with only three categories.

8.1.2 More than Two Measurements

When there are more than two measurements in a longitudinal study, the same method can be used as has been described for dichotomous outcome variables, i.e. the proportion of change can be used as a measure of total change over time. To do so, $(T - 1)r \times c$ tables[1] must be constructed (for $t = 1$ and $t = 2$, for $t = 2$ and $t = 3$, and so on), then for each table the proportion of change can be calculated. To obtain the total proportion of change, Equation 8.3 can be applied:

$$\bar{p} = \frac{1}{N(T - 1)} \sum_{i=1}^{N} c_i \qquad (8.3)$$

where $\bar{p}$ is the total proportion of change, N is the number of subjects, T is the number of measurements, and c_i is the number of changes for individual i over time.

8.1.3 Comparing Groups

In research situations in which the longitudinal development over time between several groups must be compared, the simple methods discussed for dichotomous outcome variables can also be used for categorical outcome variables, i.e. comparing the proportion of change between different groups, or comparing the proportion of change in a certain direction between different groups. When there are only two groups to compare, a 95% confidence interval can be constructed around the difference in proportions. This should be done in exactly the same way as has been described for dichotomous outcome variables (see Section 7.3).

---

[1] $r \times c$ stands for row × column, and indicates that all types of categorical variables can be analysed in this way.

8.1.4 Example

For the example, the continuous outcome variable cholesterol of the example dataset was divided into three equal groups, according to the 33rd and the 66th percentile, in order to create the categorical cholesterol variable. This was done at each of the six repeated measurements. Most of the statistical methods are suitable for situations in which there are only two measurements, and therefore the change between the first and the last repeated measurement (between $t = 1$ and $t = 6$) for the categorical outcome variable cholesterol will be considered first. In Table 8.1 the 3×3 table for cholesterol at $t = 1$ and cholesterol at $t = 6$ is presented. From Table 8.1 the Stuart–Maxwell test statistic and the proportion of change can be calculated. Output 8.1 shows the result of the Stuart–Maxwell test.

With the Stuart–Maxwell test statistic, the difference between the change over time in opposite directions is tested for significance. Because the categorisation of cholesterol was based on tertiles (i.e. fixed values), it is obvious that the Stuart–Maxwell statistic will be very low, and far from significant. The proportion of change is an indicator of the total change over time. In the example the proportion of change in cholesterol (as categorical variable) between $t = 1$ and $t = 6$ is 0.45, with a 95% confidence interval ranging from 0.37 to 0.57, indicating a highly significant change over time.

When all the measurements are included in the analysis, the only possible way to investigate the change over time in a categorical outcome variable is to calculate the overall proportion of change. To do so, all five 3×3 tables must be constructed (see Table 8.2). From the five 3×3 tables the total proportion of change can be calculated (with Equation 8.2). This proportion is equal to 0.35.

Table 8.1 3×3 table with the number of subjects for cholesterol (as categorical variable) at $t = 1$ and $t = 6$

	Cholesterol at $t = 6$			
Cholesterol at $t = 1$	0	1	2	Total
1	30	15	3	48
2	16	19	14	49
3	3	15	32	50
Total	49	49	49	147

Output 8.1 Results of a Stuart–Maxwell test to analyse the change over time in cholesterol (as categorical variable) between $t = 1$ and $t = 6$

```
- - - - - - - - - - - - - - - - - - - - - - - - - - -
cholesterol | cholesterol at t=6
at t=1      |
            |    1       2       3   Total
- - - - - -+- - - - - - - - - - - - - - - - - - -
          1 |   30      15       3    48
          2 |   16      19      14    49
          3 |    3      15      32    50
            |
     Total  |   49      49      49   147
- - - - - - - - - - - - - - - - - - - - - - - - - - -


                                            chi2      df    Prob>chi2
- - - - - - - - - - - - - - - - - - - - - - - - - - - - - - - - - -
Symmetry (asymptotic)                    |  0.07       3      0.9955
Marginal homogeneity (Stuart-Maxwell)    |  0.05       2      0.9765
- - - - - - - - - - - - - - - - - - - - - - - - - - - - - - - - - -
```

The corresponding 95% confidence interval (based on the standard error calculated with Equation 8.3) ranges from 0.32 to 0.38, i.e. a highly significant change over time.

It is also possible to compare the change over time for cholesterol (as categorical variable) between two or more groups. In the example, first, the change in cholesterol between $t = 1$ and $t = 6$ (using only those two measurements) was compared between males and females. Table 8.3 shows the two 3×3 tables. For both groups the proportion of change is exactly the same, i.e. 0.45. Around this (no) difference a 95% confidence interval can be constructed: [−0.16 to 0.16]. The width of the confidence interval provides information about the precision of the calculated difference between the two groups.

To obtain an estimation of the possible difference in change over time for the two groups by using all six measurements, the overall proportion of change must be calculated for both groups. When this is done (by creating $(T - 1)$, 3×3 tables for both groups), the overall proportion of change for males is 0.47, while for females the overall proportion of change is 0.44. Around this difference of 3% a 95% confidence interval can be calculated. To obtain a standard error for this difference, Equation 8.4 can be applied to these data, which results in a confidence interval ranging from −0.05 to 0.11, i.e. no significant difference

between the two groups in the overall proportion of change:

$$se\left(p_{g1} - p_{g2}\right) = \sqrt{\left[\frac{p_{g1}\left(1 - p_{g1}\right)}{N_{g1}}\right] + \left[\frac{p_{g2}\left(1 - p_{g2}\right)}{N_{g2}}\right]}$$

(8.4)

where se is the standard error, p_{g1} is the proportion of change in group 1, p_{g2} is the proportion of change in group 2, N_{g1} is the number of subjects in group 1, and N_{g2} is the number of subjects in group 2.

8.1.5 Regression-based Methods

In Chapters 4 and 7, it was argued that longitudinal data analysis with a continuous outcome variable is a longitudinal extension of linear regression analysis, and that longitudinal data analysis with a dichotomous outcome variable is a longitudinal extension of logistic regression analysis; i.e. both take into account the fact that the repeated observations within the subject are correlated. Analogous to this, it is obvious that longitudinal data analysis with a categorical outcome variable is a longitudinal extension of multinomial logistic regression analysis. Multinomial logistic regression analysis is the categorical extension of logistic regression analysis. With multinomial logistic regression analysis, basically multiple logistic regression analyses are

Table 8.2 Five 3 × 3 tables with the number of subjects for cholesterol (as categorical variable) between $t = 1$ and $t = 6$

	Cholesterol at $t = 2$			
Cholesterol at $t = 1$	0	1	2	**Total**
1	35	11	2	48
2	8	29	12	49
3	3	13	34	50
Total	46	53	48	147
	Cholesterol at $t = 3$			
Cholesterol at $t = 2$	0	1	2	Total
1	34	11	1	46
2	18	20	15	53
3	2	11	35	48
Total	54	42	41	147
	Cholesterol at $t = 4$			
Cholesterol at $t = 3$	0	1	2	Total
1	45	9	0	54
2	7	23	12	42
3	0	14	37	51
Total	52	46	49	147
	Cholesterol at $t = 5$			
Cholesterol at $t = 4$	0	1	2	Total
1	36	16	0	52
2	10	24	12	46
3	3	10	36	49
Total	49	50	48	147
	Cholesterol at $t = 6$			
Cholesterol at $t = 5$	0	1	2	Total
1	35	13	1	49
2	12	22	16	50
3	2	14	32	48
Total	49	49	49	147

combined into one analysis, although the method is slightly different from performing separate independent logistic regression analyses.

Multinomial logistic regression analysis for longitudinal data analysis was first described for generalised estimating equation (GEE) analysis (see for instance Liang et al., 1992; Miller et al., 1993; Lipsitz et al., 1994b). Surprisingly, the multinomial logistic GEE analysis is still not yet available in standard software packages, and will therefore not be discussed in detail. The general idea of this GEE analysis is the same as for all other GEE analyses, i.e. an adjustment for the dependency of observations is performed by assuming a certain (working) correlation structure.

From the beginning of this century, a multinomial logistic mixed model analysis has also been described (Agresti et al., 2000; Rabe-Hesketh et al.,

Table 8.3 3 × 3 table with the number of subjects for cholesterol (as categorical variable) at $t = 1$ and $t = 6$ for two groups divided by sex (males versus females)

Males	Cholesterol at t = 6			
Cholesterol at $t = 1$	0	1	2	Total
1	14	7	0	21
2	11	8	5	24
3	3	5	16	24
Total	28	20	21	69
Females	Cholesterol at t = 6			
Cholesterol at $t = 1$	0	1	2	Total
1	16	8	3	27
2	5	11	9	25
3	0	10	16	26
Total	21	29	28	78

2001a; Rabe-Hesketh and Skrondal, 2001). As with all other mixed model analyses described earlier, with a multinomial logistic mixed model analysis, all questions related to the change over time can be answered as well. Moreover, it can also be used to analyse the longitudinal relationship between a categorical outcome variable and one or more covariates. The underlying methods and the interpretation of the regression coefficients are comparable to what has been described for logistic mixed model analysis.

8.1.5.1 Example

The first step in the analysis to answer the question whether there is a relationship between cholesterol (as categorical variable) and the sum of skinfolds is to perform a multinomial logistic mixed model analysis with only a random intercept. Output 8.2 shows the result of this analysis.

The output of a multinomial logistic mixed model analysis has a slightly different structure than the outputs of linear and logistic mixed model analyses. This has to do with the fact that a multinomial logistic mixed model analysis in STATA can only be performed with the GLLAMM procedure. GLLAMM stands for Generalised Linear Latent and Mixed Models and is a very flexible method with which many complicated mixed model analyses can be performed.

In the output, first the number of level 1 units and the number of level 2 units are given. Level 1 and level 2 refers to multilevel analysis, which is another name for mixed model analysis. Level 1 refers to the repeated observations which are clustered within the subject. Level 2 refers to the subjects. So, there are 882 observations performed within 147 subjects. This was already known, because that is the structure of the example dataset. Next, the log likelihood of the model is presented (−792.87177). As for all other mixed model analyses, this number is only interesting in comparison to the log likelihood value of another model in order to perform the likelihood ratio test. In the next part of the output, the regression coefficient and standard error are given for the sum of skinfolds as well as the z-values, the corresponding p-values and the 95% confidence interval around the regression coefficient. In the example dataset, cholesterol is a categorical outcome variable with three categories (i.e. tertiles), so there are two tables with regression coefficients. In the first table the second tertile of cholesterol is compared to the first (i.e. lowest) tertile of cholesterol (which is the reference category), while in the second table the third (i.e. highest) tertile of cholesterol is compared to the lowest tertile. The interpretation of the regression coefficients is rather complicated. For the comparison between the second tertile and the reference category (i.e. the lowest tertile) the regression coefficient (0.4827596) can be transformed into an odds ratio (i.e. EXP[0.4827596] = 1.62). As for all other longitudinal regression analyses, this odds ratio has a pooled interpretation. (1) The between-subjects interpretation: a subject

Output 8.2 Results of a logistic multinomial mixed model analysis with only a random intercept to analyse the relationship between cholesterol (as categorical variable) and the sum of skinfolds

```
number of level 1 units = 882
number of level 2 units = 147


gllamm model


log likelihood = -792.87177


- - - - - - - - - - - - - - - - - - - - - - - - - - - - - - - - - - - - - - - - -
cholesterol |        Coef.  Std. Err.    z   P>|z|   [ 95% Conf. Interval]
- - - - - - - - +- - - - - - - - - - - - - - - - - - - - - - - - - - - - - - - - -
c2          |
     skinf |   .4827596  .128826   3.75  0.000    .2302654   .7352539
     _cons |  -1.174496 .5292486  -2.22  0.026   -2.211804  -.1371877
- - - - - - - - +- - - - - - - - - - - - - - - - - - - - - - - - - - - - - - - - -
c3          |
     skinf |   .7451436  .1277911  5.83  0.000    .4946777   .9956094
     _cons |  -2.20741  .5314244  -4.15  0.000   -3.248983  -1.165838
- - - - - - - - - - - - - - - - - - - - - - - - - - - - - - - - - - - - - - - - -


Variances and covariances of random effects
- - - - - - - - - - - - - - - - - - - - - - - - - - - - - - - - - - - - - - - - -


***level 2 (id)

  var(1): 6.8117255 (1.3218953)
- - - - - - - - - - - - - - - - - - - - - - - - - - - - - - - - - - - - - - - - -
```

with a one-unit higher score for the sum of skinfolds, compared to another subject, has 1.62 times higher odds of being in the second tertile compared to the odds of being in the lowest tertile. (2) The within-subjects interpretation: an increase of one unit in the sum of skinfolds within a subject is associated with 1.62 times higher odds of moving from the lowest tertile to the second tertile of cholesterol, compared to the odds of staying in the lowest tertile. The regression coefficient of the sum of skinfolds belonging to the comparison between the highest tertile and the lowest tertile (EXP[0.7451436] = 2.11) can be interpreted in the same way. (1) A subject with a one-unit higher score for the sum of skinfolds, compared to another subject, has 2.11 times higher odds of being in the highest tertile for cholesterol compared to the odds of being in the lowest tertile. (2) An increase of one unit in the sum of skinfolds within a subject is associated with 2.11 times higher odds of moving from the lowest tertile to

the highest tertile for cholesterol, compared to the odds of staying in the lowest tertile. In the last part of Output 8.2 the variance around the intercept (var(1) = 6.8117255) is provided. Again, this variance is estimated assuming a normal distribution of the intercepts. It has been mentioned before, that in a longitudinal study it is not necessary to evaluate whether or not a random intercept should be added to the model. A model without a random intercept (i.e. a naive multinomial logistic regression analysis) is theoretically wrong, because it ignores the longitudinal nature of the data.

The next step in the analysis can be to add a random slope for the sum of skinfolds to the model. Output 8.3 shows the result of the multinomial logistic mixed model analysis with both a random intercept and a random slope for the sum of skinfolds.

First of all, in Output 8.3, it can be seen that the random part of the model (variances and covariances of random effects) is extended compared to

Output 8.3 Results of a logistic multinomial mixed model analysis with a random intercept and a random slope for the sum of skinfolds to analyse the relationship between cholesterol (as categorical variable) and the sum of skinfolds

```
number of level 1 units = 882
number of level 2 units = 147

Condition Number = 69.39715

gllamm model

log likelihood = -790.51288

- - - - - - - - - - - - - - - - - - - - - - - - - - - - - - - - - - - - - - - - - -
cholesterol |       Coef.  Std. Err.      z   P>|z|   [ 95% Conf. Interval]
- - - - - - - - +- - - - - - - - - - - - - - - - - - - - - - - - - - - - - - - - - -
c2          |
      skinf |  .5687498  .1596936    3.56  0.000    .255756   .8817436
      _cons | -1.302102  .6154244   -2.12  0.034  -2.508311  -.095892
- - - - - - - - +- - - - - - - - - - - - - - - - - - - - - - - - - - - - - - - - - -
c3          |
      skinf |  .8338226  .1593379    5.23  0.000    .521526  1.146119
      _cons | -2.345778  .6188567   -3.79  0.000  -3.558715 -1.132841
- - - - - - - - - - - - - - - - - - - - - - - - - - - - - - - - - - - - - - - - - -


Variances and covariances of random effects
- - - - - - - - - - - - - - - - - - - - - - - - - - - - - - - - - - - - - - - - - -

***level 2 (id)

  var(1): 11.927035 (5.8816087)
  cov(1,2): -.94701524 (.9913524) cor(1,2): -.52829728

  var(2): .26941681 (.15834677)
- - - - - - - - - - - - - - - - - - - - - - - - - - - - - - - - - - - - - - - - - -
```

the model with only a random intercept. A random slope (var(2)) is provided as well as the covariance between the random slope and the random intercept (cov(1,2)). In the output, the correlation between the random slope and the random intercept (cor(1,2)) is also provided, although the latter is not very informative. It can also be seen that the log likelihood of the model with both a random intercept and a random slope (−790.51288) is slightly better compared to the model with only a random intercept (−792.87177). The difference between the two −2 log likelihoods equals 4.75. The improvement is, therefore, not statistically significant (the critical value of the Chi-square

distribution with two degrees of freedom equals 5.99) So, in this example, a model with only a random intercept can be used.

As has been mentioned before, the magnitude of the regression coefficient (i.e. the magnitude of the odds ratio) reflects both the between-subjects and the within-subjects relationship. The relative contribution of both parts highly depends on the proportion of subjects who move from one category to another. In the example dataset for instance, the proportion of subjects who move from the lowest to the highest category is rather low, so for the comparison between the lowest and the highest tertile, the estimated odds ratio

Output 8.4 Results of a logistic multinomial mixed model analysis to analyse the relationship between cholesterol (as categorical variable) and the individual mean value of the sum of skinfolds

```
number of level 1 units = 882
number of level 2 units = 147

Condition Number = 69.941431

gllamm model

log likelihood = -794.98068


- - - - - - - - - - - - - - - - - - - - - - - - - - - - - - - - - - - - - - - - - -
cholesterol |       Coef.  Std. Err.    z    P>|z|    [ 95% Conf. Interval]
- - - - - - - - +- - - - - - - - - - - - - - - - - - - - - - - - - - - - - - - - -
c2          |
  mean_skinf |   1.009957  .2040885   4.95  0.000    .6099512  1.409963
       _cons | -2.883731  .6723749  -4.29  0.000   -4.201561   -1.5659
- - - - - - - - +- - - - - - - - - - - - - - - - - - - - - - - - - - - - - - - - -
c3          |
  mean_skinf |  1.314746  .2030953   6.47  0.000    .9166864  1.712805
       _cons | -4.07726   .6747639  -6.04  0.000   -5.399773 -2.754747
- - - - - - - - - - - - - - - - - - - - - - - - - - - - - - - - - - - - - - - - -


Variances and covariances of random effects
- - - - - - - - - - - - - - - - - - - - - - - - - - - - - - - - - - - - - - - - -

***level 2 (id)

  var(1): 6.6572316 (1.2769519)
- - - - - - - - - - - - - - - - - - - - - - - - - - - - - - - - - - - - - - - - -
```

of 2.11 probably reflects mainly the between-subjects relationship. To verify this, a hybrid model can be analysed in which the between-subjects part of the relationship and the within-subjects part of the relationship are estimated separately. Output 8.4 shows the result of the logistic multinomial mixed model analysis to analyse the relationship between cholesterol (as categorical variable) and the individual mean value of the sum of skinfolds in order to obtain the between-subjects part of the relationship, while Output 8.5 shows the result of the logistic multinomial mixed model analysis to analyse the relationship between cholesterol (as categorical variable) and the deviation score of the sum of skinfolds in order to obtain the within-subjects part of the relationship.

From Outputs 8.4 and 8.5, it is clear that the overall relationship between cholesterol (as categorical variable) and the sum of skinfolds is mainly driven by the between-subjects part of the relationship. However, the within-subjects part of the relationship is also significant for both comparisons.

8.2 Count Outcome Variables

A special type of a categorical outcome variable is a count outcome variable (e.g. the number of asthma attacks, the number of falls in elderly people, etc.). Because of the discrete and non-negative nature of the count outcome variables, they are assumed to have a Poisson distribution. A Poisson distribution is further characterised by

Output 8.5 Results of a logistic multinomial mixed model analysis to analyse the relationship between cholesterol (as categorical variable) and the deviation score of the sum of skinfolds

```
number of level 1 units = 882
number of level 2 units = 147


Condition Number = 7.1185382


gllamm model


log likelihood = -810.98167


- - - - - - - - - - - - - - - - - - - - - - - - - - - - - - - - - - - - - - - - - - -
 cholesterol |     Coef.  Std. Err.     z  P>|z|    [ 95% Conf. Interval]
- - - - - - - - +- - - - - - - - - - - - - - - - - - - - - - - - - - - - - - - - - - - -
c2           |
   dev_skinf | .3642297  .1553568   2.34  0.019     .059736   .6687233
       _cons | .8525628  .2627121   3.25  0.001    .3376566  1.367469
- - - - - - - - +- - - - - - - - - - - - - - - - - - - - - - - - - - - - - - - - - - - -
c3           |
   dev_skinf | .5254968  .1538859   3.41  0.001    .223886   .8271075
       _cons | .8668522   .262637   3.30  0.001    .3520931  1.381611
- - - - - - - - - - - - - - - - - - - - - - - - - - - - - - - - - - - - - - - - - - -


Variances and covariances of random effects
- - - - - - - - - - - - - - - - - - - - - - - - - - - - - - - - - - - - - - - - - - -


***level 2 (id)

  var(1): 8.4114161 (1.738022)
- - - - - - - - - - - - - - - - - - - - - - - - - - - - - - - - - - - - - - - - - - -
```

equal values for the mean and the variance and therefore the Poisson distribution is skewed to the right. A longitudinal analysis with a count outcome variable is comparable to a cross-sectional Poisson regression analysis, the difference being that the longitudinal method takes into account the within-subjects correlations. It should further be noted that the longitudinal Poisson regression analysis is sometimes referred to as longitudinal log-linear regression analysis.

As for the longitudinal linear regression analysis, the longitudinal logistic regression analysis, and the longitudinal multinomial logistic regression analysis, the longitudinal Poisson regression analysis is, in fact, nothing more than an extension of the cross-sectional Poisson regression analysis, i.e. an additional adjustment for the dependency of the observations within the subject. With this analysis the longitudinal relationship between the count outcome variable and several covariates can be analysed. As in all regression analyses, the covariates can be continuous, dichotomous or categorical, although of course in the latter situation dummy coding can or must be used. As in cross-sectional Poisson regression analysis, the regression coefficient can be transformed into a rate ratio (EXP[regression coefficient]). For estimation of the regression coefficients (i.e. rate ratios) the same methods can be used as were discussed before, i.e. GEE analysis and mixed model analysis. Within GEE analysis, a correction for the within-subjects correlations is made by assuming a (working) correlation structure, while within mixed model analysis the different regression coefficients are allowed to vary between the subjects, i.e. by adding a random intercept and (if necessary) random slopes to the model. It should be realised that a longitudinal Poisson regression analysis is only valid when the count outcome variable has a Poisson distribution. It has been mentioned before that a Poisson distribution is characterised by equal values for the mean and the variance. In many research situations, however, the variance will be higher than the mean. This phenomenon is known as overdispersion and although Poisson regression analysis is still valid when the overdispersion is not that big, it is better to use an alternative method when there is overdispersion. This alternative method is known as negative binomial regression analysis and also for negative binomial regression analysis both GEE analysis and mixed model analysis are available. The interpretation of the regression coefficients obtained from a negative binomial regression analysis is exactly the same as for a Poisson regression analysis. So, also the regression coefficient from a negative binomial regression analysis has to be transformed into a rate ratio by taking EXP[regression coefficient].

8.2.1 Example

8.2.1.1 Introduction

The example chosen to illustrate the analysis of a count outcome variable is taken from the same longitudinal study which was used to illustrate most of the other methods, i.e. the Amsterdam Growth and Health Longitudinal Study (Kemper, 1995). One of the aims of this study was to investigate the possible clustering of risk factors for coronary heart disease (CHD) and the longitudinal relationship with several lifestyle covariates. To construct a measure of clustering, at each of the six repeated measurements, high-risk quartiles were formed for each of the following biological risk factors: (1) the ratio between total serum cholesterol and high-density lipoprotein cholesterol, (2) diastolic blood pressure, (3) the sum of skinfolds, and (4) cardiopulmonary fitness. At each of the repeated measurements, clustering was defined as the number of biological risk factors that occurred in a particular subject. So, if a subject belonged to the high-risk quartile for all biological risk factors, the clustering score at that particular measurement was 4, if the subject belonged to three high-risk groups, the clustering score was 3, etc. This clustering score is a count outcome variable and this outcome variable is related to the amount of physical activity, which is a time-dependent continuous covariate. Tables 8.4 and 8.5 show descriptive information about the example dataset.

Table 8.4 Number of subjects with a particular clustering score (i.e. the number of CHD risk factors) measured at six time-points

Time-point	Number of CHD risk factors				
	0	1	2	3	4
1	65	49	25	4	4
2	60	44	33	9	1
3	47	64	26	9	1
4	54	53	29	9	2
5	56	53	26	11	1
6	55	46	33	13	0

Table 8.5 Mean and standard deviation (between brackets) for the clustering score and physical activity

Time-point	Clustering	Activity
1	0.96 (0.97)	4.35 (1.9)
2	1.00 (0.90)	3.90 (1.6)
3	0.99 (0.97)	3.62 (1.7)
4	1.00 (0.97)	3.52 (1.8)
5	0.97 (0.96)	3.37 (2.1)
6	1.03 (0.98)	3.02 (2.1)

Again, the aim of the study was to investigate the longitudinal relationship between the clustering of CHD risk factors and physical activity. In the example, both GEE analysis and mixed model analysis will be used to investigate this longitudinal relationship. From the descriptive information provided in Table 8.5 it can be seen that the mean value of the clustering score is almost equal to the variance, so the variable has a nice Poisson distribution.

8.2.1.2 GEE Analysis

As with all GEE analyses, the GEE analysis with a count outcome variable requires the a priori choice of a (working) correlation structure. In principle, there are the same possibilities as has been discussed for other outcome variables (see Section 3.4.3). In the example, first an exchangeable correlation structure will be used.

Output 8.6 presents the result of the GEE analysis to analyse the relationship between clustering of CHD risk factors and physical activity. The output looks exactly the same as the output from a linear or logistic GEE analysis. The only

Output 8.6 Results of a Poisson GEE analysis to analyse the relationship between the clustering of CHD risk factors and physical activity

```
GEE population-averaged model          Number of obs    =      882
Group variable:                  id    Number of groups =      147
Link:                           log    Obs per group:
Family:                     Poisson                       min =       6
Correlation:           exchangeable                       avg =     6.0
                                                          max =       6
                                        Wald chi2(1)     =    20.15
Scale parameter:                  1     Prob > chi2      =   0.0000

                             (Std. Err. adjusted for clustering on id)
-----------------------------------------------------------------------
             |               Robust
     cluster |    Coef.    Std. Err.      z    P>|z|    [ 95% Conf. Interval]
-------------+---------------------------------------------------------
    activity |  -.085672   .0190848   -4.49   0.000    -.1230775  -.0482665
       _cons |   .2642411  .0772955    3.42   0.001     .1127447   .4157374
-----------------------------------------------------------------------
```

difference is the different link function, which is log, and the different family, which is Poisson. The other information provided in the output is exactly the same as for the linear and the logistic GEE analyses. So, the most interesting part is the last part of the output in which the regression coefficient for physical activity is given. This part of the output shows the regression coefficient, the standard error, the z-value, the corresponding p-value and the 95% confidence interval around the regression coefficient.

The scale parameter obtained from a Poisson GEE analysis has the same interpretation as the scale parameter derived from a logistic GEE analysis. This has to do with the characteristics of the Poisson distribution on which the Poisson GEE analysis is based. Within the Poisson distribution the variance is exactly the same as the mean value. So, for the Poisson GEE analysis, the scale parameter has to be one (i.e. a direct relationship between the variance and the mean).

Looking at the estimated regression coefficient, it can be seen that there is a highly significant inverse relationship between the CHD risk clustering score and physical activity. The regression coefficient of –0.085672 has to be transformed into a rate ratio by taking EXP [regression coefficient]. The rate ratio for physical

activity is therefore EXP[–0.085672] = 0.92 with a 95% confidence interval ranging from EXP[–0.1230775] = 0.88 to EXP[–0.0482665] = 0.95. As for all other longitudinal data analyses, this rate ratio has a double interpretation: (1) the between-subjects interpretation; i.e. a difference of one unit in physical activity between subjects is associated with a 9% (1/0.92 = 1.09) difference (i.e. lower) in the number of CHD risk factors and (2) the within-subjects interpretation; an increase of one unit in physical activity within a subject is associated with a 9% decrease in the number of CHD risk factors.

To investigate the influence of using a different correlation structure, the data were re-analysed with different correlation structures. The result is presented in Output 8.7, and in Table 8.6 the results of the Poisson GEE analyses with different correlation structures are summarised.

From Table 8.6, it can be seen that the results obtained with the four dependent correlation structures are only slightly different. This was also observed for the GEE analysis with a dichotomous outcome variable. In other words, for the longitudinal analysis of a count outcome variable, GEE analysis also seems to be quite robust against a wrong choice of a correlation structure. For the analysis with an independent correlation

Output 8.7 Results of a Poisson GEE analysis with different correlation structures to analyse the relationship between the clustering of CHD risk factors and physical activity

```
GEE population-averaged model              Number of obs      =        882
Group variable:                    id      Number of groups   =        147
Link:                             log      Obs per group:
Family:                       Poisson                          min =        6
Correlation:              independent                          avg =      6.0
                                                               max =        6
                                           Wald chi2(1)        =      18.62
Scale parameter:                    1      Prob > chi2         =     0.0000

Pearson chi2(882):             821.33      Deviance            =     968.54
Dispersion (Pearson):        .9312152      Dispersion          =   1.098124

                      (Std. Err. adjusted for clustering on id)
------------------------------------------------------------------
           |              Robust
   cluster |     Coef.   Std. Err.      z    P>|z|    [ 95% Conf. Interval]
-----------+------------------------------------------------------
  activity | -.0988464   .0229069   -4.32   0.000    -.143743  -.0539497
     _cons |  .3103622   .0909612    3.41   0.001    .1320815   .4886428
------------------------------------------------------------------


GEE population-averaged model              Number of obs      =        882
Group and time vars:          id time      Number of groups   =        147
Link:                             log      Obs per group:
Family:                       Poisson                          min =        6
Correlation:            stationary(5)                          avg =      6.0
                                                               max =        6
                                           Wald chi2(1)        =      22.15
Scale parameter:                    1      Prob > chi2         =     0.0000

                      (Std. Err. adjusted for clustering on id)
------------------------------------------------------------------
           |              Robust
   cluster |     Coef.   Std. Err.      z    P>|z|    [ 95% Conf. Interval]
-----------+------------------------------------------------------
  activity | -.0846262   .0179808   -4.71   0.000    -.119868  -.0493844
     _cons |  .2569902    .076354    3.37   0.001    .1073392   .4066413
------------------------------------------------------------------


GEE population-averaged model              Number of obs      =        882
Group and time vars:          id time      Number of groups   =        147
Link:                             log      Obs per group:
Family:                       Poisson                          min =        6
Correlation:                     AR(1)                          avg =      6.0
                                                               max =        6
                                           Wald chi2(1)        =      20.06
Scale parameter:                    1      Prob > chi2         =     0.0000

                      (Std. Err. adjusted for clustering on id)
------------------------------------------------------------------
```

Output 8.7 (*cont.*)

```
             |              Robust
   cluster |     Coef.   Std. Err.      z   P>|z|    [ 95% Conf. Interval]
- - - - - - - -+- - - - - - - - - - - - - - - - - - - - - - - - - - - - - - - - - - -
  activity | -.0848512   .0189464   -4.48   0.000    -.1219854   -.0477169
     _cons |  .2569211   .0799962    3.21   0.001     .1001315    .4137108
- - - - - - - - - - - - - - - - - - - - - - - - - - - - - - - - - - - - - - - - - - -


GEE population-averaged model            Number of obs      =       882
Group and time vars:        id time      Number of groups   =       147
Link:                          log       Obs per group:
Family:                    Poisson                           min =       6
Correlation:           unstructured                          avg =     6.0
                                                             max =       6
                                         Wald chi2(1)       =     20.43
Scale parameter:                 1       Prob > chi2        =    0.0000

                              (Std. Err. adjusted for clustering on id)
- - - - - - - - - - - - - - - - - - - - - - - - - - - - - - - - - - - - - - - - - - -
             |              Robust
   cluster |     Coef.   Std. Err.      z   P>|z|    [ 95% Conf. Interval]
- - - - - - - -+- - - - - - - - - - - - - - - - - - - - - - - - - - - - - - - - - - -
  activity | -.079091   .0174967   -4.52   0.000    -.1133838   -.0447981
     _cons | .2425161   .0749627    3.24   0.001     .0955919    .3894403
- - - - - - - - - - - - - - - - - - - - - - - - - - - - - - - - - - - - - - - - - - -
```

Table 8.6 Results of Poisson GEE analyses with different correlation structures

Correlation structure	Regression coefficient (se)
Exchangeable	−0.086 (0.019)
Independent	−0.099 (0.023)
5-Dependent	−0.085 (0.018)
Autoregressive	−0.085 (0.019)
Unstructured	−0.079 (0.017)

structure, the regression coefficient and the standard error was slightly higher than for the analysis with the four dependent correlation structures.

8.2.1.3 Mixed Model Analysis

The first mixed model analysis performed on this dataset is an analysis with only a random intercept.

Output 8.8 shows the result of this Poisson mixed model analysis.

The output of the Poisson mixed model analysis looks the same as the output that has been discussed earlier for the linear and logistic mixed model analyses. The left column of the first part contains general information about the model. It shows that a Poisson mixed model analysis was performed, and it gives the log likelihood of the model (−1051.6519). The right column of the first part of the output shows the information about the number of observations, the number of subjects and the number of observations within the subject. It also shows the result of a Wald test which is (again) not interesting.

The second part of the output (the fixed part of the model) shows the regression coefficient for physical activity, the standard error, the z-value, the p-value and the 95% confidence interval around the regression coefficient. Also this regression coefficient has to be transformed into a rate ratio by taking EXP[regression coefficient]. The

Output 8.8 Results of a Poisson mixed model analysis with only a random intercept to analyse the relationship between the clustering of CHD risk factors and physical activity

```
Mixed-effects Poisson regression          Number of obs     =        882
Group variable:              id           Number of groups  =        147

                                          Obs per group:
                                                        min =          6
                                                        avg =        6.0
                                                        max =          6

Integration method: mvaghermite           Integration pts.  =          7

                                          Wald chi2(1)      =      14.48
Log likelihood = -1051.6519               Prob > chi2       =     0.0001
- - - - - - - - - - - - - - - - - - - - - - - - - - - - - - - - - - - - - - -
    cluster |    Coef.   Std. Err.      z   P>|z|   [ 95% Conf. Interval]
- - - - - - - +- - - - - - - - - - - - - - - - - - - - - - - - - - - - - - - -
   activity | -.088815  .0233405   -3.81  0.000   -.1345615   -.0430684
      _cons |  .0912854 .1046205    0.87  0.383    -.113767     .2963378
- - - - - - - +- - - - - - - - - - - - - - - - - - - - - - - - - - - - - - - -
id          |
  var(_cons)|  .3901599 .0783727                   .2631837     .5783971
- - - - - - - - - - - - - - - - - - - - - - - - - - - - - - - - - - - - - - -
LR test vs. Poisson model: chibar2(01) = 126.74   Prob >= chibar2 = 0.0000
```

interpretation of the rate ratio is (as always for a time-dependent covariate) a pooled between-subjects and within-subjects interpretation.

The last part of the output shows information about the random part of the model, which contains only the variance around the intercept. Furthermore, the result of the likelihood ratio test comparing the model with a random intercept and a model without a random intercept (a naive Poisson regression analysis with physical activity) is given. This difference is 126.74, and it follows a Chi-square distribution with one degree of freedom (i.e. only a random intercept is added to the model). The corresponding p-value (prob > chi2) is very low (i.e. highly significant), so it is, also statistically, necessary to add a random intercept to the model.

Because physical activity is a time-dependent covariate, the next step in the analysis can be to add a random slope for physical activity to the model. A model with a random slope for physical activity unfortunately did not converge. Because this happens quite often when random slopes are added to the model, it is suggested to use the centred value of the continuous covariate instead of the actual observed value. The centred value for the covariate can be obtained by subtracting the overall mean value from each individual observation. It is argued that models converge better when centred values are used. However, in this particular example, a model with the centred value for physical activity including a random slope did also not converge. So, in this situation, a Poisson mixed model analysis with only a random intercept should be used.

8.2.2 Comparison between GEE Analysis and Mixed Model Analysis

When the results of the GEE analysis and the mixed model analysis are compared, it can be concluded that the differences observed for dichotomous outcome variables (see Section 7.5.2) are not observed for a count outcome variable. In fact, the observed differences between the two methods are very small, although both the regression coefficient and the standard error

Output 8.9 Results of a negative binomial GEE analysis to analyse the relationship between the clustering of CHD risk factors and physical activity

```
GEE population-averaged model           Number of obs    =     882
Group variable:                   id    Number of groups =     147
Link:                            log    Obs per group:
Family:       negative binomial(k=1)                min =       6
Correlation:           exchangeable                 avg =     6.0
                                                     max =       6
                                        Wald chi2(1)     =   19.14
Scale parameter:                   1    Prob > chi2      =  0.0000

                                  (Std. Err. adjusted for clustering on id)
- - - - - - - - - - - - - - - - - - - - - - - - - - - - - - - - - - - - - - -
              |            Semirobust
      cluster |    Coef.   Std. Err.      z    P>|z|    [ 95% Conf. Interval]
- - - - - - - + - - - - - - - - - - - - - - - - - - - - - - - - - - - - - - -
     activity | -.0840483  .0192116   -4.37   0.000    -.1217024   -.0463943
        _cons |  .2580306  .0783996    3.29   0.001     .1043702    .411691
- - - - - - - - - - - - - - - - - - - - - - - - - - - - - - - - - - - - - - -
```

obtained from a Poisson mixed model analysis are slightly higher than those obtained from a Poisson GEE analysis. The fact that the subject-specific regression coefficient and standard error derived from the Poisson mixed model analysis are slightly higher than the population-averaged coefficients derived from the Poisson GEE analysis has to do with the characteristics of the Poisson model compared to the linear model. However, the differences are far less pronounced than those discussed for the logistic model.

8.2.3 Negative Binomial Regression Analysis

As mentioned before, negative binomial regression analysis can be used as an alternative for a Poisson regression analysis when there is overdispersion in the count outcome variable (Agresti et al., 2000; Green, 2021). In the example with the clustering of CHD risk factors, the variance of the clustering variable was almost equal to the mean, so there is no need to perform a negative binomial regression analysis. However, for illustrative purposes, a negative binomial GEE analysis with an exchangeable correlation structure was performed to analyse the relationship between the clustering of CHD risk

factors and physical activity. Output 8.9 shows the result of this analysis.

From Output 8.9 it can be seen that the regression coefficient obtained from a negative binomial GEE analysis is almost the same as the coefficient obtained from a Poisson GEE analysis. Again, this is not surprising, because the outcome variable in this example (clustering of CHD risk factors) has a Poisson distribution without overdispersion. It should further be noted that a negative binomial mixed model analysis did not converge in this particular example.

To get a better feeling for the differences between longitudinal Poisson regression and longitudinal negative binomial regression on count data with overdispersion, another example is used. This second example is taken from the Longitudinal Aging Study Amsterdam (LASA). The aim of the study was to investigate the development of symptoms of loneliness over time and whether the development of symptoms of loneliness was different for males and females. In this particular dataset there were six repeated measurements and the outcome variable was a count variable theoretically ranging between 0 and 11. Figure 8.1 shows the distribution of the outcome variable (i.e. symptoms of loneliness) over all observations in the longitudinal study. The average value of symptoms of loneliness was

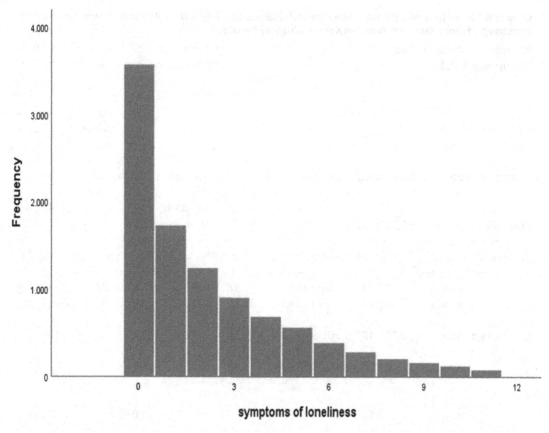

Figure 8.1 Distribution of symptoms of loneliness.

2.2, while the variance was equal to 6.8, indicating overdispersion. Both a Poisson mixed model analysis and a negative binomial mixed model analysis were used to analyse the difference in development over time in symptoms of loneliness between males and females. In the dataset males were coded 0 and females were coded 1. Outputs 8.10 and 8.11 show the results of the analyses.

From both outputs it can be seen that there are 9,937 observations within 2,539 subjects. This indicates that there is a lot of missing data in this longitudinal study. On average there are 3.9 observations for each subject. See Chapter 11 for a detailed discussion of the influence of missing data on the result of a longitudinal data analysis.

Looking at the fixed parts of both mixed model analyses it can be seen that the results are only slightly different. The regression coefficient for time indicates the linear development over time for males, while the regression coefficient

for the interaction between sex and time indicates the difference in linear development over time between females and males. Not only are the regression coefficients slightly different for the two methods, the standard errors also are. In general, the standard errors obtained from the negative binomial mixed model analysis are a bit higher than the ones obtained from the Poisson mixed model analysis. The higher standard errors estimated with the negative binomial mixed model analysis, are a better reflection of the over-dispersion in the count data. In the present example, the higher standard errors also lead to slightly lower z-values and slightly higher p-values. The result of the negative binomial mixed model analysis is not only theoretically more valid than the result of the Poisson mixed model analysis, it is also shown in the fit indicators (see Table 8.7). Both the Akaike Information Criterion (AIC) and the Bayesian Information Criterion (BIC) are much

Output 8.10 Results of a Poisson mixed model analysis to analyse the difference in development of symptoms of loneliness over time between males and females

```
Mixed-effects Poisson regression        Number of obs     =    9,937
Group variable:              id          Number of groups =    2,539

                                         Obs per group:
                                                        min =        1
                                                        avg =      3.9
                                                        max =        6

Integration method: mvaghermite          Integration pts. =        7

                                         Wald chi2(3)     =   249.80
Log likelihood = -17997.643              Prob > chi2      =   0.0000
- - - - - - - - - - - - - - - - - - - - - - - - - - - - - - - - - - - - -
  loneliness |     Coef.  Std. Err.      z  P>|z|   [ 95% Conf. Interval]
- - - - - - -+- - - - - - - - - - - - - - - - - - - - - - - - - - - - - -
        time |  .0888718  .0078256  11.36  0.000    .073534   .1042096
         sex |  .2099123  .0545349   3.85  0.000   .1030258   .3167988
             |
 c.time#c.sex| -.0233427  .0099904  -2.34  0.019  -.0429235  -.0037619
             |
       _cons |  .0421771  .0412191   1.02  0.306  -.0386109   .1229651
- - - - - - -+- - - - - - - - - - - - - - - - - - - - - - - - - - - - - -
id           |
   var(_cons)|  1.180423  .0464039                 1.092889   1.274969
- - - - - - - - - - - - - - - - - - - - - - - - - - - - - - - - - - - - -
LR test vs. Poisson model: chibar2(01) = 12473.14  Prob >= chibar2 = 0.0000
```

lower for the negative binomial mixed model analysis, indicating a better fit. As has been mentioned before, both AIC and BIC can be seen as adjusted values of the –2 log likelihood, i.e. adjusted for the number of parameters estimated by the particular model (Akaike, 1974; Schwarz, 1978).

8.2.4 Comments

As has been mentioned for the longitudinal data analyses with continuous and dichotomous outcomes, alternative models for categorical and count outcomes (such as hybrid models, time-lag models, etc.) can also be performed. In Section 8.1.5.1 the hybrid model analysis was illustrated for the analysis of the relationship between cholesterol (as categorical variable) and the sum of skinfolds. The methods are basically the same as those described in Chapters 5 and 6, so this will not be further discussed here.

One of the characteristics of a Poisson distribution is skewness to the right. When a continuous or count outcome variable is skewed to the right, normally a log transformation is performed to obtain a normal distribution. After the analysis is performed on this log transformed outcome variable, the regression coefficients have to be retransformed in order to get interpretable effect estimates. Of course, this is also possible for skewed-to-the-right longitudinal continuous or count outcomes. However, sometimes in the skewed-to-the-right longitudinal count outcome there is an excess of zeros. When there is an excess of zeros, a log transformation does not lead to a normal distribution. It has been shown

Output 8.11 Results of a negative binomial mixed model analysis to analyse the difference in development of symptoms of loneliness over time between males and females

```
Mixed-effects nbinomial regression         Number of obs      =      9,937
Overdispersion:              mean
Group variable:                id          Number of groups   =      2,539

                                           Obs per group:
                                                         min =          1
                                                         avg =        3.9
                                                         max =          6

Integration method: mvaghermite            Integration pts.   =          7

                                           Wald chi2(3)       =     209.40
Log likelihood = -17958.36                 Prob > chi2        =     0.0000
- - - - - - - - - - - - - - - - - - - - - - - - - - - - - - - - - - - - - - -
  loneliness |     Coef.   Std. Err.      z    P>|z|    [ 95% Conf. Interval]
- - - - - - -+- - - - - - - - - - - - - - - - - - - - - - - - - - - - - - - -
        time |  .0890452   .0087045   10.23   0.000    .0719846   .1061058
         sex |  .2004323   .0564515    3.55   0.000    .0897894   .3110751
             |
 c.time#c.sex | -.0200606   .0112076   -1.79   0.073    -.042027   .0019059
             |
        _cons |  .0503406   .0426286    1.18   0.238   -.0332098   .1338911
- - - - - - -+- - - - - - - - - - - - - - - - - - - - - - - - - - - - - - - -
     /lnalpha | -2.607091   .1337065  -19.50   0.000   -2.869151  -2.345032
- - - - - - -+- - - - - - - - - - - - - - - - - - - - - - - - - - - - - - - -
id           |
    var(_cons)|  1.160932   .0465391                     1.073208   1.255826
- - - - - - - - - - - - - - - - - - - - - - - - - - - - - - - - - - - - - - -
LR test vs. nbinomial model: chibar2(01) = 3550.84  Prob >= chibar2 = 0.0000
```

Table 8.7 Fit indicators for two mixed model analyses analysing the difference in development over time in symptoms of loneliness between males and females

	AIC	BIC
Poisson mixed model analysis	36005.29	36041.31
Negative binomial mixed model analysis	35928.72	35971.94

Abbreviations: AIC = Akaike Information Criterion; BIC = Bayesian Information Criterion.

that for a longitudinal count outcome, the excess of zeros is not very problematic because both a longitudinal Poisson regression analysis and a longitudinal negative binomial regression analysis can deal (to some extent) with the excess of zeros. However, sometimes the excess of zeros is related to a floor effect, which can complicate the interpretation of the result. This issue will be further discussed in Chapter 9.

Chapter 9

Outcome Variables with Floor or Ceiling Effects

9.1 Introduction

When the development over time is analysed in a particular continuous outcome variable, it is quite common that the variable reaches either a ceiling or a floor. For instance, in rehabilitation research, most of the patients will recover after a certain amount of time. On the instrument to measure the rehabilitation process, these patients cannot score any higher than the maximum. It is also possible that so-called floor effects occur. For instance, when the effect of pain medication is investigated and the outcome variable pain is measured on a visual analogue scale, some patients will report no pain after a certain amount of time. They cannot score lower than the no pain level. Also, in studies when there is some detection limit (e.g. for blood parameters), these floor effects are present. In fact, these problems always arise when a measurement instrument is used that has upper and lower limits and when some of the subjects in the study reach these upper or lower limits. When ceiling or floor effects are present in longitudinal studies it is also known as upper or lower censoring.

In most longitudinal medical studies, this upper or lower censoring is ignored. The outcome variables are analysed as if they were normally distributed over the whole period of time. This is not the case, because when patients reach the floor or ceiling, the outcome variable is not normally distributed anymore. In cross-sectional studies (especially in econometrics) the problem of upper and lower censoring is solved by using so-called tobit models, after Tobin's (1958) classical example on household expenditures. Within medical science, only a few examples are available in which cross-sectional tobit regression analysis is used (Twisk and Rijmen, 2009; Spriensma et al., 2012). However, in longitudinal medical studies tobit regression analysis is almost never used, while it has some nice theoretical advantages above standard longitudinal

data analysis. Tobit regression is an example of a so-called two-part model. The general idea behind two-part models (which are also known as mixed response models, mixed distribution models, selection models or hurdle models) is that the outcome variable has a mixed distribution, i.e. a binomial distribution for either reaching the floor or ceiling and another distribution for the part between the floor and ceiling. Within tobit regression analysis it is assumed that the distribution of the outcome variable between the floor and ceiling is approximately normal. However, in theory it can be another distribution as well. One two-part model that is used quite often is the zero-inflated Poisson regression model. A zero-inflated Poisson regression model is a two-part model that is used when a Poisson outcome variable has an excess of zeros. In this situation, the binomial distribution of being zero or not is mixed with a Poisson distribution for the non-zero part of the distribution. Within the two-part models a distinction must be made between standard two-part regression models and two-part joint regression models. In the standard two-part regression models the two processes are split and two sets of regression coefficients are obtained, which means that different sets of covariates can be included for the two processes. Zero-inflated Poisson regression is an example of a standard two-part model. With zero-inflated Poisson regression, one set of covariates is used for the binomial process (zero versus non-zero) and one set for the Poisson process. For some research questions this is a nice feature, for instance, when one is interested in the relationship between smoking behaviour and several covariates. When smoking behaviour is measured as the number of cigarettes smoked per day, smoking behaviour can be divided into two (different) processes. One process defines smoking versus non-smoking, while the other process defines the number of cigarettes smoked for a smoker. The two processes can have different relationships with the covariates.

However, in many situations one regression coefficient for each covariate would be preferable. Models that provide one set of regression coefficients are known as two-part joint regression models and tobit regression is an example of a two-part joint regression model.

9.2 Tobit Mixed Model Analysis

As has been mentioned before, tobit regression is an example of a two-part joint regression model. The general idea behind the tobit model is that the subjects that either score the lowest limit of the scale or the highest limit of the scale should not be regarded as subjects that truly all have the same score. Regarding floor effects, for some of the subjects the true score may fall beyond the scale of the measurement instrument or, regarding ceiling effects, the true score may fall above the scale of the measurement instrument. In other words, there is a certain variance between subjects at the limit that cannot be observed. In medical studies, patients who receive effective treatment over time may reach the limit of a certain scale, i.e. reach a floor or ceiling effect. When many patients reach this limit, it results in a skewed distribution of the outcome with an excess of either the lowest or the highest score on the scale of measurement. Within tobit regression, it is assumed that the true underlying distribution is a normal distribution,

but values below or above a certain threshold are not detectable, a phenomenon which is (again) also known as censoring (see Figure 9.1). Because part of the underlying normal distribution is unobserved, the assumed normal distribution within tobit regression is known as a latent normal distribution.

There are many examples of outcome variables that show floor or ceiling effects over time due to censoring. Functional ability measures, such as the Disability Index of the Health Assessment Questionnaire (HAQ-DI) (floor effect) and the Barthel index (ceiling effect), are especially prone to this phenomenon (Bruce and Fries, 2003). The problem with, for instance, the floor effect of HAQ-DI is that patients who score zero should not be regarded as patients who truly all have the same score. For some of the patients the true score may fall beyond the scale of the measurement instrument. In other words, there is a certain variance between patients at the limit that cannot be observed.

9.2.1 Example

The first example is taken from a longitudinal rehabilitation study among stroke patients (Kwakkel et al., 1999). The main purpose of the study was to analyse the development over time of the Barthel index. An outcome variable that

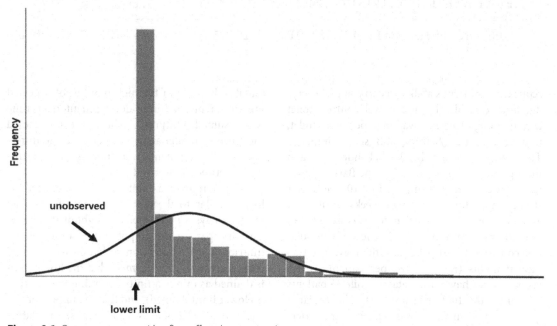

Figure 9.1 Outcome measure with a floor effect due to censoring.

Output 9.1 Results of a tobit mixed model analysis with only a random intercept to analyse the difference in development over time in the Barthel index between males and females

```
Mixed-effects tobit regression        Number of obs      =     1,646
                                       Uncensored         =     1,370
Limits: Lower = -inf                   Left-censored      =         0
        Upper = 20                     Right-censored     =       276

Group variable: id                     Number of groups   =       101
                                       Obs per group:
                                                    min =           2
                                                    avg =        16.3
                                                    max =          18

Integration method: mvaghermite        Integration pts.   =         7

                                       Wald chi2(3)       =   2957.93
Log likelihood = -3519.9879            Prob > chi2        =    0.0000
```

barthel	Coefficient	Std. err.	z	P>|z|	[95% conf. interval]	
time	.6649583	.0193571	34.35	0.000	.6270192	.7028975
sex	1.543268	1.036078	1.49	0.136	-.4874074	3.573944
time#sex	.1013071	.0265061	3.82	0.000	.0493562	.1532581
_cons	4.907955	.7778716	6.31	0.000	3.383355	6.432555

id						
var(_cons)	24.86891	3.579976			18.75526	32.97544

var(e.barthel)	6.121319	.2435694			5.662072	6.617815

```
LR test vs. tobit model: chibar2(01) = 2110.15    Prob >= chibar2 = 0.0000
```

represents a patient's ability to carry out 10 everyday tasks (i.e. bladder and bowel control, toilet use, dressing, feeding, walking, personal toilet, transfer activities, bathing and stair climbing). The lowest score for the Barthel index is 0 and the highest possible score is 20. The Barthel index was assessed weekly during the first 10 weeks after stroke onset, then every two weeks until week 20 and finally the Barthel index was assessed at week 26, week 38 and week 52. The study population consisted of 101 patients with on average 16.3 measurements (range 2–18) per patient. Forty-seven patients have a full dataset, while 33 patients only miss the first measurement. The research question to be answered was related to the difference in development over time between males and females. Because of the high number of repeated measurements, a linear development over time was assumed. Output 9.1 shows the result of a tobit mixed model analysis to analyse the difference in development over time in the Barthel index between males and females.

The output of a tobit mixed model analysis looks similar to the outputs of the other mixed model analyses performed throughout this book. The first part of the output shows some general information. It is mentioned that a mixed effects tobit regression is performed, that the lower limit is defined as minus infinity (meaning that there is no lower limit defined), and that the upper limit is equal to 20. That makes sense because the ceiling effect of the Barthel index is reached at 20. It can also be seen that in the total dataset there are 276 observations reaching the ceiling value of 20.

Furthermore, it is mentioned that there are 1,644 observations within 101 patients used in the analysis. On average there are 16.3 observations for each patient and the minimum number of observations was two and the maximum number of observations was 18. As in all mixed model analyses the log likelihood is also given, which can be used to compare different models with each other and the result of the Chi-square test relating to the covariates in the tobit mixed model (i.e. a test which is not interesting). It should be noted further that the estimation method used in the tobit mixed model analysis is the same as has been used for all mixed model analysis with a non-continuous outcome variable (i.e. the mvaghermite integration method).

The second part of the output contains the regression coefficients, standard errors, z-values, corresponding p-values and the 95% confidence intervals around the regression coefficients. The regression coefficients of the tobit mixed model analysis can be interpreted in the same way as the regression coefficients for a linear mixed model analysis. So, the regression coefficient for time (i.e. 0.6649583) indicated the difference in Barthel index with each time-point for females. This is because females are coded zero and there is an interaction between time and sex in the model. The regression coefficient for the interaction term indicates the difference in development over time between males and females, so for males the difference in Barthel index with each time-point equals $0.6649583 + 0.1013071 = 0.7662654$. The coefficient for sex gives the difference between males and females when time equals zero and is, therefore, not very informative.

The last part of the output shows the random part of the model, i.e. the random intercept variance and the residual variance. Based on the numbers it can be concluded that there is a huge correlation between the repeated observations within the subject. This is also reflected in the huge Chi-square value for the comparison between the tobit mixed model analysis with only a random intercept and the naive tobit mixed model analysis, which is given in the lowest line of the output.

As has been mentioned before, in many situations the floor or ceiling effects are ignored in longitudinal data analyses and this type of data is analysed with a linear mixed model analysis assuming a normal distribution of the outcome variable. Due to this, it is interesting to compare the result of the tobit mixed model analysis with the result of a linear mixed model analysis. Output 9.2 shows the result of a linear mixed model analysis with only a random intercept performed on the same dataset.

From Output 9.2 it can be seen that first of all the regression coefficient for the interaction term is much lower when ceiling effects are ignored. In fact, the regression coefficient obtained from the linear mixed model analysis is 10 times lower than the one obtained from the tobit mixed model analysis. Consequently, the interaction between time and sex is totally insignificant when estimated with a linear mixed model analysis. The explanation for this huge difference is the percentage of males and females that reach the ceiling in this longitudinal dataset. For females this percentage is about 8%, while for males this percentage is about 23.5% (see Figure 9.2).

It can also be seen that the log likelihood of the tobit mixed model analysis is much lower than the one obtained from the linear mixed model analysis. Although it is questionable whether the likelihood can be used to choose between the tobit mixed model analysis and the linear mixed model analysis, it gives an indication that the tobit mixed model analysis provides a better fit. This conclusion was also confirmed by the BIC values for both models; i.e. the BIC, which can be seen as an adjusted value of the -2 log likelihood and which can be used for comparing models (Schwarz, 1978) was 7929.89 for the linear mixed model analysis and 7084.412 for the tobit mixed model analysis.

The second example is taken from a hypothetical longitudinal study in 188 rheumatoid arthritis patients which are measured three times for a period of 24 weeks (measurements were taken at 8, 16 and 24 weeks after the start of treatment). The outcome variable of interest was functional ability measured by the Disability Index of the Health Assessment Questionnaire (HAQ_DI), which is prone to have a floor effect during treatment. The main objective of the study was to investigate the relationship between HAQ_DI and disease activity. Disease activity was a time-dependent continuous covariate theoretically ranging between zero and ten. Figure 9.3 shows the distribution of the outcome variable at the

Output 9.2 Results of a linear mixed model analysis with only a random intercept to analyse the difference in development over time in the Barthel index between males and females

```
Mixed-effects ML regression              Number of obs    =     1,646
Group variable: id                       Number of groups =       101

                                         Obs per group:
                                                        min =         2
                                                        avg =      16.3
                                                        max =        18

                                         Wald chi2(3)     =   2909.75
Log likelihood = -3942.7266              Prob > chi2      =    0.0000
```

barthel	Coef.	Std. Err.	z	P>|z|	[95% Conf. Interval]	
time	.6167977	.0176607	34.92	0.000	.5821833	.6514121
sex	1.842671	.9006745	2.05	0.041	.0773815	3.607961
time#sex	.0100313	.0233483	0.43	0.667	-.0357306	.0557932
_cons	5.131309	.6766974	7.58	0.000	3.805007	6.457612

Random-effects Parameters	Estimate	Std. Err.	[95% Conf. Interval]	
id: Identity				
var(_cons)	18.60101	2.674161	14.03344	24.65522
var(Residual)	5.52062	.1986321	5.144718	5.923987

```
LR test vs. linear model: chibar2(01) = 1994.73   Prob >= chibar2 = 0.0000
```

different time-points, while Output 9.3 shows the result of the tobit mixed model analysis to analyse the relationship between HAQ_DI and disease activity.

In the first part of Output 9.3, it can be seen that there are 504 observations in 188 patients. There is some missing data because the average number of observations within a patient is 2.7. It can also be seen that almost half of the observations for HAQ_DI are left censored, i.e. are equal to zero. In the second part of the output the regression coefficient for disease activity is given. The regression coefficient belongs to a time-dependent covariate, so it has a pooled interpretation; partly between-subjects and partly within-subjects. As has been mentioned before, the

regression coefficient can be interpreted in the same way as a regression coefficient in a linear mixed model analysis. A one-unit difference in disease activity is associated with a 0.2459272-unit difference in HAQ_DI (both between- and within-subjects). It can also be seen that the relationship between HAQ_DI and disease activity is highly significant.

As always, the last part of the output shows the random intercept variance and the residual variance. From the numbers it can be seen that in this example also the correlation between the repeated observations within the patient is very high.

Because disease activity is a time-dependent covariate, in the next step of the analysis it can

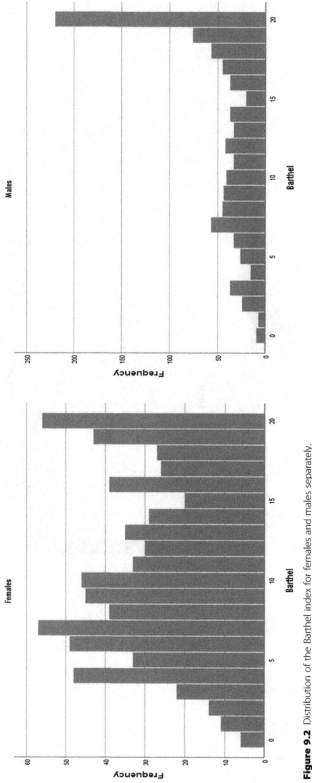

Figure 9.2 Distribution of the Barthel index for females and males separately.

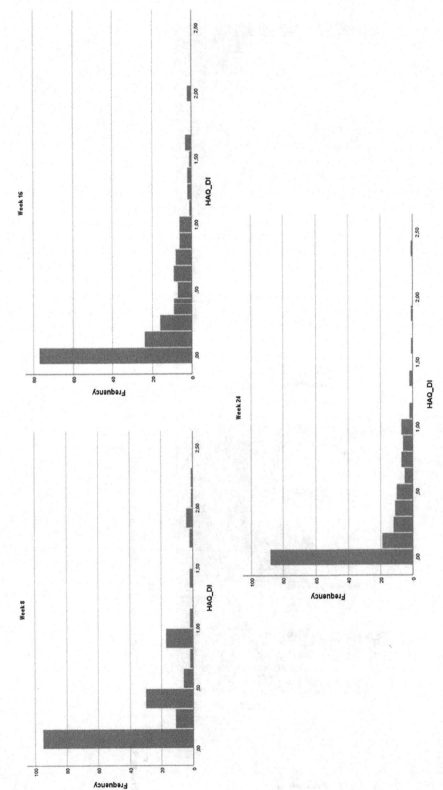

Figure 9.3 Distribution of the HAQ_DI at 8, 16 and 24 weeks after the start of treatment.

Output 9.3 Results of a tobit mixed model analysis with only a random intercept to analyse the relationship between HAQ_DI and disease activity

```
Mixed-effects tobit regression          Number of obs      =        504
                                        Uncensored         =        269
Limits: Lower = 0                       Left-censored      =        235
       Upper = +inf                     Right-censored     =          0

Group variable: id                      Number of groups   =        188
                                        obs per group:
                                                     min   =          1
                                                     avg   =        2.7
                                                     max   =          3

Integration method: mvaghermite         Integration pts.   =          7

                                        Wald chi2(1)       =     115.67
Log likelihood = -272.8182              Prob > chi2        =     0.0000
- - - - - - - - - - - - - - - - - - - - - - - - - - - - - - - - - - - - - - - -
      HAQ_DI | Coefficient  Std. err.     z   P>|z|   [ 95% conf. interval]
- - - - - - -+- - - - - - - - - - - - - - - - - - - - - - - - - - - - - - - - -
     disease |   .2459272   .0228659   10.76  0.000   .2011108   .2907435
       _cons |  -.5309732   .0742689   -7.15  0.000  -.6765376  -.3854088
- - - - - - -+- - - - - - - - - - - - - - - - - - - - - - - - - - - - - - - - -
id           |
   var(_cons)|    .275138   .0424424                  .2033506    .372268
- - - - - - -+- - - - - - - - - - - - - - - - - - - - - - - - - - - - - - - - -
var(e.HAQ_DI)|    .074088   .0082674                  .0595338   .0922003
- - - - - - - - - - - - - - - - - - - - - - - - - - - - - - - - - - - - - - - -
LR test vs. tobit model: chibar2(01) = 221.52     Prob >= chibar2 = 0.0000
```

be evaluated whether it is necessary to add a random slope for disease activity to the model. Output 9.4 shows the result of this analysis.

The necessity of adding a random slope for disease activity can be evaluated with the likelihood ratio test. To do so, the -2 log likelihood of the model with only a random intercept has to be compared to the -2 log likelihood of the model with both a random intercept, random slope for disease activity and the covariance between the random intercept and random slope. The difference between the two -2 log likelihoods equals 5.2, which is not statistically significant on a Chi-square distribution with two degrees of freedom. So, statistically, it is not necessary to add a random slope for disease activity to the model. However, because the difference between the two -2 log likelihoods is close to the critical value of 5.99, in some situations the random slope is kept in the model. Looking at the

regression coefficients of the two models, the main difference between the two is found in the standard error of the regression coefficient for disease activity, which is (as expected) a bit higher when estimated in the model with a random slope.

9.3 Longitudinal Two-part Models

Longitudinal tobit mixed model analysis is an example of a two-part joint regression model assuming a latent normal distribution. When this assumption does not hold, more flexible two-part joint regression models can be used. With the GLLAMM procedure in STATA (see Section 8.1.5.1) it is possible to mix the binomial distribution with other distributions, such as a Poisson distribution, a gamma distribution, a log normal distribution, etc. (Rabe-Hesketh et al., 2001a; Rabe-Hesketh and Skrondal, 2001).

Output 9.4 Results of a tobit mixed model analysis with both a random intercept and a random slope for disease activity to analyse the longitudinal relationship between HAQ_DI and disease activity

```
Mixed-effects tobit regression          Number of obs     =     504
                                         Uncensored        =     269
Limits: Lower = 0                        Left-censored     =     235
Upper = +inf                             Right-censored    =       0

Group variable: id                       Number of groups  =     188
                                         obs per group:
                                                     min =         1
                                                     avg =       2.7
                                                     max =         3

Integration method: mvaghermite          Integration pts. =        7

                                         Wald chi2(1)      =    78.16
Log likelihood = -270.21261              Prob > chi2       =   0.0000
- - - - - - - - - - - - - - - - - - - - - - - - - - - - - - - - - - -
         HAQ_DI| Coefficient Std. err.  z  P>|z| [ 95% conf. interval]
- - - - - - - - -+- - - - - - - - - - - - - - - - - - - - - - - - - - -
        disease | .2498791 .028265 8.84 0.000 .1944807 .3052776
          _cons | -.5348014 .0844856 -6.33 0.000 -.7003901 -.3692128
- - - - - - - - -+- - - - - - - - - - - - - - - - - - - - - - - - - - -
id              |
     var(disease)| .0144137 .0090061            .0042357 .0490488
     var(_cons) |   .38999 .1291052             .2038287 .7461765
- - - - - - - - -+- - - - - - - - - - - - - - - - - - - - - - - - - - -
id              |
cov(disease,_cons)| -.0423995 .0330067 -1.28 0.199 -.1070914 .0222924
- - - - - - - - -+- - - - - - - - - - - - - - - - - - - - - - - - - - -
     var(e.HAQ_DI)| .0646751 .0081416           .050534 .0827733
- - - - - - - - - - - - - - - - - - - - - - - - - - - - - - - - - - -
LR test vs. tobit model: chi2(3) = 226.73           Prob > chi2 = 0.0000
```

9.3.1 Example

The example is taken from the SPIRIT study (Hajos et al., 2011). This study aimed to examine the effect of initiation of insulin glargine (a long-acting insulin analogue) on general emotional well-being, diabetes symptom distress and worries about hypoglycaemia in Dutch type 2 diabetes patients who previously used oral anti-hyperglycaemic medication. Type 2 diabetes patients who used oral anti-hyperglycaemic agents were recruited from 363 Dutch primary care practices, which were spread across the country. This resulted in a total sample of 889 patients. At baseline, patients initiated insulin glargine either combined with oral

medications, a rapid-acting insulin analogue, or both at the discretion of their treating physician. Measurements were conducted at baseline, after three and after six months, and in this example the development over time in hypoglycaemic events for diabetic patients was analysed. Figure 9.4 shows the overall distribution of the number of hypoglycaemic events in the dataset used in this example. From Figure 9.4 it can be seen that the distribution is highly zero-inflated, or in other words, the distribution has a strong floor effect.

Output 9.5 shows the result of a two-part joint mixed model analysis in which a binomial distribution was used for zero versus non-zero and a Poisson

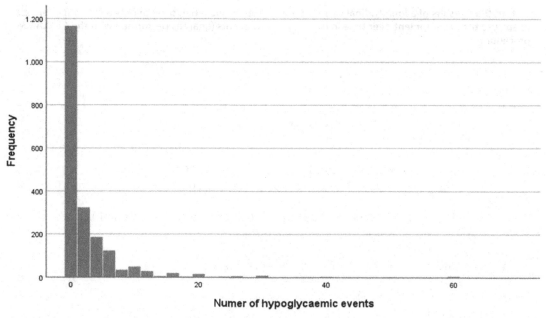

Figure 9.4 Overall distribution of the number of hypoglycaemic events in the Spirit dataset.

distribution for the non-zero part. Because there are only three fixed time-points in this study, time was treated as a categorical variable and represented by two dummy variables.

Output 9.5 is very simple and very straightforward. First the log likelihood of the model is given (i.e. −3312.5361), and after that the regression coefficients, the z-values, the corresponding p-values and the 95% confidence intervals around the regression coefficients are given. From this part of the output it can be seen that the number of hypoglycaemic events decrease gradually over time and that the difference between baseline and six months is statistically significant ($p = 0.008$). The actual interpretation of the regression coefficients for this two-part joint mixed model analysis is rather complicated and will be further discussed in Section 9.3.2. The last part of Output 9.5 shows the variance of the random intercept (i.e. 3.5673155).

In real life, a Poisson mixed model analysis is mostly used for this kind of data, but a Poisson mixed model analysis basically ignores the excess of zeroes. To compare the result of the two-part joint mixed model analysis with only a random intercept with a comparable Poisson mixed model analysis, Output 9.6 shows the result of the Poisson mixed model analysis.

When the result reported in Output 9.6 is compared with the result reported in Output 9.5, it can be seen that the regression coefficients for the time dummy variables are slightly different, especially regarding the development of hypoglycaemic events between the first measurement and the measurement after three months. Most striking, however, is the difference in the standard errors of the regression coefficients, which are much higher when estimated with the two-part mixed model analysis. Again, although it is doubtful whether the log likelihood values can be directly compared with each other, the comparison indicates that the two-part mixed model analysis provides a better fit compared to the Poisson mixed model analysis. Also in this example, this was confirmed by the Bayesian Information Criterion (BIC) values for both models, which were 6295.563 for the two-part mixed model analysis and 7983.194 for the Poisson mixed model analysis. Another way to compare the different methods with each other is to compare the observed values with the predicted values. Figure 9.5 shows, therefore, the observed versus predicted values for the two-part mixed model analysis and the Poisson mixed model analysis. The biggest difference between the two figures is found in the predicted zero values, which is (as expected) much better with the two-part mixed model analysis.

161

Output 9.5 Results of a longitudinal two-part joint mixed model analysis with only a random intercept to analyse the development over time in hypoglycaemic events (analysis performed with the GLALAMM procedure)

```
log likelihood = -3312.5361

Robust standard errors
- - - - - - - - - - - - - - - - - - - - - - - - - - - - - - - - - - - - - - - - -
         hyp |      Coef.  Std. Err.      z  P>|z|   [ 95% Conf. Interval]
- - - - - - - +- - - - - - - - - - - - - - - - - - - - - - - - - - - - - - - - - -
        time |
           2 |  -.1682755  .1210002  -1.39  0.164   -.4054316   .0688806
           3 |  -.2791713  .1050495  -2.66  0.008   -.4850646  -.073278
             |
       _cons |   .0132694  .1223562   0.11  0.914   -.2265443   .2530832
- - - - - - - - - - - - - - - - - - - - - - - - - - - - - - - - - - - - - - - - -

Variances and covariances of random effects
- - - - - - - - - - - - - - - - - - - - - - - - - - - - - - - - - - - - - - - - -

***level 2 (id)

   var(1): 3.5673155 (.30504197)
- - - - - - - - - - - - - - - - - - - - - - - - - - - - - - - - - - - - - - - - -
```

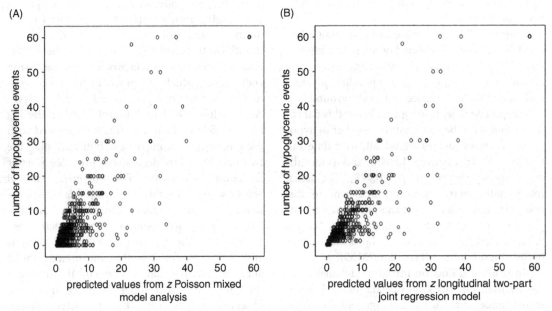

Figure 9.5 Observed versus predicted values derived from a Poisson mixed model analysis (A) and a two-part joint mixed model analysis (B).

9.3.2 Comments

In the example, the choice was made to analyse the longitudinal data with lower or upper censoring with a two-part joint mixed model analysis. An important reason why the two-part joint mixed model analysis was chosen is that the outcome variable in the example (i.e. the number of

Output 9.6 Results of a longitudinal Poisson mixed model analysis with only a random intercept to analyse the development over time in hypoglycaemic events

```
Mixed-effects Poisson regression          Number of obs      =      1984
Group variable: id                        Number of groups   =       889

                                          Obs per group: min =         1
                                                         avg =       2.2
                                                         max =         3

Integration points =  7                   Wald chi2(2)       =     38.51
Log likelihood = -3976.4112               Prob > chi2        =    0.0000

------------------------------------------------------------------------
     hyp |      Coef.  Std. Err.     z   P>|z|     [ 95% Conf. Interval]
---------+--------------------------------------------------------------
    time |
       2 |  -.1055194  .0376571  -2.80  0.005   -.1793259  -.0317129
       3 |  -.2646151   .042647  -6.20  0.000   -.3482016  -.1810286
         |
    _cons |  -.5001234  .0891871  -5.61  0.000   -.6749269    -.32532
------------------------------------------------------------------------


------------------------------------------------------------------------
Random-effects Parameters | Estimate Std. Err.   [ 95% Conf. Interval]
--------------------------+---------------------------------------------
id: Identity              |
            var(_cons) | 3.946494  .3103373   3.382799  4.604121
------------------------------------------------------------------------
LR test vs. Poisson regression: chibar2(01) = 7885.91 Prob>=chibar2 = 0.0000
```

hypoglycaemic events) can be seen as one process that cannot be split into two processes. Sometimes it is better to analyse the data with a standard two-part regression model, leading to separate regression coefficients for both parts of the process (e.g. smoking behaviour related to covariates).

The biggest problem with the two-part joint mixed model analysis is the interpretation of the regression coefficient. The general idea is that the regression coefficient pools two interpretations: (1) The difference in the outcome variable if above the limit, weighted by the probability of being above the limit; and (2) the difference in the probability of being above the limit, weighted by the expected value of the outcome variable if above the limit. Theoretically this makes sense; however, in practice, if for instance, one is interested in the magnitude of the development over time or the effect of a certain intervention, it is

difficult to get a proper interpretation of the regression coefficient.

Maybe because of the difficult interpretation of the regression coefficient, the two-part joint mixed model analysis is almost never used in longitudinal medical studies. Mostly, the floor or ceiling effects are ignored in the analysis. Other ways to analyse these kind of data are to reduce the information in the data to either a dichotomous outcome variable (mostly comparing zero to non-zero) or a categorical outcome variable (mostly comparing zero with two groups of non-zero outcome in which the two groups are divided according to the median of the non-zero part). Sometimes researchers try to transform (with a logarithmic transformation) a distribution with many zeros into a normally distributed variable. However, due to the bunch of zeros at the beginning of the distribution, this transformation will not work because it will never result in a normal distribution.

Chapter 10

Analysis of Longitudinal Intervention Studies

10.1 Introduction

In the previous chapters, all examples were taken from observational longitudinal studies. Although the same statistical methods can be used for the analysis of longitudinal intervention studies, there are some important differences. Most longitudinal intervention studies are randomised controlled trials (RCTs). In general, in an RCT, before the intervention starts (i.e. at baseline) the study population is (randomly) divided into two or more groups. In the case of two groups, one of the groups receives the intervention of interest and the other group (i.e. the control group) receives a placebo intervention, no intervention at all, or usual care. Both groups are monitored over a certain period of time, in order to find out whether the groups differ with regard to a particular outcome variable, which can be continuous, dichotomous, categorical, etc.

The simplest form of a longitudinal RCT is one in which a baseline measurement and only one follow-up measurement are performed. If the subjects are randomly assigned to the different groups, a comparison of the follow-up values between the groups will give an answer to the question of which intervention is more effective with regard to the particular outcome variable. The assumption is that random allocation at baseline will ensure that there is no difference between the groups at baseline (in fact, in this situation a baseline measurement is not even necessary). However, the assumption of no difference between the groups at baseline almost never holds. This is due to the fact that the theory behind randomisation is related to infinite sample sizes. When the group sizes are limited (which is, of course, always the case) it is expected that there

is a group difference at baseline. Therefore, in the statistical analysis, this difference between the groups at baseline should be taken into account.

In the past decade, intervention studies with only one follow-up measurement have become rare. At least one short-term follow-up measurement and one long-term follow-up measurement are performed. However, more than two follow-up measurements are usually performed in order to compare the development over time among the groups. These more complicated designs are often analysed with simple cross-sectional methods, mostly by analysing the outcome at each follow-up measurement separately, or sometimes even by ignoring the information gathered from the in-between measurements, i.e. only using the last measurement as outcome variable to evaluate the effect of the intervention. This is even more surprising, in view of the fact that there are statistical methods available which can be used to analyse the difference in development over time of the outcome variable between groups using all available data.

It is obvious that the methods that can be used for the statistical analysis of longitudinal intervention studies are exactly the same as has been discussed for observational longitudinal studies. The remainder of this chapter is devoted to extensive examples covering all aspects of the analysis of intervention studies, mostly focusing on RCTs. Like in most other chapters, separate sections will deal with continuous outcome variables and dichotomous outcome variables. Furthermore, in the examples, a distinction is made between RCTs with only one follow-up measurement and RCTs with more than one follow-up measurement. Although RCTs with only one follow-up measurement have become rare, they are theoretically very important to discuss in detail.

10.2 Continuous Outcome Variables

10.2.1 Randomised Controlled Trials with One Follow-up Measurement

When the effect of an intervention is evaluated in an RCT with only one follow-up measurement, usually the change between the baseline measurement and the follow-up measurement in the continuous outcome variable is compared between the intervention group and the control group. The effect of the intervention can then be analysed by a cross-sectional linear regression analysis (or even by an independent t-test). This is a very popular method, which greatly reduces the complexity of the statistical analysis (see Equation 10.1):

$$\Delta Y_i = Y_{it1} - Y_{it0} \tag{10.1a}$$

$$\Delta Y_i = \beta_0 + \beta_1 X_i + \varepsilon_i \tag{10.1b}$$

where Y_{it0} are observations of the outcome for subject i at baseline, Y_{it1} are observations of the outcome for subject i at the follow-up measurement, β_0 is the intercept, X_i are observations of the intervention variable for subject i, β_1 is the regression coefficient for the intervention variable, and ε_i is the error for subject i.

One of the typical problems related to the use of the change between baseline and follow-up is the phenomenon of regression to the mean. If the outcome variable at baseline is a sample of random numbers, and the outcome variable at follow-up is also a sample of random numbers, then the subjects in the upper part of the distribution at baseline are less likely to be in the upper part of the distribution at follow-up, compared to the other subjects. In the same way, the subjects in the lower part of the distribution at baseline are less likely than the other subjects to be in the lower part of the distribution at follow-up. When the change over time in a whole population is analysed, regression to the mean is not really a big problem. However, in an RCT when two groups are compared to each other, it is possible that the average baseline value of the outcome variable differs between the two groups. As has been mentioned before, the general idea of random allocation at baseline is that the average value of the two groups is the same. However, that is theoretically only the case when the (source) population is infinite. In real life practice, the two groups are of limited size and therefore it is highly possible that the average baseline value of the outcome variable differs between the two groups. When the two groups are derived from one (source) population, this difference is totally caused by chance. When the average baseline value differs between the intervention and the control group, regression to the mean becomes a problem. Suppose that the aim of a particular intervention is to decrease the outcome variable and suppose further that the intervention group has a higher average baseline value compared to the control group. When the intervention has no effect at all, due to regression to the mean, the average value of the intervention group will go down, while the average value of the control group will go up. A comparison between the intervention and the control group based on the change between baseline and follow-up will then reveal a favourable intervention effect. This is not a real effect, but an effect caused by regression to the mean.

Because of this regression to the mean problem, there are methods available which aim to adjust for regression to the mean. In many medical studies, the relative change between baseline and follow-up in the continuous outcome variable is compared between the intervention group and the control group (see Equation 10.2):

$$\Delta Y_i = \frac{(Y_{it1} - Y_{it0})}{Y_{it0}} \times 100\% \tag{10.2a}$$

$$\Delta Y_i = \beta_0 + \beta_1 X_i + \varepsilon_i \tag{10.2b}$$

where Y_{it0} are observations of the outcome for subject i at baseline, Y_{it1} are observations of the outcome variable for subject i at the follow-up measurement, β_0 is the intercept, X_i are observations of the intervention variable for subject i, β_1 is the regression coefficient for the intervention variable, and ε_i is the error for subject i.

Although most researchers believe that using this relative change adjusts for regression to the mean, this is not the case. This is illustrated in Figure 10.1.

In Figure 10.1, two situations are shown. In Figure 10.1A it can be seen that the baseline value for the intervention group is higher compared to the control group. The next column reflects the situation after the intervention period. It can be seen that the difference in outcome variable between baseline and follow-up in both groups is equal to one. However, because the

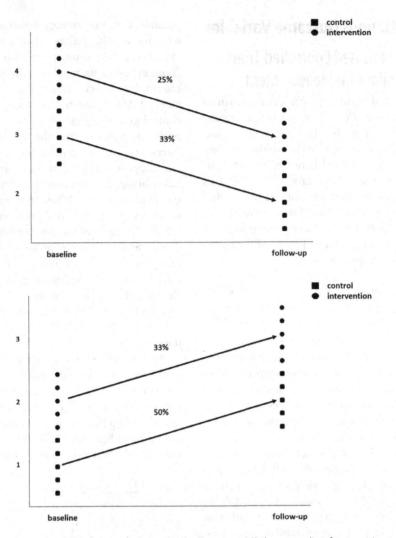

Figure 10.1 Illustration to show that the use of relative change (Equation 10.2) does not adjust for regression to the mean.

intervention group has a higher baseline value compared to the control group, due to regression to the mean, the average value of the intervention group is expected to decrease, while the average value of the control group is expected to increase. In other words, the decrease of one point in the intervention group is easier to achieve than the one-point decrease in the control group. When the relative change is calculated, the intervention group decreases by 25%, while the control group decreases by 33%. So, in this situation (when there is a decrease in the outcome variable), the use of the relative change works well.

However, Figure 10.1B shows the opposite. Again, there is a difference in baseline value between the two groups and again, the average baseline value of the intervention group is higher

compared to the control group. In the second part of the figure, however, the outcome variable increases over time. Both groups increase with one point, but because the control group has a lower value at baseline, due to regression to the mean, the one-point change is easier to achieve for the control group compared to the one-point change in the intervention group. When the relative change is calculated in this situation, the intervention group increases by 33%, while the control group increases by 50%. So, based on the difference between the two relative changes, the control group performs better than the intervention group. This is not true, because in fact, it is just the opposite; the intervention group performs better than the control group. In other words, when the outcome variable decreases over time, the use of the relative change more or less adjusts for regression to the mean, but when the outcome variable increases, it goes totally wrong.

Another method that claims to adjust for regression to the mean is known as analysis of covariance (Equation 10.3). With this method, the value of the outcome variable at the follow-up measurement is used as the outcome variable in a linear regression analysis, with the baseline value as one of the covariates.

$$Y_{it1} = \beta_0 + \beta_1 X + \beta_2 Y_{it0} + \varepsilon_i \quad (10.3)$$

where Y_{it0} are observations of the outcome for subject i at baseline, Y_{it1} are observations of the outcome for subject i at the follow-up measurement, β_0 is the intercept, X_i are observations of the intervention variable for subject i, β_1 is the regression coefficient for the intervention variable, β_2 is the regression coefficient for the baseline value and ε_i is the error for subject i.

In this model, β_1 reflects the effect of the intervention adjusted for a possible difference at baseline, i.e. adjusted for regression to the mean. Analysis of covariance is almost, but not quite, the same as the calculation of the change between baseline and follow-up (see Equation 10.1). This can be seen when Equation 10.3 is written in a slightly different way (Equation 10.4).

$$Y_{it1} - \beta_2 Y_{it0} = \beta_0 + \beta_1 X_i + \varepsilon_i \quad (10.4)$$

where Y_{it0} are observations of the outcome for subject i at baseline, Y_{it1} are observations of the outcome for subject i at the follow-up measurement, β_0 is the intercept, X_i are observations of the intervention variable for subject i, β_1 is the regression coefficient for the intervention variable, β_2 is the regression coefficient for the baseline value and ε_i is the error for subject i.

In the analysis of covariance, the change is defined relative to the value of the outcome variable at baseline. This relativity is expressed in the regression coefficient β_2, which is known as the autoregression coefficient (see also Section 5.3.3). Because of this relativity, analysis of covariance adjusts for regression to the mean. The analysis of covariance is comparable to the analysis of residual change, which was first described by Blomquist (1977). The first step in the analysis of residual change is to perform a linear regression analysis between the outcome at follow-up and the outcome at baseline. The second step is to calculate the difference between the observed

value of the outcome at follow-up and the predicted value of the outcome at follow-up (predicted by the regression model with the outcome at baseline as covariate). This difference is called the residual change, which is then used as outcome variable in a linear regression analysis with the intervention variable. The regression coefficient of the intervention variable is an estimate of the effect of the intervention adjusted for regression to the mean. Although the general idea behind the analysis of residual change is the same as for analysis of covariance, the results of both methods are not exactly the same. From the literature it is known that the analysis of residual change is not as good as the analysis of covariance (Forbes and Carlin, 2005).

Some researchers argue that the best way to estimate an intervention effect, adjusting for regression to the mean, is a combination of Equations 10.1 and 10.3. They suggest that the change between baseline and follow-up is used as the outcome in a linear regression analysis adjusting for baseline (Equation 10.5).

$$Y_{it1} - Y_{it0} = \beta_0 + \beta_1 X_i + \beta_2 Y_{it0} + \varepsilon_i \quad (10.5)$$

where Y_{it0} are observations of the outcome for subject i at baseline, Y_{it1} are observations of the outcome for subject i at the follow-up measurement, β_0 is the intercept, X_i are observations of the intervention variable for subject i, β_1 is the regression coefficient for the intervention variable, β_2 is the regression coefficient for the baseline value and ε_i is the error for subject i.

However, analysing the change, adjusting for baseline, is exactly the same as the analysis of covariance described in Equation 10.3. This can be seen when Equation 10.5 is written in another way (Equation 10.6). The only difference between the models is that the regression coefficient for the baseline value is different; i.e. the difference between the regression coefficient for the baseline value is equal to one.

$$Y_{it1} = \beta_0 + \beta_1 X_i + \beta_2 Y_{it0} + Y_{it0} + \varepsilon_i \quad (10.6a)$$

$$Y_{it1} = \beta_0 + \beta_1 X_i + (\beta_2 + 1) Y_{it0} + \varepsilon_i \quad (10.6b)$$

where Y_{it0} are observations of the outcome for subject i at baseline, Y_{it1} are observations of the outcome variable for subject i at the follow-up measurement, β_0 is the intercept, X_i are observations of the intervention variable for subject i, β_1 is the regression coefficient for the intervention variable, β_2 is the regression coefficient for the baseline value and ε_i is the error for subject i.

10.2.1.1 Example

The first example dataset is derived from an RCT, which was performed by Proper et al. (2003). The example nicely shows the influence of ignoring the regression to the mean phenomenon on the result and conclusion of an RCT. In brief, 299 civil servants working within municipal services in the Netherlands were randomised either into an intervention or a control group. All subjects randomised into the intervention group were offered seven consultations, over a period of nine months focusing primarily on the enhancement of the individual's level of physical activity. Subjects in the control group received no individual counselling. Outcome variables were assessed at baseline and directly after the completion of the last consultation. For the example, two continuous outcome variables (physical activity and total serum cholesterol) were selected. For both outcomes, differences between the intervention and control group were observed at baseline (see Table 10.1).

From Table 10.1 it can be seen that for both physical activity and total serum cholesterol, the baseline value for the intervention group is higher than for the control group.

To analyse the effect of the intervention, several methods were used. Output 10.1 shows the result for total serum cholesterol of three methods described in Section 10.2.1, i.e. the analysis of changes; the analysis of changes, adjusted for baseline; and the analysis of covariance.

From Output 10.1 it can be seen that the effect of the intervention is overestimated when the change between baseline and follow-up is compared between the intervention and control group.

Table 10.1 Mean and standard deviation (between brackets) for physical activity and cholesterol

	Baseline	Follow-up
Total serum cholesterol (mmol/l)		
Intervention group	5.51 (1.04)	5.33 (0.99)
Control group	5.35 (0.94)	5.39 (0.95)
Physical activity		
Intervention group	5.80 (1.08)	5.95 (0.95)
Control group	5.47 (1.07)	5.39 (1.04)

This overestimation is caused by the difference between the groups at baseline. Because the intervention group starts at a higher level, and the intervention is intending to decrease total serum cholesterol, regression to the mean is helping the intervention group to decrease. Analysis of covariance adjusts for the difference at baseline and therefore this analysis revealed a less strong intervention effect (i.e. −0.184309 versus −0.220306). As has been explained in Section 10.2.1, the analysis of covariance and the analysis of changes adjusted for baseline are basically the same and therefore, they reveal the same intervention effect.

Although for both total serum cholesterol and physical activity the intervention group has a higher value at baseline, for physical activity, the results show a different picture than for total serum cholesterol (see Output 10.2).

From Output 10.2, it can be seen that the analysis of changes between baseline and follow-up underestimates the effect of the intervention. Again, this is due to the difference at baseline between the intervention and the control group. The difference between the analysis of the intervention effect for total serum cholesterol and physical activity has to do with the fact that the intervention aimed to increase physical activity and to decrease total serum cholesterol. So, for physical activity, regression to the mean is helping the control group and therefore, the analysis of changes results in an underestimation of the intervention effect.

In this example with only one follow-up measurement, it is also possible to use the regression-based methods (i.e. mixed model analysis or generalised estimating equation (GEE) analysis) to estimate the intervention effect. The regression-based methods can only be used when there are correlated observations in the outcome variable, so when a regression-based method is used for the analysis of an RCT with only one follow-up measurement, it directly implies that the baseline value must be part of the outcome variable. One of the possibilities, which is often used, is given in Equation 10.7.

$$Y_{it} = \beta_0 + \beta_1 X_i + \beta_2 time + \beta_3 X_i \times time + \varepsilon_{it}$$

(10.7)

where Y_{it} are observations of the outcome for subject i at time t, β_0 is the intercept, X_i are observations of the intervention variable for subject i,

Output 10.1 Results of three methods to analyse the effect of the intervention on total serum cholesterol. (A) The analysis of changes, (B) the analysis of changes, adjusted for baseline and (C) the analysis of covariance

(A)

del_chol	Coef.	Std. Err.	t	P>|t|	[95% Conf. Interval]	
intervention	-.220306	.0888516	-2.48	0.014	-.3955283	-.0450836
_cons	.0364762	.0610664	0.60	0.551	-.0839516	.156904

(B)

del_chol	Coef.	Std. Err.	t	P>|t|	[95% Conf. Interval]	
intervention	-.184309	.0837584	-2.20	0.029	-.3494925	-.0191256
chol_base	-.2212941	.0424295	-5.22	0.000	-.304971	-.1376172
_cons	1.22021	.2341	5.21	0.000	.7585317	1.681888

(C)

chol_t1	Coef.	Std. Err.	t	P>|t|	[95% Conf. Interval]	
intervention	-.184309	.0837584	-2.20	0.029	-.3494925	-.0191256
chol_base	.7787059	.0424295	18.35	0.000	.695029	.8623828
_cons	1.22021	.2341	5.21	0.000	.7585317	1.681888

β_1 is the regression coefficient for the intervention variable, *time* is time of measurement (0 for the baseline measurement and 1 for the follow-up measurement), β_2 is the regression coefficient for time, β_3 is the regression coefficient for the interaction between the intervention variable and time, and ε_{it} is the error for subject i at time t.

The coefficient of interest in this analysis is the regression coefficient for the interaction between the intervention variable and time (i.e. β_3). The regression coefficient for the intervention variable (β_1) reflects the difference between the two groups at baseline, while the summation of the regression coefficient for the intervention variable and the regression coefficient for the interaction term $(\beta_1 + \beta_3)$ reflects the difference between the intervention and the control group at follow-up. So, the regression coefficient for the interaction term reflects the difference between the intervention and control group in the difference between baseline and follow-up, which is assumed to be an estimation of the intervention effect. Output 10.3 shows the results of the mixed model analyses for both total serum cholesterol and physical activity, using Equation 10.7.

As has been mentioned previously, the coefficients of interest from the results of the mixed model analyses shown in Output 10.3 are the regression coefficients belonging to the interaction terms. Those coefficients are assumed to reflect the effect of the intervention for the two outcome variables. For cholesterol, the effect of the intervention is −0.220306, while for physical activity, the effect of the intervention is 0.2473911. When these results are compared to the results obtained from the three methods presented in Outputs 10.1 and 10.2, it is obvious that the estimated intervention effects are exactly the same as the ones obtained from the analysis of changes.

So, in the analyses performed in this way there is no adjustment for the difference at baseline between the two groups and therefore, the estimated

Output 10.2 Results of three methods to analyse the effect of the intervention on physical activity. (A) The analysis of changes, (B) the analysis of changes, adjusted for baseline and (C) the analysis of covariance

(A)

del_act	Coef.	Std. Err.	t	P>|t|	[95% Conf. Interval]	
intervention	.2473911	.096712	2.56	0.011	.0566673	.4381149
_cons	-.0904762	.0664688	-1.36	0.175	-.221558	.0406056

(B)

del_act	Coef.	Std. Err.	t	P>|t|	[95% Conf. Interval]	
intervention	.3328238	.0887946	3.75	0.000	.1577083	.5079392
act_base	-.2675616	.0408708	-6.55	0.000	-.3481645	-.1869587
_cons	1.375379	.2319074	5.93	0.000	.9180252	1.832734

(C)

act_t1	Coef.	Std. Err.	t	P>|t|	[95% Conf. Interval]	
intervention	.3328238	.0887946	3.75	0.000	.1577083	.5079392
act_base	.7324384	.0408708	17.92	0.000	.6518355	.8130413
_cons	1.375379	.2319074	5.93	0.000	.9180252	1.832734

intervention effects are not correct. An alternative solution for this problem is a comparable analysis without the intervention variable in the model (Equation 10.8).

$$Y_{it} = \beta_0 + \beta_1 time + \beta_2 X_i \times time + \varepsilon_{it} \qquad (10.8)$$

where Y_{it} are observations of the outcome for subject i at time t, β_0 is the intercept, $time$ is time of measurement (0 for the baseline measurement and 1 for the follow-up measurement), β_1 is the regression coefficient for time, X_i are observations of the intervention variable for subject i, β_2 is the regression coefficient for the interaction between the intervention variable and time, and ε_{it} is the error for subject i at time t.

Because the intervention variable is not in the model, the baseline value for both groups is assumed to be equal and is reflected in the intercept of the model (i.e. β_0). In this model, the coefficient of interest is, again, the regression coefficient for the interaction between the intervention

variable and time (β_2), because this coefficient reflects the intervention effect. Output 10.4 shows the results of the mixed model analyses based on this method for both total serum cholesterol and physical activity.

From Output 10.4 it can be seen that the intervention effects estimated with this method are slightly different from the intervention effects estimated with the analysis of covariance. For total serum cholesterol the effect estimates were −0.1871102 and −0.184309 respectively, while for physical activity the effect estimates were 0.3146177 and 0.3328238. This was not really expected because both methods adjust for the difference at baseline. However, when a mixed model analysis is used with both a random intercept and a random slope for time, the effect estimates were exactly the same as the ones estimated with the analysis of covariance (see Output 10.5). This is despite the fact that the estimation of the random part of the model is estimated with a huge error.

Output 10.3 Results of a mixed model analysis to analyse the effect of the intervention on (A) total serum cholesterol and (B) physical activity, using Equation 10.7

```
(A)
Mixed-effects ML regression              Number of obs     =        398
Group variable: id                       Number of groups  =        199

                                         Obs per group:
                                                        min =          2
                                                        avg =        2.0
                                                        max =          2

                                         Wald chi2(3)      =       8.72
Log likelihood = -454.04432              Prob > chi2       =     0.0333

---------------------------------------------------------------------
     cholesterol |    Coef.  Std. Err.    z   P>|z| [ 95% Conf. Interval]
-----------------+---------------------------------------------------
    intervention | .1626657 .138033   1.18 0.239  -.107874  .4332053
          1.time | .0364762 .0607588  0.60 0.548  -.0826088 .1555612
                 |
time#intervention |
               1 | -.220306 .088404  -2.49 0.013  -.3935746 -.0470374
                 |
           _cons | 5.349143 .0948681 56.39 0.000  5.163205  5.535081
---------------------------------------------------------------------


---------------------------------------------------------------------
 Random-effects Parameters | Estimate Std. Err.  [ 95% Conf. Interval]
---------------------------+-----------------------------------------
id: Identity               |
            var(_cons)     | .7511852 .0855751    .6008666  .939109
---------------------------+-----------------------------------------
           var(Residual)   | .1938106 .0194297    .1592369  .2358909
---------------------------------------------------------------------
LR test vs. linear model: chibar2(01) = 198.87   Prob >= chibar2 = 0.0000

(B)

Mixed-effects ML regression              Number of obs     =        398
Group variable: id                       Number of groups  =        199

                                         Obs per group:
                                                        min =          2
                                                        avg =        2.0
                                                        max =          2

                                         Wald chi2(3)      =      17.07
Log likelihood = -483.02277              Prob > chi2       =     0.0007

---------------------------------------------------------------------
```

Output 10.3 *(cont.)*

```
      activity |   Coef. Std. Err.    z  P>|z| [ 95% Conf. Interval]
- - - - - - - - - - - -+- - - - - - - - - - - - - - - - - - - - - - - - - - - - - - - -
  intervention | .3193009 .1470612  2.17 0.030  .0310663 .6075355
        1.time |-.0904762  .066134 -1.37 0.171 -.2200964  .039144
               |
time#intervention |
            1 | .2473911 .0962248  2.57 0.010  .0587939 .4359883
               |
         _cons | 5.478571 .1010731 54.20 0.000 5.280472 5.676671
- - - - - - - - - - - - - - - - - - - - - - - - - - - - - - - - - - - - - - - - - - -


- - - - - - - - - - - - - - - - - - - - - - - - - - - - - - - - - - - - - - - - - - -
Random-effects Parameters | Estimate Std. Err.  [ 95% Conf. Interval]
- - - - - - - - - - - - - - - -+- - - - - - - - - - - - - - - - - - - - - - - - - - -
id: Identity                  |
          var(_cons) | .8430361 .0967123    .6732822   1.05559
- - - - - - - - - - - - - -+- - - - - - - - - - - - - - - - - - - - - - - - - - - -
        var(Residual) | .2296193 .0230195    .1886577   .2794745
- - - - - - - - - - - - - - - - - - - - - - - - - - - - - - - - - - - - - - - - - - -
LR test vs. linear model: chibar2(01) = 191.34   Prob >= chibar2 = 0.0000
```

Table 10.2 summarises the results of the different analyses performed to evaluate the effect of the intervention on total serum cholesterol and physical activity.

From the results reported in Table 10.2 it can be seen that the estimation of the intervention effect highly depends on the method used. And although there is some debate about whether or not an adjustment for baseline must be performed, it is more or less accepted that the adjustment has to be done (Steyerberg et al., 2000; Vickers and Altman, 2001; Twisk and Proper, 2004; Lingsma, 2010; Twisk et al., 2018; Twisk, 2022). In other words, it is strongly advised to use analysis of covariance to estimate the effect of an intervention in an RCT with only one follow-up measurement.

It is essential to realise that whether the difference between the groups at baseline is statistically significant is not important. It is a huge misunderstanding to believe that an adjustment for baseline is only necessary when there is a significant difference in baseline value between the groups. Also, a non-significant difference at baseline can lead to regression to the mean. So, an adjustment for baseline is always necessary.

10.2.2 Randomised Controlled Trials with More than One Follow-up Measurement

The example dataset used in this section is taken from an RCT in which a new treatment is compared to placebo with regard to the development of systolic blood pressure (Vermeulen et al., 2000). In this RCT, three measurements were carried out: one baseline measurement and two follow-up measurements with equally spaced time intervals. Table 10.3 gives descriptive information about the variables used in the study. It should be noted that the main purpose of the treatment under study was not to lower systolic blood pressure; this was investigated as a side-effect. That is one of the reasons why the number of subjects at baseline was lower than the number of subjects at the first follow-up measurement. In the next sections, the results of many different analyses will be shown. It should be realised that some of the analyses are not really appropriate. However, because these (wrong) analyses are often used in real life practice, it is important to show the impact of the use of such inappropriate analyses.

Output 10.4 Results of a mixed model analysis to analyse the effect of the intervention on (A) total serum cholesterol and (B) physical activity, using Equation 10.8

```
(A)
Mixed-effects ML regression                Number of obs      =        398
Group variable: id                         Number of groups   =        199

                                           Obs per group:
                                                         min =          2
                                                         avg =        2.0
                                                         max =          2

                                           Wald chi2(2)       =       7.33
Log likelihood = -454.73672                Prob > chi2        =     0.0256

------------------------------------------------------------------------------
 cholesterol |      Coef.  Std. Err.     z   P>|z|   [ 95% Conf. Interval]
-------------+----------------------------------------------------------------
        time |   .0207958  .0592975   0.35   0.726   -.0954251    .1370167
    time_int |  -.1871102  .0838021  -2.23   0.026   -.3513593   -.0228612
       _cons |    5.42598  .0691071  78.52   0.000    5.290532    5.561427
------------------------------------------------------------------------------


------------------------------------------------------------------------------
 Random-effects Parameters |  Estimate  Std. Err.   [ 95% Conf. Interval]
---------------------------+--------------------------------------------------
id: Identity               |
             var(_cons)    |  .7564342  .0861727     .6050657    .9456703
---------------------------+--------------------------------------------------
            var(Residual)  |  .1939479  .0194559     .1593298    .2360876
------------------------------------------------------------------------------
LR test vs. linear model: chibar2(01) = 198.87   Prob >= chibar2 = 0.0000

(B)
Mixed-effects ML regression                Number of obs      =        398
Group variable: id                         Number of groups   =        199

                                           Obs per group:
                                                         min =          2
                                                         avg =        2.0
                                                         max =          2

                                           Wald chi2(2)       =      12.22
Log likelihood = -485.3575                 Prob > chi2        =     0.0022

------------------------------------------------------------------------------
    activity |      Coef.  Std. Err.     z   P>|z|   [ 95% Conf. Interval]
-------------+----------------------------------------------------------------
        time |  -.1222315  .0645477  -1.89   0.058   -.2487427    .0042797
    time_int |   .3146177  .0911307   3.45   0.001    .1360048    .4932306
       _cons |   5.629397  .0741206  75.95   0.000    5.484123    5.774671
------------------------------------------------------------------------------
```

Output 10.4 *(cont.)*

```
----------------------------------------------------------------
Random-effects Parameters |  Estimate  Std. Err.  [ 95% Conf. Interval]
--------------------------+-------------------------------------
id: Identity             |
             var(_cons)  |  .8630965   .099009    .6893104  1.080697
--------------------------+-------------------------------------
           var(Residual) |  .2301825   .0231269   .1890385   .2802814
----------------------------------------------------------------
LR test vs. linear model: chibar2(01) = 191.36    Prob >= chibar2 = 0.0000
```

Output 10.5 Results of a mixed model analysis with both a random intercept and random slope for time to analyse the effect of the intervention on (A) total serum cholesterol and (B) physical activity, using Equation 10.8

(A)

```
Mixed-effects ML regression                     Number of obs    =      398
Group variable: id                              Number of groups =      199

                                                Obs per group:
                                                           min =        2
                                                           avg =      2.0
                                                           max =        2

                                                Wald chi2(2)    =     7.29
Log likelihood = -454.60514                     Prob > chi2     =   0.0261

----------------------------------------------------------------
cholesterol |   Coef.   Std. Err.    z    P>|z|    [ 95% Conf. Interval]
------------+---------------------------------------------------
       time |  .0194728  .0589978   0.33  0.741  -.0961608   .1351064
   time_int | -.1843094  .0828422  -2.22  0.026  -.3466771  -.0219417
      _cons |  5.42598   .0698616  77.67  0.000   5.289054   5.562906
----------------------------------------------------------------


----------------------------------------------------------------
Random-effects Parameters |  Estimate  Std. Err.  [ 95% Conf. Interval]
--------------------------+-------------------------------------
id: Unstructured          |
              var(time)   |  .2000262  15.29588    1.62e-66   2.47e+64
             var(_cons)   |  .8772897   7.648724   3.33e-08   2.31e+07
         cov(time,_cons)  | -.1209703   7.648175  -15.11112  14.86918
--------------------------+-------------------------------------
           var(Residual)  |  .0939592   7.647949   4.88e-71   1.81e+68
----------------------------------------------------------------
LR test vs. linear model: chi2(3) = 199.13          Prob > chi2 = 0.0000
```

Output 10.5 *(cont.)*

(B)

```
Mixed-effects ML regression                 Number of obs    =        398
Group variable: id                          Number of groups =        199

                                            Obs per group:
                                                         min =          2
                                                         avg =        2.0
                                                         max =          2

                                            Wald chi2(2)    =      14.88
Log likelihood = -483.79738                 Prob > chi2     =     0.0006
```

activity	Coef.	Std. Err.	z	P>|z|	[95% Conf. Interval]
time	-.130831	.0633416	-2.07	0.039	-.2549783 -.0066838
time_int	.3328232	.0871659	3.82	0.000	.1619811 .5036653
_cons	5.629397	.0768869	73.22	0.000	5.478702 5.780092

Random-effects Parameters	Estimate	Std. Err.	[95% Conf. Interval]
id: Unstructured			
var(time)	.2385996	24.59686	4.25e-89 1.34e+87
var(_cons)	1.065177	12.2992	1.58e-10 7.18e+09
cov(time,_cons)	-.2035301	12.29869	-24.30852 23.90146
var(Residual)	.1112289	12.29843	8.51e-96 1.45e+93

```
LR test vs. linear model: chi2(3) = 194.48          Prob > chi2 = 0.0000
```

10.2.2.1 Simple Analysis

The simplest way to answer the question of whether the treatment is more effective than placebo is to compare systolic blood pressure values at the two follow-up measurements between the two groups. In this example, a distinction can be made between the short-term effect and the long-term effect. To analyse the short-term effect, the mean systolic blood pressure measured at the first follow-up can be compared between the treatment group and placebo group. For the long-term effect, the systolic blood pressure measured at the second follow-up can be compared between the groups. The difference between the two groups can be analysed with an independent samples *t*-test. Table 10.4 shows the results of these analyses.

From the results in Table 10.4, it can be seen that there is both a significant short-term and a significant long-term effect in favour of the treatment group, but that the long-term difference between the two groups is smaller than the short-term difference. This indicates that the short-term effect is stronger than the long-term effect. A slightly different method is not to analyse the systolic blood pressure values at the first and the second follow-up, but to analyse the short-term and long-term changes in systolic blood pressure. For this purpose, the changes in systolic blood pressure between baseline and the first follow-up and between baseline and the second follow-up were calculated. Obviously, the change in scores for treatment and placebo can be compared to each

Table 10.2 Regress and standard deviation (between brackets) for physical activity and cholesterol

	Effect (se)
Total serum cholesterol (mmol/l)	
Changes	−0.22 (0.09)
Changes adjusted for baseline	−0.18 (0.08)
Analysis of covariance	−0.18 (0.08)
Mixed model analysis not adjusted for baseline	−0.22 (0.09)
Mixed model analysis adjusted for baseline[1]	−0.18 (0.08)
Physical activity	
Changes	0.25 (0.10)
Changes adjusted for baseline	0.33 (0.09)
Analysis of covariance	0.33 (0.09)
Mixed model analysis not adjusted for baseline	0.25 (0.10)
Mixed model analysis adjusted for baseline[1]	0.33 (0.09)

[1] With a random intercept and a random slope for time.

Table 10.3 Mean and standard deviation (between brackets) of systolic blood pressure at the three time-points

	Placebo group			Treatment group		
	Baseline	Follow-up 1	Follow-up 2	Baseline	Follow-up 1	Follow-up 2
N	71	74	66	68	69	65
Systolic blood pressure	130.7 (17.6)	129.1 (16.9)	126.3 (14.2)	126.5 (12.5)	122.5 (11.2)	121.6 (12.1)

Table 10.4 Results of independent samples t-tests to obtain a short-term and long-term effect of the new treatment by comparing the mean systolic blood pressure at both follow-up measurements between the treatment and placebo group

	Effect	95% CI	P-value
Short-term effect	−6.57	−11.34 to −1.80	0.007
Long-term effect	−4.69	−9.26 to −0.11	0.044

other with an independent samples t-test. Table 10.5 shows the results of these analyses.

The results presented in Table 10.5 show a different picture to the results in Table 10.4; i.e. the analysis of the changes between baseline and follow-up measurements show a non-significant beneficial effect of treatment compared with placebo. Although the changes for the treatment group were slightly greater than the changes for the placebo group in all comparisons, the independent samples t-test did not produce any significant difference. In conclusion, most of the assumed effect of the treatment was already present at baseline. So this effect could not be attributed to the new treatment.

In Section 10.2.1 it was shown that both analyses performed (i.e. the comparison of the follow-up measurements and the comparison of the changes between baseline and the follow-up measurements) are not appropriate in an RCT when the baseline value of the groups is different. From the descriptive information (Table 10.3) it was shown that the baseline blood pressure of the two groups differed from each other (130.7 mmHg for the placebo group versus 126.5 mmHg for the treatment group). To adjust for baseline, analyses of covariance should be performed to obtain a short-term and long-term effect of the intervention. Table 10.6 shows the result of these analyses.

Table 10.5 Results of independent samples t-tests to obtain a short-term and long-term effect of the new treatment by comparing the changes in systolic blood pressure between the treatment and placebo group

	Treatment	Placebo	Effect	95% CI	P-value
Short-term difference[1]	3.38	0.64	-2.74	-6.84 to 1.37	0.189
Long-term difference[2]	4.23	3.13	-1.10	-5.46 to 3.25	0.616

[1] Systolic blood pressure at baseline − systolic blood pressure at first follow-up.
[2] Systolic blood pressure at baseline − systolic blood pressure at second follow-up.

Table 10.6 Results of analyses of covariance to obtain a short-term and long-term effect of the new treatment

	Effect	95% CI	P-value
Short-term effect	-4.38	-8.11 to -0.65	0.022
Long-term effect	-2.96	-6.77 to 0.85	0.127

Table 10.7 Examples of summary statistics which are frequently used in intervention studies

The mean of all follow-up measurements
The highest (or lowest) value during follow-up
The time needed to reach the highest value or a certain predefined level
The area under the curve

As expected, from Table 10.6, it can be seen that the long-term effect is less strong than the short-term effect. Furthermore, both effects are a bit stronger than the effects estimated with the comparison between the changes between baseline and the follow-up measurements. This has to do with regression to the mean; because the baseline value of the treatment group is lower than the baseline value of the control group, it is more difficult for the treatment group to decrease its systolic blood pressure (see also Section 10.2.1).

10.2.2.2 Summary Statistics

There are many summary statistics available with which to estimate the effect of an intervention in an RCT with more than one follow-up measurement. Depending on the research question to be addressed and the characteristics of the outcome variable, different summary statistics can be used. The general idea of a summary statistic is to express the longitudinal development of a particular outcome variable as one quantity. Therefore, the longitudinal problem is reduced to a cross-sectional problem. To evaluate the effect of the intervention, the summary statistics of the groups under study are compared to each other. Table 10.7 shows a few examples of summary statistics.

One of the most frequently used summary statistics is the area under the curve (AUC). The AUC is calculated as shown in Equation 10.9.

$$AUC = \frac{1}{2}\sum_{t=1}^{T}(t_{t+1} - t_t)(Y_{it} + Y_{it+1}) \quad (10.9)$$

where AUC is the area under the curve, T is the number of measurements, and Y_{it} are the observations of the outcome variable for subject i at time t.

The unit of the AUC is the multiplication of the unit used for the outcome variable and the unit used for time. This is often rather difficult, and therefore the AUC is often divided by the total time period under consideration in order to obtain a weighted average over the whole time period. When the AUC is used as a summary statistic, the AUC must first be calculated for each subject; this is then used as an outcome variable to evaluate the effect of the intervention under study. Again, this comparison can be performed with an independent samples t-test. Table 10.8 shows the results of this analysis.

From Table 10.8 it can be seen that a highly significant difference was found between the AUC values of the two groups. This will not directly indicate that the treatment has an effect on the outcome variable. In the calculation, the difference in baseline value between the two groups is not taken into account. So, again, a difference in baseline value between groups can cause a difference in AUC.

When the time intervals are equally spaced (like in the example dataset), the AUC is comparable to the overall mean. The AUC becomes more

Table 10.8 Area under the curve for systolic blood pressure between baseline and the second follow-up measurement; a comparison between treatment and placebo and p-value derived from an independent samples t-test

	Treatment	Placebo	Effect	95% CI	P-value
Area under the curve	246.51	259.23	-12.72	-21.98 to -3.47	0.007

interesting when the time intervals in the longitudinal study are unequally spaced, because then the AUC reflects the weighted average in a certain outcome variable over the total follow-up period.

10.2.2.3 Generalised Linear Model for Repeated Measures

With the simple methods described in Section 10.2.2.1, separate analyses for short-term and long-term effects were performed. The purpose of summary statistics, such as the AUC, is to summarise the total development of the outcome variable, in order to make a cross-sectional analysis possible. Another way to analyse the total development of the outcome variable over time and to answer the question of whether the intervention has an effect on a certain continuous outcome variable, is to use a generalised linear model (GLM) for repeated measures (see Chapter 2). Output 10.6 shows the results of the GLM for repeated measures to analyse the difference in development over time in systolic blood pressure between treatment and placebo.

The output of the GLM for repeated measures reveals that for systolic blood pressure there is an overall treatment effect ($p = 0.011$), and an overall time effect ($p = 0.002$), but no significant interaction between treatment and time ($p = 0.283$). In particular, the information regarding the interaction is important, because this indicates that the observed overall group effect does not change over time. This means that from the result of the GLM for repeated measures it can be concluded that the two groups on average differ over time (a significant overall treatment effect), but that this difference is present along the whole longitudinal period, including the baseline measurement. So, there is no real treatment effect. From Figure 10.2 it can be seen that there is a decrease in systolic blood pressure over time for both groups.

10.2.2.4 Generalised Linear Model for Repeated Measures Adjusted for Baseline

When the baseline value of the outcome variable is different in the groups to be compared, it is often suggested that a GLM for repeated measures

should be performed, adjusting for baseline. It should be noted that when this analysis, which is also known as multivariate analysis of covariance (MANCOVA) for repeated measures is performed, the baseline value is both an outcome variable and a covariate. In some software packages (such as SPSS) this is not possible, and therefore an exact copy of the baseline value must be added to the model. Output 10.7 shows the result of the GLM for repeated measures adjusted for baseline.

It should be noted that in a GLM for repeated measures adjusted for baseline, the overall group effect is an indication of the effect of the new treatment. This has to do with the adjustment for baseline (see Figure 10.3). From Output 10.7 it can be seen that there is a significant treatment effect ($p = 0.018$). In addition, the interaction between time and treatment (obtained from this analysis) does not provide information about the overall treatment effect. The treatment by time interaction provides information about whether the observed treatment effect is stronger at the beginning or at the end of the follow-up period. From the result it can be seen that the time by treatment interaction is almost significant ($p = 0.062$), but it is not clear during which part of the follow-up period the effect is the strongest. Therefore, the graphical representation of the GLM result is needed (see Figure 10.3). From Figure 10.3 it can be seen that in the first part of the follow-up period, the treatment effect is the strongest. It should further be noted that the adjustment for baseline leads to equal starting points for both groups.

10.2.2.5 Regression-based Methods

In the discussion regarding the modelling of time (Chapter 4) it has already been mentioned that the questions answered by a GLM for repeated measures could also be answered by regression-based methods, such as mixed model analysis or GEE analysis. The advantage of the regression-based methods is that all available data are included in the analysis, while with a GLM for

Output 10.6 Results of a generalised linear model for repeated measures to analyse the difference in development over time in systolic blood pressure between treatment and placebo[1]

Tests of within-subjects effects

Measure: MEASURE_1

Source		Type III sum of squares	df	Mean square	F	Sig.
Time	Sphericity assumed	816.415	2	408.207	6.430	.002
	Greenhouse–Geisser	816.415	1.957	417.209	6.430	.002
	Huynh–Feldt	816.415	2.000	408.207	6.430	.002
	Lower-bound	816.415	1.000	816.415	6.430	.013
Time * treatment	Sphericity assumed	160.953	2	80.476	1.268	.283
	Greenhouse–Geisser	160.953	1.957	82.251	1.268	.283
	Huynh–Feldt	160.953	2.000	80.476	1.268	.283
	Lower-bound	160.953	1.000	160.953	1.268	.263
Error (time)	Sphericity assumed	14854.683	234	63.482		
	Greenhouse–Geisser	14854.683	228.951	64.881		
	Huynh–Feldt	14854.683	234.000	63.482		
	Lower-bound	14854.683	117.000	126.963		

Tests of between-subjects effects

Measure: MEASURE_1
Transformed variable: Average

Source	Type III sum of squares	df	Mean square	F	Sig.
Intercept	5701685.315	1	5701685.315	12039.101	.000
Treatment	3122.558	1	3122.558	6.593	.011
Error	55410.881	117	473.597		

[1]Only the univariate estimation procedure is presented.

repeated measures (both with and without an adjustment for baseline) only those subjects with a complete dataset are included. In the present example, both GLM for repeated measures were carried out for 118 patients, whereas with the regression-based methods all available data from the 152 patients can be used. Another limitation of GLM for repeated measures is that the method is merely based on statistical testing, while regression-based methods on the other hand, are merely based on the estimation of the magnitude of the treatment effect.

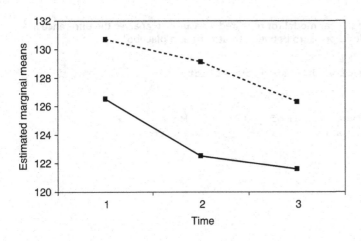

Figure 10.2 Graphical representation of the result of the generalised linear model for repeated measures (—— placebo, – – – treatment).

Output 10.7 Results of a generalised linear model for repeated measures to analyse the difference in development over time in systolic blood pressure between treatment and placebo, adjusted for baseline[1]

Tests of within-subjects effects

Measure: MEASURE_1

Source		Type III sum of squares	df	Mean square	F	Sig.
Time	Sphericity assumed	1959.230	2	979.615	18.057	.000
	Greenhouse–Geisser	1959.230	1.953	1003.326	18.057	.000
	Huynh–Feldt	1959.230	2.000	979.615	18.057	.000
	Lower-bound	1959.230	1.000	1959.230	18.057	.000
Time * treatment	Sphericity assumed	304.692	2	152.346	2.808	.062
	Greenhouse–Geisser	304.692	1.953	156.033	2.808	.064
	Huynh–Feldt	304.692	2.000	152.346	2.808	.062
	Lower-bound	304.692	1.000	304.692	2.808	.096
Error (time)	Sphericity assumed	12586.272	232	54.251		
	Greenhouse–Geisser	12586.272	226.517	55.564		
	Huynh–Feldt	12586.272	232.000	54.251		
	Lower-bound	12586.272	116.000	108.502		

(cont.)

Tests of between-subjects effects					
Measure: MEASURE_1 Transformed variable: average					
Source	Type III sum of squares	df	Mean square	F	Sig.
Intercept	3599.882	1	3599.882	38.534	.000
Treatment	539.478	1	539.478	5.775	.018
Error	10836.937	116	93.422		

[1]Only the univariate estimation procedure is presented.

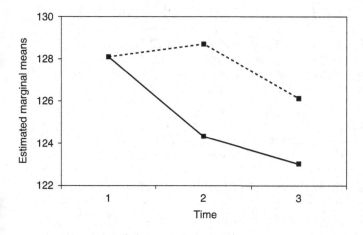

Figure 10.3 Graphical representation of the result of the generalised linear model for repeated measures adjusted for baseline (——— placebo, – – – treatment).

There are many possibilities to use the regression-based methods to evaluate the effect of an intervention in an RCT with more than one follow-up measurement. The different possibilities will be discussed step by step. Again, it should be noted that not all possibilities are equally appropriate.

To analyse the effects of an intervention, first, a longitudinal analysis of covariance can be used (Equation 10.10):

$$Y_{it} = \beta_0 + \beta_1 X_i + \beta_2 Y_{it0} + \varepsilon_{it} \qquad (10.10)$$

where Y_{it} are the observations of the outcome for subject i at time t, β_0 is the intercept, X_i are observations of the intervention variable for subject i, β_1 is the regression coefficient for the intervention variable, Y_{it0} are observations of the outcome for subject i at baseline, β_2 is the regression coefficient for the baseline value, and ε_{it} is the error for subject i at time t.

This model is an extension of analysis of covariance used for an RCT with one follow-up measurement. In the longitudinal analysis of covariance, the outcome is longitudinal including all follow-up measurements. It is important to realise that the regression coefficient for the intervention variable reflects the overall intervention effect on average over time. The model looks similar to the autoregressive model which was described in Chapter 5 (Section 5.3.3), but it is slightly different. In an autoregressive model, an adjustment is made for the value of the outcome variable at $t - 1$ (Equation 10.11), while in the analysis of covariance, an adjustment is made for baseline.

$$Y_{it} = \beta_0 + \beta_1 X_i + \beta_2 Y_{it-1} + \varepsilon_{it} \qquad (10.11)$$

where Y_{it} are observations of the outcome for subject i at time t, β_0 is the intercept, X_i are observations of the intervention variable for subject i, β_1 is the regression coefficient for the intervention variable, Y_{it-1} are observations of the outcome for subject i at $t - 1$, β_2 is the autoregression coefficient, and ε_{it} is the error for subject i at time t.

Output 10.8 Results of a mixed model analysis to analyse the effect of the new treatment on systolic blood pressure using a longitudinal analysis of covariance

```
Mixed-effects ML regression            Number of obs     =      249
Group variable: id                     Number of groups  =      130

                                       Obs per group:
                                                     min =        1
                                                     avg =      1.9
                                                     max =        2

                                       Wald chi2(2)      =   159.71
Log likelihood = -929.0358             Prob > chi2       =   0.0000

-----------------------------------------------------------------------
    systolic |     Coef.  Std. Err.     z   P>|z|   [ 95% Conf. Interval]
-------------+---------------------------------------------------------
   treatment | -3.708809  1.568446  -2.36  0.018   -6.782906  -.6347113
    baseline |  .6145549  .0516282  11.90  0.000    .5133654   .7157443
       _cons |  48.4137   6.829042   7.09  0.000    35.02903   61.79838
-----------------------------------------------------------------------


-----------------------------------------------------------------------
Random-effects Parameters | Estimate  Std. Err.   [ 95% Conf. Interval]
--------------------------+--------------------------------------------
id: Identity              |
             var(_cons) |  42.02991  11.28599    24.83084   71.14192
--------------------------+--------------------------------------------
            var(Residual) |  67.89443   9.06958    52.25497   88.21464
-----------------------------------------------------------------------
LR test vs. linear model: chibar2(01) = 16.31     Prob >= chibar2 = 0.0000
```

Output 10.8 shows the results of the mixed model analysis based on a longitudinal analysis of covariance, while Output 10.9 shows the results of an autoregressive mixed model analysis.

When the result obtained from a longitudinal analysis of covariance is compared to the result obtained from an autoregressive analysis, it can be seen that the treatment effect obtained from a longitudinal analysis of covariance is higher than the one obtained from an autoregressive analysis (−3.708809 versus −2.276566). So, the question is, which of the two methods is better? As has been mentioned before, in the autoregressive model, the first follow-up measurement is adjusted for baseline, but the second follow-up measurement is adjusted for the value at the first follow-up measurement. In Section 10.2.1 it was explained that an adjustment for baseline is necessary to take into account regression to the mean. It was indicated

that in an RCT the difference in the baseline value between the groups was totally due to chance. Therefore, it makes sense to adjust both follow-up measurements for baseline. In an autoregressive model, the second follow-up measurement is adjusted for the first follow-up measurement. It is, however, highly questionable whether the difference between the groups observed at the first follow-up measurement are due to chance. It is more likely that the difference at the first follow-up measurement are partly (or maybe totally) caused by the treatment itself (Boshuizen, 2005; Twisk and Proper, 2005). An adjustment for the value at the first follow-up measurement, therefore, partly (or maybe totally) adjusts the treatment effect at the second follow-up measurement for the treatment effect at the first follow-up measurement and that is wrong. So, therefore, it is highly recommended to use longitudinal analysis of

Output 10.9 Results of a mixed model analysis to analyse the effect of the new treatment on systolic blood pressure using an autoregressive analysis

```
Mixed-effects ML regression              Number of obs     =      261
Group variable: id                       Number of groups  =      142

                                         Obs per group:
                                                       min =        1
                                                       avg =      1.8
                                                       max =        2

                                         Wald chi2(2)      =   248.43
Log likelihood = -975.67735              Prob > chi2       =   0.0000


------------------------------------------------------------------------
   systolic |     Coef.  Std. Err.       z   P>|z|   [ 95% Conf. Interval]
------------+-----------------------------------------------------------
  treatment | -2.276566  1.284747    -1.77   0.076   -4.794624   .2414915
 systolic_1 |  .6458443  .0430679    15.00   0.000    .5614328   .7302558
      _cons |  44.06264  5.677741     7.76   0.000    32.93447   55.1908
------------------------------------------------------------------------


-------------------------------------------------------------------------
Random-effects Parameters | Estimate Std. Err.   [ 95% Conf. Interval]
--------------------------+----------------------------------------------
id: Identity              |
            var(_cons) |  4.28e-21  1.62e-20    2.57e-24   7.13e-18
--------------------------+----------------------------------------------
          var(Residual) |  103.3972  9.051242    87.0955   122.7501
-------------------------------------------------------------------------
LR test vs. linear model: chibar2(01) = 0.00     Prob >= chibar2 = 1.0000
```

covariance to estimate the intervention effect in an RCT with more than one follow-up measurement. It should be noted that when the overall treatment effect on average over time is estimated, the time variable is not included in the model. For some readers, this may be strange. However, an adjustment for the time variable does not make sense, because both groups are measured at the same time-points. Therefore, time is not related to treatment and, therefore, time cannot be a confounder in the estimation of the overall treatment effect on average over time.

After the total intervention effect over time is estimated, in the next step of the analysis, the effect of the intervention at the different follow-up measurements can (or maybe must) be estimated. This can be done by adding time and the interaction between intervention and time to the longitudinal analysis of covariance (Equation 10.12). Because in an RCT the time-points are more or less fixed, when there are more than two follow-up measurements, time can be treated as a categorical variable and therefore represented by dummy variables.

$$Y_{it} = \beta_0 + \beta_1 X_i + \beta_2 time + \beta_3 X_i \times time + \beta_4 Y_{it0} + \varepsilon_{it}$$
$$(10.12)$$

where Y_{it} are observations of the outcome for subject i at time t, β_0 is the intercept, X_i are observations of the intervention variable for subject i, β_1 is the regression coefficient for the intervention variable, β_2 is the regression coefficient for time, β_3 is the regression coefficient for the interaction between the intervention variable and time, Y_{it0} are observations of the outcome for subject i at baseline, β_4 is the regression coefficient for the baseline value, and ε_{it} is the error for subject i at time t.

Output 10.10 Results of a mixed model analysis to analyse the effect of the new treatment on systolic blood pressure at the two follow-up measurements using a longitudinal analysis of covariance

```
Mixed-effects ML regression              Number of obs     =      249
Group variable: id                       Number of groups  =      130

                                         Obs per group:
                                                       min =        1
                                                       avg =      1.9
                                                       max =        2

                                         Wald chi2(4)      =   162.61
Log likelihood = -926.90682              Prob > chi2       =   0.0000

- - - - - - - - - - - - - - - - - - - - - - - - - - - - - - - - - - - - - - - - -
   systolic |      Coef.  Std. Err.     z   P>|z|    [ 95% Conf. Interval]
- - - - - - -+- - - - - - - - - - - - - - - - - - - - - - - - - - - - - - - - - -
  treatment |  -4.57607  1.850071  -2.47  0.013   -8.202142  -.9499968
     2.time |  -2.872997 1.448173  -1.98  0.047   -5.711363  -.0346307
            |
      time#|
  treatment |
          2 |  1.900896  2.063158   0.92  0.357   -2.142819   5.94461
            |
   baseline |  .6132101  .0518268  11.83  0.000    .5116315   .7147887
      _cons |  49.91222  6.893055   7.24  0.000   36.40208   63.42236
- - - - - - - - - - - - - - - - - - - - - - - - - - - - - - - - - - - - - - - - -


- - - - - - - - - - - - - - - - - - - - - - - - - - - - - - - - - - - - - - - - -
Random-effects Parameters | Estimate  Std. Err.  [ 95% Conf. Interval]
- - - - - - - - - - - - - - -+- - - - - - - - - - - - - - - - - - - - - - - - - -
id: Identity               |
            var(_cons) |  44.23749   11.3064     26.8063   73.00356
- - - - - - - - - - - - - - -+- - - - - - - - - - - - - - - - - - - - - - - - - -
          var(Residual) |  64.92999  8.692522    49.94483   84.41123
- - - - - - - - - - - - - - - - - - - - - - - - - - - - - - - - - - - - - - - - -
LR test vs. linear model: chibar2(01) = 18.34     Prob >= chibar2 = 0.0000
```

Output 10.10 shows the result of the mixed model analysis based on a longitudinal analysis of covariance including time and the interaction between treatment and time.

In the analysis reported in Output 10.10, the first follow-up measurement is used as reference time-point. Because of that, the regression coefficient for treatment (i.e. −4.57607) indicates the difference between the two groups at the first follow-up measurement. Furthermore, because the baseline value is added to the model as a covariate, the analysis is adjusted for baseline and, therefore, adjusted for regression to the

mean. Based on Output 10.10 it is also possible to calculate the difference between the two groups at the second follow-up measurement. Therefore, the regression coefficient for the interaction term (i.e. 1.900896) has to be added to the regression coefficient for treatment (i.e. −4.57607). This leads to a treatment effect of −2.675174. The problem is, however, that in this way it is only possible to obtain the effect estimate, while it is also necessary to report the 95% confidence interval around the effect estimate and the corresponding p-value. To obtain these, the same analysis has to be redone with the second follow-up

Output 10.11 Results of a mixed model analysis to analyse the effect of the new treatment on systolic blood pressure at the two follow-up measurements using a longitudinal analysis of covariance with the second follow-up measurement as reference category

```
Mixed-effects ML regression                 Number of obs    =      249
Group variable: id                          Number of groups =      130

                                            Obs per group:
                                                        min =        1
                                                        avg =      1.9
                                                        max =        2

                                            Wald chi2(4)     =   162.61
Log likelihood = -926.90682                 Prob > chi2      =   0.0000


- - - - - - - - - - - - - - - - - - - - - - - - - - - - - - - - - - - - - - -
   systolic |      Coef.  Std. Err.      z   P>|z|    [ 95% Conf. Interval]
- - - - - - - +- - - - - - - - - - - - - - - - - - - - - - - - - - - - - - - -
  treatment | -2.675174  1.917198  -1.40   0.163   -6.432813   1.082465
     1.time |  2.872997  1.448173   1.98   0.047    .0346307   5.711363
            |
      time# |
  treatment |
          1 | -1.900896  2.063158  -0.92   0.357    -5.94461   2.142819
            |
   baseline |  .6132101  .0518268  11.83   0.000    .5116315   .7147887
      _cons |  47.03922  6.893941   6.82   0.000    33.52735    60.5511
- - - - - - - - - - - - - - - - - - - - - - - - - - - - - - - - - - - - - - -


- - - - - - - - - - - - - - - - - - - - - - - - - - - - - - - - - - - - - - -
Random-effects Parameters | Estimate  Std. Err.    [ 95% Conf. Interval]
- - - - - - - - - - - - - - - - - +- - - - - - - - - - - - - - - - - - - - - -
id: Identity                      |
               var(_cons) |  44.23749   11.3064      26.8063   73.00356
- - - - - - - - - - - - - - - - - +- - - - - - - - - - - - - - - - - - - - - -
             var(Residual) |  64.92999  8.692522     49.94483   84.41123
- - - - - - - - - - - - - - - - - - - - - - - - - - - - - - - - - - - - - - -
LR test vs. linear model: chibar2(01) = 18.34      Prob >= chibar2 = 0.0000
```

measurement as reference time-point. Output 10.11 shows the results of this analysis.

In Output 10.11 it can be seen that indeed the regression coefficient for treatment equals −2.675174. It can also be seen that the 95% confidence interval around the effect estimate ranges from −6.432813 to 1.082465 and that the corresponding p-value equals 0.163. It should be noted that in this particular analysis it is not really interesting whether the p-value of the interaction term is statistically significant. This is different from standard regression analysis with an interaction term, in which significance of the regression coefficient of the interaction term determines whether stratified results should be reported. In the analysis of intervention studies, the research question is not whether the effects at the different follow-up measurements are significantly different from each other, the research question is directly related to effect estimates at the different follow-up measurements.

A method which is often used to evaluate the effect of an intervention at the different follow-up measurements is also known as the repeated measures method (Twisk et al., 2018; Twisk, 2022). In this method a longitudinal regression analysis is performed in which all measurements are used as outcome (including the baseline measurement) including time (represented as dummy variables) and the interaction between the intervention variable and time (Equation 10.13, i.e. a longitudinal extension of Equation 10.7).

$$Y_{it} = \beta_0 + \beta_1 X_i + \beta_2 time_1 + \beta_3 time_2$$
$$+ \beta_4 X_i \times time_1 + \beta_5 X_i \times time_1 + \varepsilon_{it}$$
$$(10.13)$$

where Y_{it} are observations of the outcome for subject i at time t, β_0 is the intercept, X_i are observations the intervention variable for subject i, β_1 is the regression coefficient for the intervention variable, $time_1$ is the first dummy variable for time, β_2 is the regression coefficient for the first dummy variable for time, $time_2$ is the second dummy variable for time, β_3 is the regression coefficient for the second dummy variable for time, β_4 is the regression coefficient for the interaction between the intervention variable and the first dummy variable for time, β_5 is the regression coefficient for the interaction between the intervention variable and the second dummy variable for time and ε_{it} is the error for subject i at time t.

In this model, the β_1 coefficient reflects the difference between the two groups at baseline, $\beta_1 + \beta_4$ reflects the difference at the first follow-up measurement, while $\beta_1 + \beta_5$ reflects the difference between the two groups at the second follow-up measurement. Although this is a nice way of analysing the effect of the intervention at the different time-points, it does not adjust for the baseline difference between the groups, or in other words, it does not adjust for possible regression to the mean. Output 10.12 shows the output of the repeated measures method to analyse the effect of the new treatment on systolic blood pressure.

From Output 10.12, it can be seen that at baseline the treatment group had a lower systolic blood pressure compared to the control group (−4.146645 mmHg). At the first follow-up measurement there is a bigger difference between the groups (−4.146645 + −2.940018 = −7.086663). At the second follow-up measurement the difference between the groups is somewhat less than estimated at the first follow-up measurement (i.e. −4.146645 + −1.050144 = −5.196789). Due to

missing values in the dataset, the differences between the treatment group and the control group at the two follow-up measurements are not exactly the same as the observed differences between the average values at the two follow-up measurements (see Table 10.3), but they are close. However, again, the repeated measures method does not adjust for the difference observed at baseline and therefore, this method is not appropriate to analyse data from an RCT.

To make a proper adjustment for baseline (and therefore, for regression to the mean), the model shown in Equation 10.13 without the intervention variable can be used (Equation 10.14, i.e. a longitudinal extension of Equation 10.8)

$$Y_{it} = \beta_0 + \beta_1 time_1 + \beta_2 time_2 + \beta_3 X_i$$
$$\times time_1 + \beta_4 X_i \times time_1 + \varepsilon_{it} \qquad (10.14)$$

where Y_{it} are observations of the outcome for subject i at time t, β_0 is the intercept, $time_1$ is the first dummy variable for time, β_1 is the regression coefficient for the first dummy variable for time, $time_2$ is the second dummy variable for time, β_2 is the regression coefficient for the second dummy variable for time, X_i are observations of the intervention variable for subject i, β_3 is the regression coefficient for the interaction between the intervention variable and the first dummy variable for time, β_4 is the regression coefficient for the interaction between the intervention variable and the second dummy variable for time and ε_{it} is the error for subject i at time t.

Without the intervention variable, the baseline value for the two groups is assumed to be equal and is reflected in the intercept of the model. Output 10.13 shows the results of the mixed model analysis based on Equation 10.14 to analyse the effect of the new treatment on systolic blood pressure.

The result shown in Output 10.13 indicate that the intervention effect at the first follow-up measurement is −4.304897 and at the second follow-up is 2.415109. As has been mentioned before, the analysis based on Equation 10.14 is basically the same as a longitudinal analysis of covariance, although the result is slightly different. The difference between the two methods was also observed in the analysis of an RCT with only one follow-up measurement (see Section 10.2.1.1).

Output 10.12 Results of a mixed model analysis to analyse the effect of the new treatment on systolic blood pressure at the different follow-up measurements using the repeated measures method (see Equation 10.13)

```
Mixed-effects ML regression              Number of obs     =      388
Group variable: id                       Number of groups  =      139

                                         Obs per group:
                                                       min =        1
                                                       avg =      2.8
                                                       max =        3

                                         Wald chi2(5)      =    22.47
Log likelihood = -1503.3301              Prob > chi2       =   0.0004

-----------------------------------------------------------------------
 systolic |     Coef.  Std. Err.     z   P>|z|   [ 95% Conf. Interval]
----------+------------------------------------------------------------
treatment | -4.146645  2.452393  -1.69  0.091   -8.953247   .6599575
          |
     time |
        1 | -.6333109  1.435063  -0.44  0.659   -3.445984   2.179362
        2 | -3.491867  1.493045  -2.34  0.019   -6.418182  -.5655524
          |
    time# |
treatment |
        1 | -2.940018  2.059911  -1.43  0.154    -6.97737   1.097334
        2 | -1.050144  2.125544  -0.49  0.621   -5.216132   3.115845
          |
    _cons |  130.6761  1.715288  76.18  0.000    127.3142    134.038
-----------------------------------------------------------------------


-----------------------------------------------------------------------
Random-effects Parameters | Estimate Std. Err.  [ 95% Conf. Interval]
--------------------------+--------------------------------------------
id: Identity              |
             var(_cons) |   139.253  20.06486   104.9918   184.6943
--------------------------+--------------------------------------------
            var(Residual) |  69.64419  6.248278   58.41408   83.03329
-----------------------------------------------------------------------
LR test vs. linear model: chibar2(01) = 163.59   Prob >= chibar2 = 0.0000
```

10.3 Dichotomous Outcome Variables

10.3.1 Introduction

The example of an RCT with a dichotomous outcome variable uses a hypothetical dataset from a study in which a new treatment was applied on patients with low back pain. Treatment duration was one month, and patients were seen at three follow-up visits. The first follow-up visit was directly at the end of the treatment period (after one month) and the two long-term follow-up visits were scheduled at six and 12 months after the start of the treatment. In this RCT, the treatment is compared to usual care, and 60 patients were included in each of the two groups. The dichotomous outcome variable of interest was

Output 10.13 Results of a mixed model analysis to analyse the effect of the new treatment on systolic blood pressure at the different follow-up measurements using the repeated measures method (see Equation 10.14)

```
Mixed-effects ML regression              Number of obs     =     388
Group variable: id                       Number of groups  =     139

                                         Obs per group:
                                                         min =       1
                                                         avg =     2.8
                                                         max =       3

                                         Wald chi2(4)      =   19.49
Log likelihood = -1504.75                Prob > chi2       =  0.0006

--------------------------------------------------------------------
    systolic |    Coef.   Std. Err.      z    P>|z|    [95% Conf. Interval]
-------------+------------------------------------------------------
       time1 |  .0353962  1.380497     0.03   0.980   -2.670328    2.74112
       time2 | -2.823212  1.440867    -1.96   0.050    -5.64726   .0008363
  treat_time1| -4.304897  1.894967    -2.27   0.023   -8.018965  -.5908295
  treat_time2| -2.415109  1.96634     -1.23   0.219   -6.269064   1.438846
        _cons|  128.6475  1.234181   104.24   0.000    126.2285   131.0664
--------------------------------------------------------------------


--------------------------------------------------------------------
Random-effects Parameters |  Estimate  Std. Err.   [95% Conf. Interval]
--------------------------+-----------------------------------------
id: Identity              |
              var(_cons)  |  141.9214  20.47283     106.969   188.2945
--------------------------+-----------------------------------------
            var(Residual) |  69.8037   6.274467    58.52834   83.25123
--------------------------------------------------------------------
LR test vs. linear model: chibar2(01) = 163.62      Prob >= chibar2 = 0.0000
```

self-reported recovery, which was reversible, so it is possible that, for instance, patients could be recovered after one month, but not recovered at later follow-up measurements. There was no missing data, so all 120 patients had a full follow-up. Figure 10.4 shows the proportion of patients who were recovered at the different follow-up measurements.

10.3.2 Simple Analysis

The classical way to analyse the result of such an RCT is to analyse the difference in proportion of patients experiencing recovery between treatment and usual care at each of the three follow-up measurements, by simply applying a Chi-square test. Furthermore, at each of the follow-up measurements, the effect of the new treatment can be estimated by calculating the relative risk (and corresponding 95% confidence interval). The relative risk is defined as the proportion of subjects recovered in the treatment group, divided by the proportion of subjects recovered in the usual care group. Table 10.9 summarises the results of the analyses.

From the results in Table 10.9 it can be seen that during the treatment period of one month both the treatment group and the usual care group show quite a high proportion of patients who recover, and although in the treatment group this proportion is slightly higher, the difference is not statistically significant ($p = 0.20$). After the

Table 10.9 Results of an RCT to investigate the effect of a new treatment, i.e. the number of patients recovered, the relative risks and 95% confidence intervals (between brackets) for the treatment group and the corresponding *p*-values at each of the follow-up measurements

	Recovery after one month		Recovery after six months		Recovery after 12 months	
	Yes	No	Yes	No	Yes	No
Treatment	35	25	39	21	60	10
Placebo	28	32	29	31	30	30
Relative risk	1.28 (0.87–1.88)		1.48 (0.97–2.53)		3.00 (1.61–5.58)	
P-value	0.20		0.07		< 0.01	

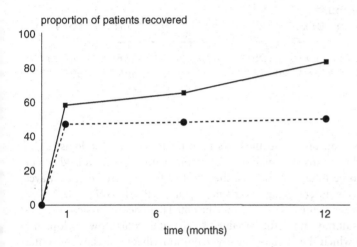

proportion of patients recovered

time (months)

Figure 10.4 The proportion of patients recovered in an RCT to investigate the effect of a new treatment for patients with low back pain (■ —— treatment, • – – – usual care).

treatment period, in both groups there is an increase in the number of patients who recovered, but in the treatment group this increase is more pronounced, which results in a significant difference between the treatment group and the usual care group after 12 months of follow-up with a relative risk of 3.0, which indicates that in the treatment group the probability of recovery is three times as high compared to the usual care group.

10.3.3 Regression-based Methods

It is, of course, also possible to estimate the effect of the new treatment with either a logistic GEE analysis or a logistic mixed model analysis. The first thing that should be realised is that within a logistic GEE analysis or a logistic mixed model analysis, odds ratios are estimated. Odds ratios can be interpreted as relative risks, but they are not the same. Due to the mathematical background of odds ratios and relative risks, odds ratios always reveal stronger effects compared to

Table 10.10 Odds ratios, 95% confidence intervals (between brackets) and *p*-values as a result of an RCT to analyse the effect of a new treatment on recovery

	One month	Six months	12 months
Odds ratio	1.60 (0.78–3.29)	1.99 (0.95–4.13)	5.00 (2.14–11.66)
P-value	0.20	0.07	< 0.01

relative risks. This difference between the two becomes larger as the proportion of cases (i.e. recovered patients) increases. To illustrate this, the odds ratios for treatment versus usual care were calculated at each of the follow-up measurements (see Table 10.10).

From the results in Table 10.10 it can be seen that the odds ratios are bigger than the relative risks shown in Table 10.9, and that the confidence intervals are wider, but that the significance levels are the same. So, when a logistic GEE analysis or a

Output 10.14 Results of a logistic GEE analysis with an exchangeable correlation structure to analyse the effect of a new treatment on recovery on average over a period of 12 months

```
GEE population-averaged model          Number of obs    =      360
Group variable:                  id    Number of groups =      120
Link:                         logit    Obs per group:
Family:                    binomial                     min =        3
Correlation:           exchangeable                     avg =      3.0
                                                        max =        3
                                       Wald chi2(1)     =     8.71
Scale parameter:                  1    Prob > chi2      =   0.0032

                              (Std. Err. adjusted for clustering on id)
- - - - - - - - - - - - - - - - - - - - - - - - - - - - - - - - - - - -
             |              Robust
   recovery  |    Coef.   Std. Err.     z   P>|z|   [ 95% Conf. Interval]
- - - - - - -+- - - - - - - - - - - - - - - - - - - - - - - - - - - - -
  treatment  |  .8616212  .2919719   2.95  0.003    .2893669   1.433876
      _cons  | -.0666914  .1983756  -0.34  0.737   -.4555004   .3221177
- - - - - - - - - - - - - - - - - - - - - - - - - - - - - - - - - - - -
```

logistic mixed model analysis is carried out, one must realise that the results (i.e. odds ratios) obtained from such an analysis have to be interpreted with caution, and cannot be directly interpreted as relative risks. Output 10.14 presents the results of a logistic GEE analysis (assuming an exchangeable correlation structure), in which the effect of the new treatment on average over time is analysed.

From Output 10.14, it can be seen that the new treatment is highly successful over the total follow-up period. To obtain the odds ratio, EXP[regression coefficient] has to be taken. In the present example, the odds ratio is EXP[0.8616212] = 2.37. This can be interpreted as on average over time, the odds for recovery in the treatment group is 2.37 as high as the odds for recovery in the usual care group. To obtain the 95% confidence interval around the odds ratio, EXP[0.2893669] and EXP [1.433876] have to be taken; the 95% confidence interval around the odds ratio of 2.37 ranges therefore from 1.34 to 4.19. Although logistic GEE analysis is the best way to estimate the effect of the new treatment (see Section 7.2.5), the same analysis can also be performed with a logistic mixed model analysis. To illustrate the difference between the two methods, Output 10.15 shows the results of the logistic mixed model analysis.

As expected, the odds ratio obtained from the logistic mixed model analysis is higher compared

to the odds ratio obtained from the logistic GEE analysis. Estimated with logistic mixed model analysis, the effect of the new treatment on average over time equals EXP[1.415927] = 4.12.

It should be noted that there is no need to adjust for baseline. As all patients had low back pain at baseline (by definition), there is no baseline difference between the groups. Every patient in both groups is not recovered at baseline This is mostly the case when a dichotomous outcome variable is considered in an RCT. So, the whole discussion about how and when to adjust for baseline is mostly not relevant for dichotomous outcome variables.

The odds ratios obtained from the analyses performed are interpreted as the effect of the new treatment on average over time. This is an interesting effect measure, but it is also interesting to investigate the effect of the treatment at different time-points. Therefore, a logistic GEE analysis can be performed with time and an interaction between treatment and time in the model. Because fixed time-points are used, time can be treated as a categorical variable and represented by dummy variables. Output 10.16 shows the results of the logistic GEE analysis to estimate the effect of the new treatment at the different time points.

From Output 10.16 the effects of the new treatment at the different time-points can be derived. The coefficient for the treatment variable

Output 10.15 Results of a logistic mixed model analysis to analyse the effect of a new treatment on recovery on average over a period of 12 months

```
Mixed-effects logistic regression        Number of obs    =        360
Group variable:              id          Number of groups =        120

                                         Obs per group:
                                                    min =          3
                                                    avg =        3.0
                                                    max =          3

Integration method: mvaghermite          Integration pts. =          7

                                         Wald chi2(1)     =       8.44
Log likelihood = -214.78798              Prob > chi2      =     0.0037
-------------------------------------------------------------------------
   recovery |      Coef.  Std. Err.     z   P>|z|    [ 95% Conf. Interval]
------------+------------------------------------------------------------
  treatment |   1.415927  .4874143   2.90  0.004     .4606122   2.371241
       _cons|  -.0966625  .3254968  -0.30  0.766    -.7346245   .5412995
------------+------------------------------------------------------------
id          |
  var(_cons)|   3.924528  1.359409                   1.990406   7.738081
-------------------------------------------------------------------------
LR test vs. logistic model: chibar2(01) = 42.95   Prob >= chibar2 = 0.0000
```

(i.e. 0.4700036) can be transformed into an odds ratio, which reflects the effect of the new treatment at the first follow-up measurement (i.e. at month one). The odds ratio at the first follow-up measurement is therefore equal to 1.60. The intervention effect at the second follow-up measurement (i.e. at month six) can be calculated by adding up the regression coefficient for treatment and the regression coefficient for the interaction between treatment and the first dummy variable for time (i.e. 0.4700036 + 0.215727 = 0.6857306), which gives an odds ratio of 1.99. In the same way, the odds ratio at the last follow-up measurement (i.e. at month 12) can be calculated (i.e. 0.4700036 + 1.139434 = 1.6094376), which gives an odds ratio of 5.00. To obtain the 95% confidence intervals around the odds ratios at the different time-points the time dummy variables for time should be recoded. The odds ratios (and 95% confidence intervals) derived in this way are exactly the same as the odds ratios derived from three separate analyses, the results of which were shown in Table 10.10. This has to do with the fact that there is no missing data in the example RCT. With missing data (which is normally the case),

the results would not have been exactly the same. Output 10.17 shows the results of the logistic GEE analyses to obtain the effects of the new treatment at the different follow-up measurements including the 95% confidence intervals and corresponding p-values. In the outputs, the odds ratios are given instead of the regression coefficients.

10.3.4 Other Methods

Besides a longitudinal logistic regression analysis, a survival analysis can also be used to analyse the data from the present example. Regarding survival analysis, Cox regression for recurrent events can be used. Although there are different estimation methods available (Kelly and Lim, 2003) the general idea behind Cox regression for recurrent events is that the different time periods are analysed separately and adjusted for the fact that the time periods within a subject are dependent of each other (Glynn et al., 1993). The idea of this adjustment is that the standard error of the regression coefficient of interest is increased proportional to the correlation of the observations within the subject. One of the problems with

Output 10.16 Results of a logistic GEE analysis with an exchangeable correlation structure to analyse the effect of a new treatment on recovery at different time-points

```
GEE population-averaged model          Number of obs    =     360
Group variable:                 id     Number of groups =     120
Link:                        logit     Obs per group:
Family:                   binomial                     min =       3
Correlation:         exchangeable                      avg =     3.0
                                                       max =       3
                                       Wald chi2(5)     =   18.94
Scale parameter:                1      Prob > chi2      =  0.0020


                                 (Std. Err. adjusted for clustering on id)
- - - - - - - - - - - - - - - - - - - - - - - - - - - - - - - - - - - - - -
             |              Robust
    recovery |    Coef.  Std. Err.     z   P>|z|   [ 95% Conf. Interval]
- - - - - - -+- - - - - - - - - - - - - - - - - - - - - - - - - - - - - - -
intervention | .4700036  .3696954   1.27  0.204   -.254586   1.194593
             |
        time |
           6 |   .06684  .3075189   0.22  0.828  -.5358859   .6695659
          12 | .1335314  .3416822   0.39  0.696  -.5361533   .8032161
             |
       time#|
intervention |
           6 |  .215727  .4051391   0.53  0.594   -.578331   1.009785
          12 | 1.139434  .5097866   2.24  0.025    .140271   2.138598
             |
        _cons | -.1335314  .2598596  -0.51  0.607  -.6428468   .3757841
- - - - - - - - - - - - - - - - - - - - - - - - - - - - - - - - - - - - - -
```

using Cox regression for recurrent events is the question of how to define the time at risk. This is especially so in the present example, because the events under study are not short-lasting events, but can be long lasting and can be considered as states, i.e. the events can continue over more than one repeated measurement. In general, the time at risk can be defined in three different ways (see Figure 10.5): (1) The counting method; each time period is analysed separately assuming that all patients are at risk at the beginning of each period, irrespective of the situation at the end of the foregoing period. (2) The total time method; this method is comparable to the counting method, however, in the total time method, the starting point for each period is the beginning of the study. (3) The time to event method; in this method only the transitions from no treatment success to treatment success are taken into account. So, if for a patient treatment is successful after

three months and stays successful at all repeated measurements, only the first measurement is taken into account in the analysis. When, for another patient, treatment is successful after three months, and not successful at six months, that particular patient is again at risk from three months onwards until treatment for that patient is successful for the second time, or until the follow-up period ends.

Output 10.18 shows the result of a Cox regression analysis for recurrent events when the time at risk is defined according to the counting method.

From Output 10.18 it can be seen that the hazard ratio for treatment compared to usual care is 1.43 with a 95% confidence interval that ranges between 1.12 and 1.81. The treatment effect is much lower than the one estimated with the logistic GEE analysis. This is not surprising, because the hazard ratio can be interpreted as an average relative risk over time and (as has been mentioned

Output 10.17 Results of a logistic GEE analysis with an exchangeable correlation structure to analyse the effect of a new treatment on recovery at different time-points. (Odds ratios are shown instead of regression coefficients.)

```
GEE population-averaged model              Number of obs     =      360
Group variable:                    id      Number of groups  =      120
Link:                           logit      Obs per group:
Family:                      binomial                 min =         3
Correlation:              exchangeable                 avg =       3.0
                                                       max =         3
                                           Wald chi2(5)      =    18.94
Scale parameter:                    1      Prob > chi2       =   0.0020

                                   (Std. Err. adjusted for clustering on id)
-------------------------------------------------------------------------
                 |             Robust
        recovery | Odds Ratio Std. Err.   z    P>|z|  [ 95% Conf. Interval]
-----------------+-------------------------------------------------------
       treatment |       1.6  .5915126  1.27  0.204  .7752374  3.302214
                 |
            time |
               6 |  1.069124 .3287759  0.22  0.828  .5851507  1.953389
              12 |  1.142857 .3904939  0.39  0.696  .5849942   2.23271
                 |
 time#c.treatment |
               6 |  1.240764 .5026818  0.53  0.594  .5608336  2.745011
              12 |     3.125 1.593083  2.24  0.025  1.150586  8.487526
                 |
           _cons |      .875 .2273771 -0.51  0.607  .5257934  1.456133
-------------------------------------------------------------------------

GEE population-averaged model              Number of obs     =      360
Group variable:                    id      Number of groups  =      120
Link:                           logit      Obs per group:
Family:                      binomial                 min =         3
Correlation:              exchangeable                 avg =       3.0
                                                       max =         3
                                           Wald chi2(5)      =    18.94
Scale parameter:                    1      Prob > chi2       =   0.0020

                                   (Std. Err. adjusted for clustering on id)
-------------------------------------------------------------------------
                 |             Robust
        recovery | Odds Ratio Std. Err.   z    P>|z|  [ 95% Conf. Interval]
-----------------+-------------------------------------------------------
       treatment | 1.985222  .7459188  1.83  0.068  .9505657  4.146063
                 |
            time |
               1 |  .9353448 .2876362 -0.22  0.828  .5119307  1.708962
              12 |  1.068966 .2146099  0.33  0.740  .7212287  1.584362
                 |
 time#c.treatment |
```

Output 10.17 *(cont.)*

```
       1 |   .8059553   .326524   -0.53  0.594     .3642973   1.78306
      12 |    2.51861  .9345178    2.49  0.013     1.217102  5.211888
         |
    _cons |   .9354839  .2426885   -0.26  0.797     .5626169  1.555463
```
```
GEE population-averaged model              Number of obs      =      360
Group variable:                     id     Number of groups  =      120
Link:                            logit     Obs per group:
Family:                       binomial                  min =        3
Correlation:              exchangeable                  avg =      3.0
                                                        max =        3
                                           Wald chi2(5)      =    18.94
Scale parameter:                    1      Prob > chi2       =   0.0020

                        (Std. Err. adjusted for clustering on id)
                   |            Robust
         recovery | Odds Ratio  Std. Err.    z   P>|z| [ 95% Conf. Interval]
         ----------+----------------------------------------------------------
        treatment |        5   2.169305   3.71  0.000  2.136323  11.70235
                  |
             time |
              1 |     .875   .2989719  -0.39  0.696  .4478862  1.709419
              6 | .9354839   .1878116  -0.33  0.740  .6311689  1.386523
                  |
 time#c.treatment |
              1 |      .32   .1631317  -2.24  0.025    .11782  .8691227
              6 | .3970443   .1473213  -2.49  0.013   .191869   .821624
                  |
            _cons |        1  .2592815   0.00  1.000   .601588  1.662267
```

before) a relative risk always gives a milder effect compared to an odds ratio estimated on the same data. In the example study the difference between the two is relatively big, because the prevalence of the outcome of interest (i.e. recovery) is quite high (around 60%).

It should be realised that Cox regression for recurrent events is especially useful for short-lasting events, such as asthmatic attacks, falls, etc. In all three ways the time at risk can be defined, it is assumed that directly after an event occurs, the subject is at risk to get another event. As has been mentioned before, in the present example, this is not really the case, i.e. the events are long lasting and can be considered as states. Therefore, in the present example it is not recommended to use Cox regression for recurrent events.

There are also other possibilities to model recurrent events data, such as the continuous-time Markov process model for panel data (Berkhof et al., 2009) or the conditional frailty model (Box-Steffensmeier et al., 2006). However, most of those alternative methods are mathematically complicated and not used extensively in practice. Therefore, they are beyond the scope of this book.

Output 10.18 Results of a Cox regression for recurrent events to analyse the effect of a new treatment on recovery when time at risk is defined according to the counting method

```
Cox regression - Breslow method for ties

No. of subjects    =      360          Number of obs   =       360
No. of failures    =      211
Time at risk       =     2280
                                        Wald chi2(1)    =      8.40
Log pseudolikelihood =  -1123.2464      Prob > chi2     =    0.0037

               (Std. Err. adjusted for 120 clusters in id)
- - - - - - - - - - - - - - - - - - - - - - - - - - - - - - - - - - - - - - -
           |             Robust
        _t | Haz. Ratio  Std. Err.    z   P>|z|    [ 95% Conf. Interval]
- - - - - -+- - - - - - - - - - - - - - - - - - - - - - - - - - - - - - - - -
 treatment |  1.425287   .1742538   2.90  0.004      1.121594   1.811212
- - - - - - - - - - - - - - - - - - - - - - - - - - - - - - - - - - - - - - -
```

● *No treatment success*
■ *Treatment success*

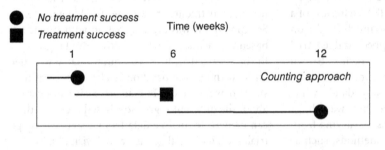

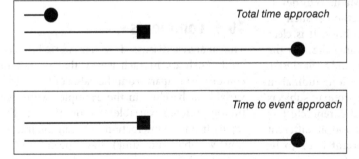

Figure 10.5 Possible definitions of the time at risk to be analysed with Cox regression for recurrent events for a patient whose treatment was not successful at week one, successful at week six and not successful at week 12.

10.4 Stepped Wedge Designs

In the RCTs discussed so far, the intervention variable was time-independent, which means that a subject who is allocated to the intervention group stays within the intervention group over the whole follow-up period. It is also possible that the intervention variable is time-dependent, i.e. the subject is allocated to both the intervention and the control condition. This study design is known as a cross-over design. In a cross-over design, mostly two groups receive both the intervention and the control condition in a different order. The analysis of data from a cross-over design is not much different from the analysis of data from a regular intervention study (Twisk, 2022). A combination of a regular design and a cross-over design is the stepped wedge design. The stepped wedge design is known as a one-way cross-over design in which several arms start with the intervention at different time points (see Table 10.11). Due to the fact that, after receiving the intervention, the subjects do not go back to the control condition, it is a one-way

Table 10.11 Schematic illustration of a stepped wedge trial design with four arms and five repeated measurements

	Time				
Arm	Baseline	2	3	4	5
1	0	X	X	X	X
2	0	0	X	X	X
3	0	0	0	X	X
4	0	0	0	0	X

Key: 0 = control; X = intervention.

cross-over design. The starting point of the intervention is randomised and although this randomisation can be on the subject level, it is mostly on a cluster level, such as hospitals, nursery homes, etc. Although there is some debate about the usefulness of a stepped wedge design (Kotz et al., 2012), it is increasingly popular as an alternative to the RCT.

Besides the discussion about the usefulness of a stepped wedge design, there is also much confusion about the way data from a stepped wedged trial should be analysed. In a systematic review, Brown and Lilford (2006) mentioned that "no two studies use the same method in analysing data", while Mdege et al. (2011) concluded that there was a huge variation in statistical methods used, varying from simple cross-sectional statistical methods, such as independent samples t-tests or Mann-Whitney U tests to more complicated methods, such as regression-based longitudinal methods. It is clear that there is no consensus regarding the way the data from a stepped wedge trial should be analysed.

Most stepped wedge trials are longitudinal in nature. This means that the same group of subjects is followed over time and that the different (clusters of) subjects receive the intervention at different points in time. The most important issue to be considered in the analysis of data from a longitudinal stepped wedge trial is the one-way cross-over nature of the design. Because of that, the effect of the intervention can be measured partly within the subjects (each subject moves at a certain point in time from the control condition to the intervention condition) and partly between the subjects (at a certain point in time, the intervention group can be compared to the control group). Ideally, these two aspects of the intervention effect should be combined in one analysis. Because of this, it is necessary that data from a stepped wedge trial is analysed with a method that is capable to combine

these effects; i.e., a linear mixed model analysis for continuous outcomes or a logistic GEE analysis for dichotomous outcomes.

Besides the combination of the between- and within-subjects effects, in the analysis of data from a stepped wedge trial the time variable can also play an important role. It has already been mentioned that in a standard intervention study, an adjustment for the time variable is not necessary, because the control group and the intervention group are measured at the same time-points and therefore, adjustment for time cannot influence the estimated intervention effect. In a stepped wedge trial this is different, because all (clusters of) subjects start with the intervention at different time-points and the effects of the intervention are also measured at different time-points. Therefore, the intervention variable becomes time-dependent and, therefore, time can influence the estimated intervention effect. Finally, it should be evaluated whether or not an adjustment for baseline should be made. In Section 10.2 it was argued that an adjustment for baseline is necessary to take into account regression to the mean. It is, however, questionable whether an adjustment for baseline is also necessary in a stepped wedge trial. For an extensive discussion about the different regression-based methods than can be used to analyse data from a stepped wedge trial, see Twisk et al. (2016) and Twisk (2022).

10.5 Comments

The analyses discussed so far were limited to crude analyses, in such a way that no potential confounders (apart from the value of the outcome variable at baseline in the examples with a continuous outcome variable) and/or effect modifiers (apart from the interaction between the intervention variable and time) have been discussed. Potential effect modifiers can be interesting if one wishes to investigate whether the intervention effect is different for subgroups of the population under study. The way confounders and effect modifiers are treated in longitudinal data analysis is, however, exactly the same as in cross-sectional regression analysis.

It is recommended that statistical analysis to evaluate the effect of an intervention should always start with descriptive statistics. This not only provides insight into the data, but can also provide (important) information regarding the effect of the intervention. After descriptive statistics, it is (highly) recommended to apply regression-based methods, especially for the analysis of continuous outcomes for which it is necessary to adjust for baseline. Furthermore, it is also important to use regression-based methods when the number of repeated measurements differs between subjects, and/or when there is (a lot of) missing data.

10.6 Beyond the Randomised Controlled Trial

Although the RCT is the best way to estimate intervention effects, in some situations it is not possible to perform an RCT. Furthermore, due to the increasing availability of real word data, it is also important to evaluate intervention effects in real-life observational studies. In Section 6.3.1, G-methods were introduced as methods to evaluate causal relationships when time-varying covariates were present in longitudinal data. G-methods are also suitable to evaluate the effect of different intervention strategies seen in observational data. It has already been mentioned that the outcome variables that can be used in G-methods are either a dichotomous outcome measured at the end of the study or a survival outcome. When the outcome is longitudinal (i.e. measured at different time-points) or when the outcome variable is continuous, G-methods cannot be used. One of the key issues in estimating intervention effects in observational data is the difference in all kinds of covariates between the groups being compared. In an RCT this difference is in general small due to the randomisation process. However, in observational data, there is no randomisation, so there will be differences between the groups. In other words, there are many possible confounders that should be taken into account. The challenge of all methods dealing with the estimation of intervention effects in observational studies is to take these differences, i.e. these confounders, into account. It should be realised that a possible confounder in the estimation of an intervention effect must not only be different between the intervention groups, but that the possible confounder must also be related to the particular outcome. The simplest way to deal with the confounding problem is to adjust for the confounders in a standard way by adding these possible confounders to the regression model. However, in some situations (for instance when the number of possible confounders is very high) a standard adjustment is not really possible. Therefore, other methods are developed to deal with this problem. In Section 6.3.1, for instance, it was mentioned that marginal structural models use inverse probability weighting for the estimation. With inverse probability weighting, an artificial population is generated in which exposures are independent of possible confounders. Also, the whole theory behind propensity score adjustment and the use of instrumental variables are related to this problem.

Although in real-life observational data an adjustment has to be made for (many) possible confounders, it is, however, questionable whether an adjustment has to be made for the baseline difference in the outcome variable between the groups. In an RCT, an adjustment for baseline has to be made to take into account regression to the mean. In an RCT this is necessary because the difference between the groups at baseline is due to chance. However, when observational data is used to estimate an intervention effect, the baseline difference in the outcome variable between the groups is (in general) not due to chance. In most situations, the baseline difference in the outcome variable between the groups is a real difference and is mostly related to the intervention provided to the subjects. When this is the case, an adjustment for baseline should not be performed.

Another key issue in the estimation of intervention effects in observational studies is the fact that in real-life observational data, usually the intervention can change over time. Although in standard longitudinal data analysis the intervention can be time-dependent, in Section 6.3.1 it was shown that G-methods (including marginal structural models) can also deal with this issue.

A relatively new method that can be used to estimate intervention effects in an observational study is the difference in difference method (see Section 10.6.1). Most methods (including the G-methods and the difference in difference method) that claim to estimate (causal) intervention effects in observational studies are related to counterfactuals or potential outcomes. The general idea behind this is that for a particular subject, the observed outcome under a certain intervention must be compared with the hypothetical situation that that particular subject did not receive the intervention. That hypothetical situation is not observed and should, therefore, be simulated. Although the whole idea of counterfactuals or potential outcomes theoretically makes sense, in practice the result of an analysis based on counterfactuals or potential outcomes is the same as the result obtained from a standard (longitudinal) regression analysis comparing the two groups with each other.

10.6.1 Difference in Difference Method

The application of the difference in difference method is relatively simple. Basically, the difference between the groups at baseline is compared to the difference between the groups at the follow-up measurement(s). Nevertheless, the literature regarding the difference in difference method is rather complicated. Because the difference in difference method is supposed to be used in evaluating intervention effects in observational studies, the key issue in the theory is about the possible confounding. One of the most important assumptions for using the difference in difference method is the so-called common trend assumption. This assumption includes that possible confounders varying across the groups are time-independent and that possible confounders that are time-dependent are independent of the groups. It goes beyond the scope of this book to explain in detail all the theoretical concepts behind the difference in difference method. A good overview of the difference in difference method can be found in Wing et al. (2018).

10.6.1.1 Example

To illustrate the general idea behind the difference in difference method, the same example is given which has been used to illustrate the estimation of an intervention effect in an intervention study with more than one follow-up measurement (see Table 10.3). Although in this study a baseline measurement and two follow-up measurements were performed, first a difference in difference analysis was performed using only the first follow-up measurement. It should be realised that in the long data structure used for the difference in difference analysis, the baseline value is included. Output 10.19 shows the results of this analysis.

Output 10.19 Results of a difference in difference analysis to analyse the effect of the new treatment on systolic blood pressure using only the first follow-up measurement

```
DIFFERENCE-IN-DIFFERENCES ESTIMATION RESULTS
Number of observations in the DIFF-IN-DIFF: 269
              Before      After
    Control: 71          67         138
    Treated: 68          63         131
             139        130

- - - - - - - - - - - - - - - - - - - - - - - - - - - - -
Outcome var.  | sys      | S. Err. |  |t|  | P>|t|
- - - - - - - +- -- -- -+- - - - - +- - - - +- - - - - - -
Before        |          |         |       |
  Control     | 130.676  |         |       |
  Treated     | 126.529  |         |       |
  Diff (T-C)  | -4.147   | 2.582   | -1.61 | 0.110
After         |          |         |       |
  Control     | 130.060  |         |       |
  Treated     | 122.571  |         |       |
  Diff (T-C)  | -7.488   | 2.531   | 2.96  | 0.004***
              |          |         |       |
Diff-in-Diff  | -3.342   | 2.101   | 1.59  | 0.114
- - - - - - - - - - - - - - - - - - - - - - - - - - - - -
R-square:  0.04
* Means and Standard Errors are estimated by linear regression
** Clustered Std. Errors
** Inference: *** p<0.01; ** p<0.05; * p<0.1
```

Output 10.20 Results of a difference in difference analysis to analyse the effect of the new treatment on systolic blood pressure using both follow-up measurements

```
DIFFERENCE-IN-DIFFERENCES ESTIMATION RESULTS
Number of observations in the DIFF-IN-DIFF: 388
          Before    After
  Control: 71       127      198
  Treated: 68       122      190
           139       249
- - - - - - - - - - - - - - - - - - - - - - - - - - - - -
Outcome var.  | sys      | S. Err.|  |t|   | P>|t|
- - - - - - - -+- - - — -+- - - - -+- - - --+- - - - - -
Before        |          |         |       |
  Control     | 130.676 |         |       |
  Treated     | 126.529 |         |       |
  Diff (T-C)  | -4.147  | 2.577  | -1.61 | 0.110
After         |          |         |       |
  Control     | 128.717 |         |       |
  Treated     | 122.123 |         |       |
  Diff (T-C)  | -6.594  | 2.255  | 2.92  | 0.004***
              |          |         |       |
Diff-in-Diff  | -2.447  | 1.947  | 1.26  | 0.211
- - - - - - - - - - - - - - - - - - - - - - - - - - - - -
R-square:   0.05
* Means and Standard Errors are estimated by linear regression
**Clustered Std. Errors
**Inference: *** p<0.01; ** p<0.05; * p<0.1
```

The first part of Output 10.19 shows the number of observations used for the analysis. In the second part, the result of the analysis is given. First the difference in systolic blood pressure between the two groups at baseline is given. This difference is equal to −4.147. Second, the difference in systolic blood pressure between the two groups at the first follow-up measurement is given. This difference is equal to −7.488. After that the final result of the analysis is given, i.e. the difference between the two differences, which is equal to −3.342. In the last part of Output 10.19 it is mentioned that the result is obtained from linear regression analysis and that clustered standard errors are estimated. The latter indicates that the standard errors are adjusted for the dependency of the observations within the subject. It should be realised that this adjustment for the dependency of the observations only influences the standard error and not the effect estimate, which is a (strong) limitation of the analysis. For the difference in difference analysis including

both follow-up measurements, it is important to realise that the time variable must be coded 1 for both follow-up measurements. Output 10.20 shows the results of the analysis.

In the first part of Output 10.20 it can be seen that in this analysis more observations are used, while in the second part of the analysis the difference between the groups at baseline is given and between the groups on average over the two follow-up measurements. Furthermore, the second part of the output shows the difference in the difference, which is equal to –2.447.

10.6.1.2 Comments

Based on the literature, the theory behind the difference in difference method seems to be rather complicated, but basically the method is relatively simple and calculates the difference in the difference between the groups at baseline and the difference between the groups at the follow-up measurement (s). An important limitation of the method is the rather simple adjustment for the correlated observations within the subject, which only influences the standard error. Furthermore, it should be realised that exactly the same analyses can be performed with regression-based longitudinal methods, such as mixed model analysis. The latter is preferable due to the more sophisticated adjustment for the dependency of the observations.

Missing Data in Longitudinal Studies

11.1 Introduction

One of the main methodological problems in longitudinal studies is missing data, i.e. the (unpleasant) situation when not all subjects have data on all repeated measurements. When subjects have missing data at the end of a longitudinal study they are referred to as drop-outs. It is, however, also possible that subjects miss one particular measurement, and then return to the study at the next follow-up. This type of missing data is referred to as intermittent missing data (Figure 11.1). It should be noted that, in practice, drop-outs and intermittent missing data usually occur together.

Besides the distinction regarding the missing data pattern (i.e. intermittent missing data versus drop-outs), in the statistical literature a distinction is made regarding the missing data mechanism. Rubin (1976) was the first to develop a framework of different missing data mechanisms. The three missing data mechanisms are missing completely at random (MCAR), missing at random (MAR) and missing not at random (MNAR). MCAR means that missing values are randomly distributed over the data sample. The reason for missing data is not related to relevant outcomes and/or covariates. For example, suppose a study in which people with familial hypertension are invited to come to the research centre where blood pressure and several covariates are measured in order to investigate which covariates are related to blood pressure in this particular population. When data on blood pressure is missing, because some people were not able to visit the research centre due to, for instance, a strike on public transport, this missing data is MCAR. Missing at random (MAR) means that the probability of missing data is related to other variables. For example, when more data on blood pressure is missing of people with high body mass index (BMI) this missing data is MAR. Missing not at random (MNAR) is when the probability of missing data is dependent on the values

of the variable itself. This is the case when people with the highest values for blood pressure do not visit the research centre. This situation is problematic because you never know whether this is the case or not. Although the above-mentioned distinction between the three different types of missing data is important, it is rather theoretical. For a correct interpretation of the result of a longitudinal data analysis, two issues must be considered. First of all, it is important to investigate whether or not missing data on the outcome variable at a certain time-point is dependent on the values of the outcome variable observed one (or more) time-point(s) earlier or later. In other words, it is important to investigate whether or not missing data depends on earlier or later observations of the outcome variable. Secondly, it is important to determine whether or not particular covariates are related to the occurrence of missing data. For example, are males more likely to have missing data than females? In general, it is preferable to make a distinction between non-informative missing data (i.e. when missing is not dependent on other observations of the outcome variable and/or covariates) and informative missing data (i.e. when missing is dependent on other observations of the outcome variable and/or covariates).

11.2 Informative or Non-informative Missing Data

Although there is an abundance of statistical literature describing (complicated) methods that can be used to investigate whether or not one is dealing with informative or non-informative missing data in a longitudinal study (see, for instance, Diggle, 1989; Ridout, 1991; Potthoff, et al., 2006; Enders, 2010), it is basically quite easy to investigate this matter. It can be done by comparing the group of subjects with data at a certain time-point with the group of subjects with missing data at that certain time-point. First of all, this

intermittent missing data

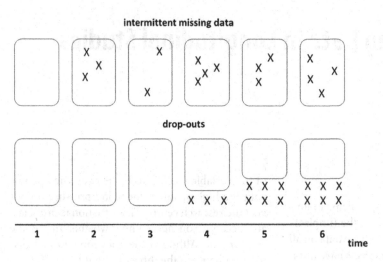

Figure 11.1 Illustration of intermittent missing data and drop-outs. (X indicates a missing data point.)

drop-outs

comparison can concern the particular outcome variable of interest measured one time-point earlier or later. Depending on the distribution of that particular variable, an independent sample *t*-test (for continuous variables) or a Chi-square test (for dichotomous and categorical outcome variables) can be carried out. Secondly, the influence of covariates on the occurrence of missing data can be investigated. This can be done by means of a standard logistic regression analysis, with missing or non-missing at each of the repeated measurements as a dichotomous outcome variable.

Up to now, a distinction has been made between missing data dependent on other values of the outcome variable and missing data dependent on values of covariates. Of course, this distinction is not really necessary, because in practice they both occur together and can both be investigated with a logistic regression analysis, with both values of the outcome variable and covariates as possible determinants for the missing data.

When there are only a few (repeated) measurements, and when the amount of missing data at each of the (repeated) measurements is rather high, the above-mentioned methods are highly suitable to investigate whether one is dealing with informative or non-informative missing data. However, when the amount of missing data at a particular measurement is rather low, the power to detect differences between the subjects with data and the subjects without data at a particular time-point can be too low. Although the possible significance of the differences is not the most important issue in determining whether or not the pattern of missing data is informative or non-informative, it

can be problematic to interpret the observed differences correctly. Therefore, the information about missing data at different time-points can be combined. This can be done in a relatively simple way in which the population is divided into two groups; i.e. the subjects without any missing data over the longitudinal period and the subjects with missing data at one or more of the repeated measurements. The two groups are then compared to each other regarding the values of the outcome variable and/or the covariates at the first measurement. This is done because in practice, mostly all subjects are measured at the first measurement. There are also more complicated methods available to combine the information about missing data at different time-points (Diggle, 1989; Ridout, 1991). However, the statistical techniques involved are seldom used in practice.

11.3 Example

11.3.1 Generating Datasets with Missing Data

The dataset used to illustrate the influence of missing data on the result of a statistical analysis is the same example dataset which has been used throughout this book (see Section 1.5).

From the complete dataset, four datasets with missing data were created. In all datasets, the first measurement is complete for all subjects. The second measurement was made missing for 15 subjects (approximately 10%). The third to sixth measurements were made missing for 25 (17%), 35 (24%), 45 (30%) and 55 (37%) subjects

Table 11.1 Mean value and standard deviation (between brackets) of cholesterol at the different time-points in the different datasets with missing data[1]

Time	Complete mean (sd)	MCAR mean (sd)	MAR_1 mean (sd)	MAR_2 mean (sd)	MNAR mean (sd)	N[2]
1	4.4 (0.7)	4.4 (0.7)	4.4 (0.7)	4.4 (0.7)	4.4 (0.7)	147
2	4.3 (0.7)	4.3 (0.7)	4.3 (0.7)	4.2 (0.6)	4.2 (0.5)	132
3	4.3 (0.7)	4.3 (0.7)	4.3 (0.7)	4.1 (0.6)	4.0 (0.5)	122
4	4.2 (0.7)	4.2 (0.7)	4.1 (0.6)	3.9 (0.5)	3.9 (0.5)	112
5	4.7 (0.8)	4.7 (0.8)	4.6 (0.8)	4.3 (0.6)	4.3 (0.5)	102
6	5.1 (0.9)	5.2 (0.9)	5.1 (0.9)	4.7 (0.8)	4.5 (0.5)	92
N[3]	147	43	73	81	75	

[1] See Section 11.3.1 for the description of the datasets with different types of missing data.
[2] Number of observations in the datasets with missing data.
[3] Number of complete cases.

respectively. In the MCAR dataset, all missing data was randomly selected from the complete dataset. Regarding MAR, two datasets were created; one in which missing data was related to sex and one in which the missing data was related to the outcome variable cholesterol measured one time-point earlier. In the first MAR dataset (MAR_1), missing data at the different time-points was randomly selected from the males, while in the second MAR dataset (MAR_2), all observations were made missing for subjects with the highest values for cholesterol measured one time-point earlier. Finally, in the MNAR dataset, all observations were made missing for subjects with the highest values for cholesterol at that particular time-point. For all missing datasets, when the outcome variable is made missing, also the time-dependent covariate sum of skinfolds is made missing. This is comparable to missing data observed in a real-life study, because when a certain subject does not attend a particular visit in a longitudinal study, all data to be collected at that measurement is generally missing. Furthermore, the missing datasets contain both intermittent missing data and dropouts. Table 11.1 shows descriptive information for the outcome variable cholesterol in the complete dataset and in the datasets with missing data.

11.3.2 Analysis of Determinants for Missing Data

As has been mentioned in the introduction of this chapter, it is important to investigate whether or not the missing data is informative or non-informative. This knowledge can have important implications for the interpretation of the results of a longitudinal study with missing data.

As previously stated, it is quite simple to investigate whether the missing data is dependent on other values of the outcome variable cholesterol. This can be done by comparing the subjects with data at a certain time-point with the subjects with missing data at that time-point. The comparison is then performed on, for instance, the value of cholesterol one time-point earlier. The difference between the two groups can be tested with an independent samples t-test.

Besides the analyses at each time-point, an analysis can also be performed in which the subjects with complete data (i.e. data at all six measurements) are compared with the subjects with missing data at, at least, one of the measurements. The two groups can be compared to each other regarding cholesterol at the first measurement.

To illustrate the latter, in Table 11.2, the results of the independent samples t-tests comparing the group with missing data with the group without missing data are given for the four datasets with missing data.

Because the missing datasets are forced to be of a certain type, the results are as expected. In the MNAR and MAR_2 datasets, missing was related to the outcome variable (either at the time of missing or one time-point earlier) and therefore, for these two datasets the outcome variable cholesterol at the first measurement is significantly

Table 11.2 Results of independent samples t-tests to compare subjects with missing data[1] with subjects without missing data regarding the value of cholesterol at the first measurement

		N	Cholesterol[2]	p-value
MCAR				
	Missing	104	4.4	0.35
	Not missing	43	4.5	
MAR_1				
	Missing	74	4.4	0.78
	Not missing	73	4.5	
MAR_2				
	Missing	66	4.8	< 0.01
	Not missing	81	4.1	
MNAR				
	Missing	72	4.8	< 0.01
	Not missing	75	4.0	

[1] See Section 11.3.1 for the description of the datasets with different types of missing data.
[2] Measured at the first time-point.

Table 11.3 Regression coefficients and p-values of logistic regression analyses to investigate possible determinants of missing data[1]

	Sex	Sum of skinfolds[2]
MCAR	−0.49 (p=0.22)	0.24 (p=0.12)
MAR_1	[3]	0.08 (p=0.83)
MAR_2	−0.50 (p=0.19)	−0.61 (p<0.01)
MNAR	−0.44 (p=0.25)	−0.65 (p<0.01)

[1] See Section 11.3.1 for the description of the datasets with different types of missing data.
[2] Measured at the first time-point.
[3] Not applicable, because there were no complete cases for males.

different between subjects with complete data compared to subjects with missing data. For the MCAR and MAR_1 datasets no significant differences were found between subjects with complete data compared to subjects with missing data. Also, this is not very surprising, because in both datasets, missing data was not (forced to be) related to (earlier) values of cholesterol.

The independent samples t-tests are only performed to determine whether the missing data are dependent on the outcome variable cholesterol. It is also of interest to analyse the relationship between the occurrence of missing data and other covariates. This information can also be important for correct interpretation of the result of a longitudinal analysis performed on a dataset with missing data. To illustrate this, logistic regression analyses were performed, with complete versus non complete as the dichotomous outcome variable. The values of two covariates in the example dataset (sex and sum of skinfolds) at the first measurement were analysed as potential determinants for the missing data. Table 11.3 summarises the results of the logistic regression analyses.

From the results presented in Table 11.3 it can be seen that it is only in the MAR_2 and MNAR datasets that subjects with higher values of sum of skinfolds at the first measurement seem to have a higher probability of having missing data. This is not really surprising, because from earlier analyses of the example dataset it is already known that cholesterol and sum of skinfolds are strongly associated with each other. So, when missing data is found to be dependent on the value of cholesterol at the first measurement, it can be expected that this is also the case for the sum of skinfolds.

The analyses described in this section illustrate how to investigate possible determinants of missing data. In the example datasets these analyses were not really interesting, because the datasets with missing data were forced to be of a certain type. However, in practice it is necessary to perform these analyses, because interpretation of the result can depend on the missing data mechanism.

11.4 Analysis Performed on Datasets with Missing Data

In the foregoing sections it was stressed that it is important to investigate whether one is dealing with informative or non-informative missing data. First of all, it is important to invoke a correct interpretation of the result of a longitudinal analysis performed on a dataset with missing data. Secondly, it is also important because the regression-based methods to analyse longitudinal data (i.e. generalised estimating equations (GEE) analysis and mixed model analysis) differ in the way in which they treat missing data. In fact, in the literature it is often argued that one of the most important differences

Table 11.4 Regression coefficients and standard errors (between brackets) derived from GEE analyses (with an exchangeable correlation structure) and mixed model analyses (with only a random intercept) performed on a complete dataset and several datasets with missing data[1] to analyse the relationship between cholesterol and the sum of skinfolds

		GEE analysis	Mixed model analysis
Complete dataset		0.186 (0.020)	0.186 (0.018)
Missing data			
	MCAR	0.176 (0.023)	0.175 (0.020)
	MAR_1	0.202 (0.025)	0.202 (0.021)
	MAR_2	0.154 (0.023)	0.158 (0.020)
	MNAR	0.115 (0.019)	0.116 (0.018)

[1] See Section 11.3.1 for the description of the datasets with different types of missing data.

between GEE analysis and mixed model analysis is found in the analysis of datasets with missing data. The difference is that within GEE analysis the missing data is assumed to be missing completely at random (MCAR), and that within mixed model analysis the missing data is assumed to be missing at random (MAR) (Little, 1995; Albert, 1999; Omar et al., 1999). When GEE analysis is performed on a dataset with informative missing data, the calculation of the working correlation structure is assumed to be biased, and therefore the calculation of the regression coefficients is also assumed to be biased. However, from the literature it is not clear how important this bias really is (see also Section 11.6). It is therefore interesting to analyse the missing datasets with both GEE analysis and mixed model analysis, and to compare the results. Table 11.4 shows the results of both a linear mixed model analysis and a linear GEE analysis performed on the different datasets. With both methods the relationship between cholesterol and the sum of skinfolds was analysed.

From Table 11.4 it can be seen that almost the same result was obtained for a GEE analysis and a mixed model analysis, even when data are MAR or MNAR. This is remarkable because, as has been mentioned before, in the literature it is argued that GEE analysis is only valid when missing data are MCAR, while mixed model analysis is

assumed to be valid also on MAR datasets. These results show again that the difference between GEE analysis and mixed model analysis on datasets with missing data is slightly more subtle than often suggested. In Section 11.6 this issue will be further discussed.

Because a few decades ago generalised linear model (GLM) for repeated measures was the only available method for the analysis of longitudinal data, imputation methods had to be used in order to create complete datasets. In the following sections, several of the available imputation methods to replace missing data will be discussed, and the influence of different imputation methods on the results of statistical analyses will be illustrated.

11.5 Imputation Methods

11.5.1 Continuous Variables

Historically, imputation methods can be divided into cross-sectional and longitudinal imputation methods. Both can be used to replace missing data in longitudinal studies. The cross-sectional methods described here are the mean or median of series method, the hot-deck method and the cross-sectional linear regression method. Longitudinal imputation methods which are described are the last value carried forward or last observation carried forward method, the linear interpolation method and the longitudinal linear regression method. Besides these historical methods, a lot of attention will be given to multiple imputation, which is the state-of-the-art method for imputing missing data.

11.5.1.1 Cross-sectional Imputation Methods

All variants of the mean or median of the series imputation method involve calculation of the mean or median of the available data for a particular variable at a particular time-point. The mean or median is imputed for the missing value. Because of its simplicity, it was by far the most frequently used imputation method in practice. A somewhat different method is called the hot-deck imputation method. With this method, the mean or median value of a sub-set of comparable subjects (e.g. subjects with the same gender, age, etc.) is imputed for the missing value. The minimum number of subjects in the sub-set can be one, and the maximum number can be the total population (which makes the hot-deck method the same as the mean or median of series method). With cross-sectional regression methods, a linear regression with all available (possible) covariates at a certain time-point is used to provide predicted values for the variable with missing data at that particular time-point. This predicted value is then used for the imputation.

11.5.1.2 Longitudinal Imputation Methods

The simplest longitudinal imputation method is called the last value carried forward (LVCF) or last observation carried forward (LOCF) method. In this method the value of a variable at ($t = 1$) for a particular subject is imputed for a missing value for that subject at ($t = 2$). Another longitudinal imputation method is the linear interpolation method. With this method, for a missing value at ($t = 2$) the average of the values at ($t = 1$) and ($t = 3$) is imputed, assuming a linear development over time of the variables with missing data. Comparable, but somewhat more sophisticated, is the longitudinal regression imputation method. With this method, a linear regression analysis between the time-dependent variable with missing data and time is assessed for each subject with a missing value. The predicted value for the time-point of the missing value is then used for the imputation.

11.5.1.3 Comments

The biggest problem with imputation methods based on average values or predicted values from a cross-sectional or longitudinal regression analy-sis is that the standard deviation of the imputed variable is artificially decreased. When a statistical analysis is performed on such an imputed dataset, the standard error of the effect estimate will be decreased as well and, therefore, the corresponding p-value will be too low. This problem can be solved by making a random draw from a distribution around the average value or around the value predicted by the cross-sectional or longitudinal regression analysis. This will add some noise to the imputed data, leading to more realistic standard deviations and therefore, to more realistic standard errors and p-values.

All imputation methods discussed so far are known as single imputation methods. Nowadays, however, it is generally accepted that multiple imputation must be used instead of single imputation.

11.5.1.4 Multiple Imputation

With multiple imputation, various (say M) imputation values are calculated for every missing value. With the M imputations, M complete datasets are developed, and on each dataset created in this way, a statistical analysis is performed. The M complete dataset summary statistics (e.g. regression coefficients) can be combined (i.e. pooled) to form one summary statistic (see Figure 11.2).

The point estimate of the summary statistic is calculated as the average of the M imputations, while the standard error of the summary statistic is usually calculated from two components (i.e.

imputation   analysis

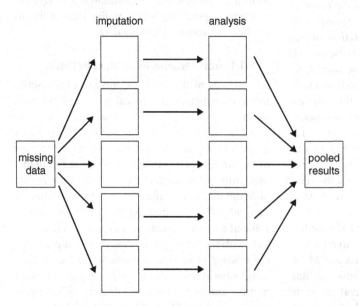

Figure 11.2 Illustration of multiple imputation.

two variances). One component reflects the within-imputation variance (the average of the variances of the summary statistics of the M imputations) and the other component reflects the between-imputation variance (the difference between the summary statistic of each imputation and the average of the summary statistics of the M imputations). Equation 11.1 shows a possible way in which the overall variance is calculated:

$$var_w = \frac{\sum_{i=1}^{M} var_i}{M} \tag{11.1a}$$

$$var_b = \frac{\sum_{i=1}^{M} (b_i - \overline{b})^2}{M} \tag{11.1b}$$

$$var = var_w + \frac{M+1}{M} var_b \tag{11.1c}$$

where var_w is the within-imputation variance, var_i is the variance of imputation i, M is the number of imputations, var_b is the between-imputations variance, b_i is the parameter of interest calculated with imputation i, and $\overline{b}$ is the average of the parameter of interest calculated with M imputations.

The major advantage of multiple imputation is that the combined standard error is greater than the standard error obtained from a single imputation. This greater standard error accounts for the uncertainty introduced by estimating the missing values. In principle, the M imputations of the missing values are M repetitions from the posterior predictive distribution of the missing values. The posterior predictive distribution is related to a model for missing data which can (or in fact must) be based on the information derived from the simple analyses discussed in Sections 11.2 and 11.3. When the missing data is known to be dependent on the observed values of the outcome variable and/or several covariates, these variables can or must be used (for instance in a regression analysis) to create the posterior predictive distribution of the missing values (see the example in Section 11.5.3.1). In the literature it is suggested that five imputations should be enough to obtain a valid result (Rubin, 1987; Schafer, 1999). However, it is questionable whether that is true (see Section 11.5.3.3). For extensive information on multiple imputation, reference is made to several other publications (e.g. Rubin, 1987, 1996; Schafer, 1999; Royston, 2004; Kenward and Carpenter, 2007;

Royston et al., 2009; Buuren van, 2018; Austin et al., 2021; Lee et al., 2021).

11.5.2 Dichotomous and Categorical Variables

For dichotomous and/or categorical variables, a commonly used cross-sectional method is imputation of the category with the highest frequency for the subject(s) with missing data. This can either be based on the total population (mean or median of series method) or on a particular subset (hot-deck method). The most frequently used longitudinal imputation method available for dichotomous and categorical missing data is the LVCF method. Linear interpolation can be used, but the average value of the outcome variable at the two surrounding time-points has to be rounded off. For dichotomous variables, cross-sectional and longitudinal logistic regression can also be used to predict missing data. However, in these situations, the predicted values also have to be rounded off, which makes the use of these techniques slightly complicated.

11.5.3 Example

11.5.3.1 Continuous Variables

The example deals with the influence of the imputation of missing data on the result of a mixed model analysis. Both the use of LVCF and multiple imputation will be illustrated. It is questionable whether or not it is necessary to perform multiple imputation in combination with a mixed model analysis, because it is suggested that performing a mixed model analysis without any imputation is valid when missing data is either MCAR or MAR. However, because many researchers are not aware of the differences between a mixed model analysis on a dataset with missing values and a mixed model analysis on multiple imputed datasets, these differences will be illustrated in this example. For multiple imputation, in this example, Data Augmentation (DA) was used. DA is an iterative Markov Chain Monte Carlo (MCMC) method to generate the imputed values assuming a multivariate normal distribution. DA is recognised as one of the state-of-the-art methods for imputing arbitrary missing data patterns (i.e. for longitudinal data with both intermittent missing data and drop-outs)

Table 11.5 The relationship between cholesterol and the sum of skinfolds estimated with a linear mixed model analysis with only a random intercept with and without imputation on datasets with different missing data mechanisms[1]

	Regression coefficient	Standard error
Complete dataset	0.186	0.018
MCAR		
Without imputing	0.175	0.020
LVCF	0.172	0.018
Multiple imputation[2]	0.177	0.022
MAR_1		
Without imputing	0.201	0.021
LVCF	0.181	0.018
Multiple imputation[2]	0.223	0.034
MAR_2		
Without imputing	0.158	0.020
LVCF	0.174	0.018
Multiple imputation[2]	0.155	0.032
MNAR		
Without imputing	0.116	0.018
LVCF	0.111	0.016
Multiple imputation[2]	0.104	0.025

[1] See Section 11.3.1 for the description of the datasets with different types of missing data.
[2] For multiple imputation, five imputations were used.

(Barnard and Meng, 1999; Fairclough et al., 2008; STATA, 2009). Furthermore, for all multiple imputation models, the observed values of the outcome variable cholesterol at the different timepoints as well as the covariate used in the mixed model analyses (i.e. sum of skinfolds) were used to predict the missing values. For all multiple imputations, the first five imputations were used.

Table 11.5 shows the results of the analyses to analyse the relationship between cholesterol and the sum of skinfolds on the complete dataset, the datasets with missing data and the imputed datasets.

From Table 11.5, it can be seen that for the MCAR datasets, mixed model analyses without imputation only provided slightly different results compared to LVCF and multiple imputation. The regression coefficients obtained from multiple imputation were a bit closer to the regression coefficient obtained from the complete dataset compared to the dataset without imputations and the LVCF imputed dataset. The standard errors obtained from the analyses with and without multiple imputation were, as expected, slightly higher compared to the analysis on the complete dataset. The standard error obtained from the mixed model analysis on the LVCF imputed dataset is the same as the one obtained from the complete dataset. Although this seems to be an advantage, it is not. Due to the artificial increase in the number of observations in an LVCF imputed dataset with missing data, the standard error of the regression coefficient decreases. Also, in the multiple imputation method, the number of observations is artificially increased, but the decrease in standard error due to the higher number of observations is compensated with the higher standard error based on the combination of two variances (see Equation 11.1).

For the MAR datasets, regarding the regression coefficients, the analyses led to comparable results for the mixed model analyses with and without imputation. However, they were different from the regression coefficient obtained from the complete dataset. Regarding the uncertainty of the estimates, the standard errors of the analyses with or without multiple imputation were quite different. Surprisingly, the regression coefficient obtained from a mixed model analysis on an LVCF imputed dataset were relatively close to the regression coefficient obtained from the complete dataset. The standard error, again, is underestimated.

For the MNAR datasets, the regression coefficients obtained from the different analyses are more or less the same, but they are totally different from the analysis on the complete dataset without missing data. The comparison of standard errors shows the same picture as for all other analyses.

In general, the results of the example show that the results obtained from the imputed and non-imputed datasets are different. More specifically, the standard errors of the regression coefficients are different and in general somewhat larger when they are obtained from mixed model analyses with multiple imputation than obtained from mixed model analyses without multiple imputation. Regarding the regression coefficients, the results are not straightforward in favour of one of the methods.

In the example, the standard errors of the mixed model analyses with multiple imputation were higher than the standard errors obtained from the mixed model analyses without multiple imputation. The remaining question is whether the standard error resulting from the mixed model analysis without multiple imputation is an underestimation or whether the standard error obtained from the mixed model analysis with multiple imputation is an overestimation. In the literature, most evidence is given for the fact that the two methods lead to similar results when the data are either MCAR and MAR, which is, however, not the case in the present example. There are authors who suggest that a mixed model analysis without multiple imputation leads to an underestimation of the standard error (Kenward and Carpenter, 2007; Mazumdar et al., 2007), while Enders on the other hand states that the imputation phase can use an unnecessarily complex model to deal with the missing data and that this additional complexity can add a small amount of noise to the resulting estimations (Enders, 2010), which leads to an overestimation of the standard error. Furthermore, Robins and Wang suggest that the combination rule shown in Equation 11.1c leads to an overestimation of the standard error (Robins and Wang, 2000). In their theoretical paper they suggest an alternative method to obtain the pooled standard error.

However, that alternative method has never been used in applied (medical) studies.

11.5.3.2 Multiple Imputation in Combination with Mixed Model Analysis?

Because the comparison of regression coefficients and standard errors in the example does not give a straight answer to the question whether or not multiple imputation should be used in combination with a mixed model analysis, other arguments must be used to provide an answer to that question. A mixed model analysis without multiple imputation is definitely less complicated because only one dataset has to be analysed, while with multiple imputation, multiple datasets have to be analysed. So, it is computationally more efficient to perform a mixed model analysis without multiple imputation than a mixed model analysis with multiple imputation.

Besides this, with multiple imputation, basically two maximum likelihood estimations have to be performed to obtain the final result; one maximum likelihood estimation to impute the missing data and one maximum likelihood estimation to estimate the regression coefficients. With a mixed model analysis, only one maximum likelihood estimation has to be performed to obtain the final result. Because both multiple imputation and mixed model analysis use the same information for the estimations, it is obvious that mixed model analysis without multiple imputation is more efficient (see Figure 11.3).

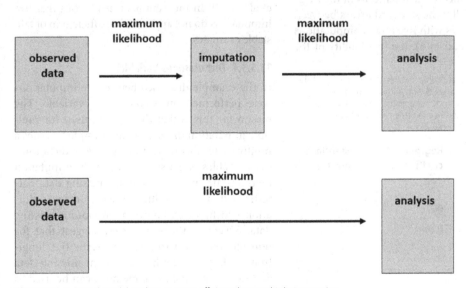

Figure 11.3 Mixed model analysis is more efficient than multiple imputation.

In addition, the results of the example show that the results obtained from a mixed model analysis with multiple imputation can be quite unstable (see also Section 11.5.3.3). So, based on these arguments, it can be concluded that in general it is not necessary to perform multiple imputation before performing a mixed model analysis.

Although in the example, performing multiple imputation in combination with a mixed model analysis did not lead to a more valid result, there are situations in which multiple imputation potentially holds an advantage (Enders, 2010). When auxiliary variables (i.e. variables that are related to the missing data mechanism but not used in the model to answer the research question) are measured, they can be included in predicting the missing data, without being included in the mixed model analysis, which probably increases the efficiency. Also, in a situation when only covariates are missing, performing multiple imputation before a mixed model analysis seems to be better. However, the latter hardly exists in longitudinal studies, because in these studies most data to be collected at a visit is missing for a particular subject.

11.5.3.3 Additional Analyses

Because there is ongoing discussion in the literature regarding the number of imputations needed to obtain a stable result, for all multiple imputations performed in the present example, the use of 50 imputations was evaluated. Table 11.6 shows the results of these analyses.

Based on the inconsistent patterns in the magnitude of (especially) the standard errors between some of the analyses with five and 50 imputations (see Tables 11.5 and 11.6), the (in)stability of the

Table 11.6 The relationship between cholesterol and the sum of skinfolds, estimated with a linear mixed model analysis with only a random intercept on datasets with different missing data mechanisms[1] with multiple imputation with 50 imputations

	Regression coefficient	Standard error
MCAR	0.183	0.024
MAR_1	0.213	0.029
MAR_2	0.168	0.027
MNAR	0.113	0.021

[1] See Section 11.3.1 for the description of the datasets with different types of missing data.

mixed model analyses with multiple imputation was further investigated. In the additional analyses to evaluate the relationship between cholesterol and the sum of skinfolds, all multiple imputations were repeated 100 times. Figure 11.4 summarises the (in)stability of the different multiple imputations for both the regression coefficient and the standard error. Figure 11.5 shows the distribution of the standard errors of the 100 analyses performed on the MAR_2 dataset. It is clear that using five imputations lead to very unstable results in all datasets, but especially for the MAR_2 dataset. For the latter even the use of 50 imputations is somewhat unstable.

The (in)stability of multiple imputation is in contrast with most basic multiple imputation literature (Rubin, 1987; Kenward and Carpenter, 2007), which suggests that five imputations should be sufficient to obtain a valid result. However, Graham recognised that some analyses may require much more imputations to obtain a valid result (Graham, 2009). Literature with formal recommendations on how to choose the optimal number of imputations is scarce. It is sometimes argued that the number of imputations must be at least equal to the percentage of missing data. So, when the missing data percentage is around 20%, at least 20 imputed datasets must be created. Royston and co-workers discuss the impact of the number of imputations on the precision of the estimates and suggests ways of determining the required number of imputations by evaluating the sampling error of the multiple imputation estimates (Royston, 2004; Royston et al., 2009). In the example it is obvious that five imputations do not appear to be sufficient to obtain stable estimates.

11.5.3.4 Dichotomous Variables

In the example discussed before, the imputations were performed on a continuous variable. The reason for this is that the method used for multiple imputation in the present example assumes a multivariate normal distribution. For dichotomous variables, sophisticated multiple imputation methods are only available for missing data patterns without intermittent missing data; a situation which is also known as monotone missing data. Several authors, however, suggest that for non-monotone missing data patterns (i.e. longitudinal data with both intermittent missing data and drop-outs) the same methods can be used as for continuous variables (Bernaards et al., 2007;

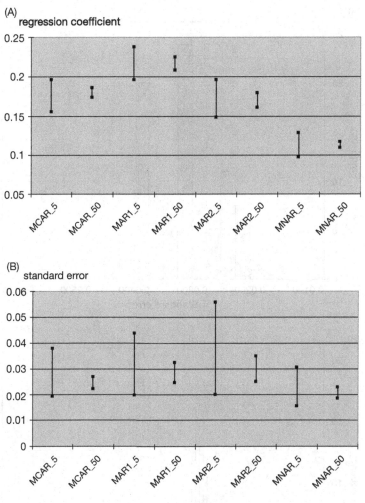

Figure 11.4 (A) Range in regression coefficients and (B) range in standard errors obtained from 100 mixed model analyses, after multiple imputation for different types of missing data with either 5 or 50 imputations, analysing the relationship between cholesterol and the sum of skinfolds.

Demirtas et al., 2008). One major problem for dichotomous data is the rounding of the imputed values (Yucel et al., 2008). Although it is not expected that the conclusions based on logistic mixed model analyses with and without multiple imputation would be different from the ones based on the linear mixed model analyses, Table 11.7 shows the results of logistic mixed model analyses on imputed datasets (both LVCF and multiple imputation) to analyse the relationship between the dichotomous outcome variable hypercholesterolemia and the sum of skinfolds.

From Table 11.7 it can be seen that multiple imputation only seems to work well for the MAR_1 dataset. On the other hand, for the MAR_2 dataset, LVCF seems to be the most appropriate. This is rather surprising because it is generally accepted that multiple imputation is better than any single imputation method. The fact that the standard errors of the effect estimates are not lower than the ones obtained from the logistic mixed model analyses on either the dataset with missing values or the multiple imputed datasets is rather strange. Due to the artificial increase in the number of observations, it was expected that the standard errors would be comparable to the one obtained from the complete dataset.

It should be realised, however, that the comparison is based on only one dataset with very typical missing data mechanisms and that the

(A)

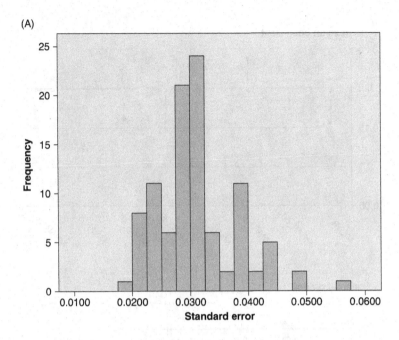

(B)

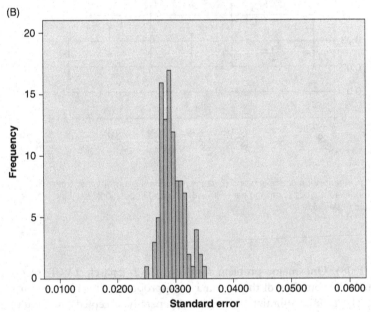

Figure 11.5 Distribution of the standard errors obtained from 100 mixed model analyses after multiple imputation analysing the relationship between cholesterol and the sum of skinfolds, performed on the MAR_2 dataset with either (A) five or (B) 50 imputations.

results of a logistic mixed model analysis should be interpreted with caution (see Chapter 7).

11.5.4 Comments

The present example shows that mixed model analyses with or without multiple imputation do not lead to valid results when performed on a MNAR dataset. Both methods behave equally unsatisfactorily when the results are compared with the result of the analysis on the complete dataset without missing data. This is as expected because both multiple imputation and mixed model analysis use the observed data for the estimations. Because of that, for both mixed model analysis and multiple

Table 11.7 The relationship between hypercholesterolemia and the sum of skinfolds estimated with a logistic mixed model analysis with only a random intercept with and without imputation on datasets with different missing data mechanisms[1]

	Regression coefficient	Standard error
Complete dataset	0.560	0.106
MCAR		
Without imputing	0.602	0.121
LVCF	0.597	0.120
Multiple imputation[2]	0.478	0.103
MAR_1		
Without imputing	0.663	0.127
LVCF	0.695	0.129
Multiple imputation[2]	0.546	0.113
MAR_2		
Without imputing	0.442	0.122
LVCF	0.586	0.137
Multiple imputation[2]	0.367	0.132
MNAR		
Without imputing	0.114	0.122
LVCF	0.115	0.135
Multiple imputation[2]	0.160	0.124

[1] See Section 11.3.1 for the description of the datasets with different types of missing data.
[2] For multiple imputation, five imputations were used.

imputation, the assumption is that the methods are only valid when the missing data is either MAR of MCAR (Hogan et al., 2004; Kristman et al., 2005; Kenward and Carpenter, 2007). A big problem, however, is that in real-life data it is not possible to evaluate whether missing data is MAR or MNAR (Potthoff et al., 2006; Kenward and Carpenter, 2007; Enders, 2010), which means that it is never known whether the results obtained from the mixed model analysis (either with or without multiple imputation) provides a valid result. Furthermore, in real-life data, missing data

is never totally MCAR, MAR or MNAR. Some missing observations will be totally random, while other missing observations will depend on either observed data or unobserved data. Surprisingly, even in the MCAR datasets, the results of the mixed model analyses were different from the results obtained from the complete dataset without missing data. This is probably to do with the fact that only one MCAR dataset was created, which makes it possible that the created MCAR dataset was not completely MCAR (Burton et al., 2006).

11.6 Alternative Methods

Although in the literature most researchers use a mixed model analysis with or without multiple imputation, there are some alternative methods available to deal with missing data in longitudinal studies. These alternative methods include selection models and pattern mixture models (Little, 1993, 1994; Demirtas and Schafer, 2003; Yang and Shoptaw, 2008). Both are frequently used in econometrics and are supposed to provide valid results even on MNAR datasets. The general idea of a selection model is that the analysis is split into two parts. The first part is the regression analysis of interest and the second part is a regression analysis that predicts the response probabilities. Within a pattern mixture model, first, subgroups of subjects with the same missing data pattern are created. In the next step, the regression coefficients are estimated within the different subgroups. In the last step, the subgroup specific coefficients are combined to get one regression coefficient that accounts for missing data being MNAR. Although both methods have some potential in adequately dealing with missing values, they also have some disadvantages (i.e. computational complexity and their reliance on knowledge about the missing data mechanism) and are therefore not used extensively in real-life medical studies.

In the literature, some other alternative methods are also suggested (e.g. Fitzmaurice et al., 1994; Greenland and Finkle, 1995; Little, 1995; Hogan and Laird, 1997; Shis and Quan, 1997; Molenberghs et al., 1998; Kenward, 1998; Haan et al., 1999; Kenward and Molenberghs, 1999; Chen et al., 2000; Verbeke and Molenberghs, 2000; Sun and Song, 2001), but unfortunately most of them are very technical and difficult to understand for non-statisticians.

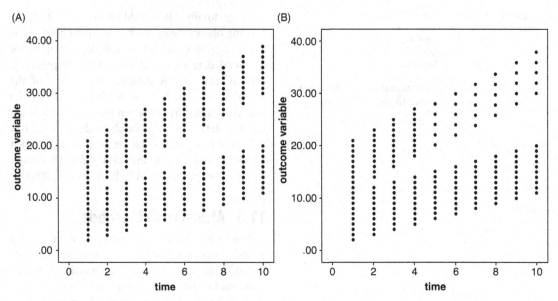

Figure 11.6 Simple longitudinal dataset used to illustrate the difference between GEE analysis and mixed model analysis regarding the analysis of a dataset with missing data; (A) complete dataset and (B) dataset with missing data.

11.7 GEE Analysis or Mixed Model Analysis for the Analysis of Datasets with Missing Data?

In the literature there is some discussion about the use of GEE analysis in datasets with missing data. It has already been mentioned that it is argued that GEE analysis only provides a valid result when missing data is MCAR. Mixed model analysis on the other hand provides a valid result when missing data is MAR. However, from Table 11.4 it could be seen that the results of a GEE analysis on datasets with missing values were comparable to the results of a mixed model analysis even when missing data is MAR or MNAR. To explore the difference between GEE analysis and mixed model analysis on datasets with missing data a bit further, a very simple example dataset will be used, in which 20 subjects were measured 10 times. Half of the subjects show an increase of one unit per time-interval, while the other half show an increase of two units per time-interval (see Figure 11.6A). When this data is analysed by either GEE analysis or mixed model analysis, both will give the same regression coefficient of 1.5. Figure 11.6B shows a situation in which there is missing data. From the subjects with an increase of two units per time-interval, half of them dropped out after the fifth

measurement. When this data is analysed with a GEE analysis, the regression coefficient will be 1.357. A mixed model analysis with only a random intercept will also give a regression coefficient of 1.357. However, when a random slope is added to the mixed model analysis, the regression coefficient returned to 1.5. So, in general, only if the missing values can be predicted perfectly by observed data (when the missing values are perfectly MAR), and only when a mixed model analysis is performed with a correctly specified model (i.e. including random slopes and the appropriate covariances between the random intercept and slopes) a mixed model analysis will provide a valid result whereas GEE analysis will provide an invalid result. However, when missing values are not perfectly MAR, GEE analysis and mixed model analysis will both provide (comparable) invalid results.

11.8 Conclusions

For continuous outcome variables, the use of imputation methods is recommended when GLM for repeated measures is used to analyse a longitudinal dataset with missing data. When mixed model analysis is used to analyse a longitudinal dataset with missing data, no imputations at all may be better than applying any of the imputation methods. If a decision is made to impute missing values, longitudinal methods are generally pre-ferred above cross-sectional methods and multiple imputation is preferred above single imputation.

Beyond the question of whether or not to use imputations, it is of utmost importance to describe as well as possible the missing data mechanisms in the study dataset, because this can have important implications for the interpretation of the results of the statistical analysis performed.

12 Sample Size Calculations

12.1 Introduction

Before performing a longitudinal (intervention) study, it is necessary to calculate the number of subjects needed to ensure that a certain predefined effect will be statistically significant. Sample size calculations are also a prerequisite for research grants and are used by (medical) ethical committees in their evaluation of study design protocols. Besides this, sample size calculations are part of the CONSORT statement, meaning that without a sample size calculation, a paper reporting the result of an intervention study will not be published. The importance of sample size calculations is basically a very strange phenomenon. First of all, sample size calculations are based on many assumptions which can easily be changed, in which case the calculated number of subjects will be totally different. Secondly, sample size calculations are related to the importance of significance levels (how many subjects are needed to make a certain effect significant?) and that is strange because in medical research the importance of significance testing is becoming more and more questionable. Nevertheless, there is a large amount of literature discussing sample size calculations for longitudinal studies (e.g. Lui and Cumberland, 1992; Snijders and Bosker, 1993; Lee and Durbin, 1994; Lipsitz and Fitzmaurice, 1994; Liu and Liang, 1997; Hedeker et al., 1999; Basagaña and Spiegelman, 2010; Guo et al., 2013; Guo and Pandis, 2015).

In general, the sample size calculations used for a longitudinal intervention study are the same as for standard intervention studies. It should be noted that the standard sample size calculations are developed for intervention studies with one follow-up measurement. In fact, with the standard sample size calculations, the difference in a certain outcome variable between several groups at the first follow-up measurement is used as an effect size. This assumes that the baseline values for the groups to be compared are equal, which seems to

be a reasonable assumption in a randomised trial, but which is not always true (see Chapter 10). Equation 12.1 shows how the sample size can be calculated in an intervention study with one follow-up measurement for a continuous outcome variable.

$$N = \frac{\left(Z_{(1-\alpha/2)} + Z_{(1-\beta)}\right)^2 \times \sigma^2 \times 2}{v^2} \quad (12.1)$$

where N is the sample size in either the intervention or control group, $Z_{(1-\alpha/2)}$ is the $(1 - \alpha/2)$ percentile point of the standard normal distribution, $Z_{(1-\beta)}$ is the $(1 - \beta)$ percentile point of the standard normal distribution, σ is the standard deviation of the outcome variable and v is the difference in mean value of the outcome variable between the groups.

For dichotomous outcome variables, a comparable equation can be used (Equation 12.2).

$$N = \frac{\left(Z_{(1-\alpha/2)} + Z_{(1-\beta)}\right)^2 \times \bar{p}(1 - \bar{p}) \times 2}{(p_1 - p_0)^2}$$

$$(12.2a)$$

$$\bar{p} = \frac{p_1 + p_0}{2} \quad (12.2b)$$

where N is the sample size in either the intervention or control group, $Z_{(1-\alpha/2)}$ is the $(1 - \alpha/2)$ percentile point of the standard normal distribution, $Z_{(1-\beta)}$ is the $(1 - \beta)$ percentile point of the standard normal distribution, $\bar{p}$ is the weighted average of p_0 and p_1, p_1 is the proportion of cases in the intervention group, and p_0 is the proportion of cases in the control group.

In the standard sample size calculations, it is assumed that the number of subjects in the intervention group is equal to the number of subjects in the control group. Although an equal number of subjects in both groups is the most efficient way to divide the population under study into two groups, it is also possible to have unequal numbers in both groups. When that is the case, the number 2 in the numerator of the standard sample size calculation equation must be replaced by $r + 1$, where r is the ratio in the number of subjects in the two groups. Furthermore, r should be multiplied by the effect size (either v^2 or $(p_1 - p_0)^2$) in the denominator of the standard sample size equation.

When more than one follow-up measurement is carried out, and the purpose of the study is to estimate the effect of the intervention on average over the total follow-up period, Equation 12.3 can be applied.

$$N = \frac{\left(Z_{(1-\alpha/2)} + Z_{(1-\beta)}\right)^2 \times \sigma^2 \times 2 \times [1 + (T-1) \times \rho]}{v^2 \times T}$$

(12.3)

where N is the sample size in either the intervention or control group, $Z_{(1-\alpha/2)}$ is the $(1 - \alpha/2)$ percentile point of the standard normal distribution, $Z_{(1-\beta)}$ is the $(1 - \beta)$ percentile point of the standard normal distribution, σ is the standard deviation of the outcome variable, T is the number of follow-up measurements, ρ is the (average) correlation coefficient between the repeated measurements, and v is the difference in mean value of the outcome variable between the groups.

To illustrate how many subjects are needed to make a certain difference between groups statistically significant, Equation 12.3 is applied to several research situations with different effect sizes, different correlation coefficients between the repeated measurements and either two or three follow-up measurements (see Table 12.1).

For sample size calculations in longitudinal intervention studies with a dichotomous outcome variable, Equation 12.4 can be applied.

$$N = \frac{\left(Z_{(1-\alpha/2)} + Z_{(1-\beta)}\right)^2 \times \bar{p}(1-\bar{p}) \times 2 \times [1 + (T-1) \times \rho]}{(p_1 - p_0)^2 \times T}$$

(12.4)

where N is the sample size in either the intervention or control group, $Z_{(1-\alpha/2)}$ is the $(1 - \alpha/2)$ percentile point of the standard normal distribution, $Z_{(1-\beta)}$ is the $(1 - \beta)$ percentile point of the standard normal distribution, $\bar{p}$ is the weighted average of p_0 and p_1 (Equation 12.2b), T is the

Table 12.1 Sample sizes needed to make a certain difference in a continuous outcome variable statistically significant on a 5% level with a power of 80%; studies with different expected differences and different (average) correlation coefficients (ρ) between the repeated measurements

	Expected difference (in standard deviation units)			
	0.1	0.2	0.5	1
Two follow-up measurements				
$\rho = 0$	785	196	31	8
$\rho = 0.25$	981	245	39	10
$\rho = 0.5$	1178	294	47	12
$\rho = 0.75$	1374	343	55	14
Three follow-up measurements				
$\rho = 0$	523	130	21	5
$\rho = 0.25$	785	196	31	8
$\rho = 0.5$	1047	262	42	10
$\rho = 0.75$	1308	327	52	13

number of follow-up measurements, ρ is the (average) correlation coefficient between the repeated measurements, p_1 is the proportion of cases in the intervention group, and p_0 is the proportion of cases in the control group.

Based on Equation 12.4, a sample size table for the same research situations with a dichotomous outcome variable can also be constructed (see Table 12.2).

All sample size equations presented in this section can be used to estimate the sample size needed for a particular intervention study or to calculate the power of that particular study. Here again it should be noted that for the calculation of sample sizes or power, several unknown values have to be filled in, i.e. the expected (relevant) difference between the groups, the standard deviation of the outcome variable of interest, and the (average) correlation coefficient between the repeated measurements. Furthermore, in the equations, a specific significance level (usually 5%) is essential, and as has been mentioned before, the importance of significance testing is becoming more and more questionable. Caution is therefore strongly advised in the use of sample size calculations.

Table 12.2 Sample sizes needed to make a certain difference in a dichotomous outcome variable statistically significant on a 5% level with a power of 80%; studies with different expected differences and different (average) correlation coefficients (ρ) between the repeated measurements

	Expected proportion of intervention group[1]		
	0.4	0.3	0.2
Two follow-up measurements			
$\rho = 0$	194	47	20
$\rho = 0.25$	243	59	25
$\rho = 0.5$	291	71	30
$\rho = 0.75$	340	82	35
Three follow-up measurements			
$\rho = 0$	130	31	13
$\rho = 0.25$	194	47	20
$\rho = 0.5$	259	59	26
$\rho = 0.75$	324	78	33

[1] The expected proportion in the reference category is assumed to be 0.5.

Table 12.3 Information needed for the sample size calculation of the RCT regarding decrease in systolic blood pressure

Number of follow-up measurements	2
Average difference to be detected	5 mmHg
Assumed standard deviation	14 mmHg
Assumed correlation between repeated measures	0.6
power	80%
Significance	0.05
Ratio of the number of observations in the groups to be compared	1

12.2 Example

The way a required sample size is calculated in a longitudinal intervention study will be illustrated for the two examples, which were explained in detail in Chapter 10. The first example was a randomise controlled trial (RCT) with two follow-up measurements aiming to reduce systolic blood pressure (see Section 10.2.2).

Table 12.3 shows the information that is needed to perform a sample size calculation for the longitudinal intervention study with a continuous outcome variable, i.e. systolic blood pressure.

The first step in the sample size calculation is to apply the standard sample size calculation formula (see Equation 12.1)

$$N_1 = \frac{7.85 \times 14^2 \times 2}{5^2} = 123$$

So, with 123 subjects, a difference of 5 mmHg will be statistically significant with a significance level of 0.05 and a power of 80%, assuming a standard deviation of 14 mmHg. When this number is calculated, it is common practice to take into

account the fact that some of the subjects will drop out during the study and because of that, the required sample size is slightly increased. In this case, the sample size per group can be increased to 135 subjects, assuming a drop-out percentage of around 10%.

In the next step, it must be taken into account that there are two follow-up measurements and that there is an assumed correlation of 0.6 between the two follow-up measurements (see Table 10.1). To do that, Equation 12.3 can be applied to obtain the multiplication factor.

$$\frac{[1 + (2 - 1) \times 0.6]}{2} = 0.8$$

$$0.8 \times 135 = 108$$

So, taken into account the fact that there are two follow-up measurements with a correlation of 0.6, the number of subjects needed in this RCT reduces to 108 subjects per group.

A similar sample size calculation can be performed for the example with a dichotomous outcome variable, i.e. recovery from lower back pain (see Section 10.3.1). Table 12.4 shows the information that is needed to perform a sample size calculation for this RCT.

The first step in the sample size calculation is to apply the standard sample size calculation formula (see Equation 12.2).

$$N_1 = \frac{7.85 \times 0.585 \times 0.415 \times 2}{0.13^2} = 226$$

So, with 226 subjects a difference of 13% in recovery between the two groups will be statistically significant with a significance level of 0.05 and a

Table 12.4 Information needed for the sample size calculation of the RCT regarding recovery from lower back pain

Number of follow-up measurements	3
Proportion recovered in usual care group	52%
Expected proportion recovered in treatment group	65%
Assumed (average) correlation between repeated measures	0.4
power	80%
Significance	0.05
Ratio of the number of observations in the groups to be compared	1

power of 80%, assuming a recovery percentage of 52% in the usual care group. Assuming a drop out percentage of around 10%, around 250 patients are needed for each group.

In the next step, it must be taken into account that there are three follow-up measurements and that there is an (average) assumed correlation of 0.4 between the three follow-up measurements. To do that, Equation 12.4 can be applied to obtain the multiplication factor.

$$\frac{[1 + (3 - 1) \times 0.4]}{3} = 0.6$$

$$0.6 \times 250 = 150$$

So, taken into account the fact that there are three follow-up measurements with an (average) correlation of 0.4 between the repeated measurements, the number of subjects needed in this RCT reduces to 150 subjects per group.

12.3 Comment

It should be realised that the sample size calculations performed in this way use the difference between the groups on average over time as effect estimate. When the differences between the groups at the different time-points are used as effect estimates, the multiplication factor cannot be used. In that case, the standard sample size calculation formula must be used.

13 | Software for Longitudinal Data Analysis

13.1 Introduction

In the previous chapters, many methods for the analysis of longitudinal data have been discussed. In the examples, the generalised linear model (GLM) for repeated measures was performed with SPSS, while the regression-based methods were performed with STATA. This chapter provides an overview of a few major software packages (i.e. SPSS, SAS and R) and their ability to perform regression-based longitudinal data analysis. In this chapter, only generalised estimating equation (GEE) analysis and mixed model analysis will be discussed in detail. GLM for repeated measurements can be performed with all major software packages, and can usually be found under the repeated measures option of the GLM or as an extension of the (M)ANOVA procedure. The emphasis of this overview lies on the output and syntax of the regression-based longitudinal data analysis in the different software packages, and on the comparison of the results obtained with the different packages. In this overview, only the analyses used to evaluate the relationship between cholesterol and the sum of skinfolds and the relationships between hypercholesterolemia and the sum of skinfolds will be discussed. Because STATA was used in the examples throughout this book, the STATA outputs will not be repeated here.

13.2 GEE Analysis with a Continuous Outcome Variable

13.2.1 STATA

The syntax needed to perform a linear GEE analysis is very simple:

```
xtgee chol skinf, i(id) corr(exch)
robust
```

First the STATA procedure is specified (i.e. xtgee), directly followed by the outcome variable

and the covariates. After the comma, additional information is supplied, i.e. the subject identifier (id) and the working correlation structure (exch). Because an exchangeable correlation structure is the default in STATA, the syntax will also run without this additional information. It should be noted that in STATA, the default procedure for the estimation of the standard errors is so-called model based. This is rather strange, because it is generally accepted that a robust estimation of the standard error is preferred; see Section 3.4.3 for details of the robust estimation of the standard error within GEE analysis.

13.2.2 SAS

In SAS, the genmod procedure can be used to perform a GEE analysis. Output 13.1 shows part of the output of a linear GEE analysis performed with the genmod procedure.

From Output 13.1 it can first be seen that a linear GEE analysis has been performed (i.e. a normal distribution and an identity link function). Furthermore, it can be seen that an exchangeable correlation structure is used and that the value of the (exchangeable) correlation is equal to 0.515210383. At the end of the output, the parameter estimates are given, i.e. the regression coefficients, the standard errors, the 95% confidence intervals around the regression coefficients, the z-values and the corresponding p-values.

The syntax needed to perform a linear GEE analysis in SAS is slightly more complicated than the syntax for STATA:

```
proc genmod data=chol_long;
class id;
model chol = skinf;
repeated subject=id/type=exch;
run;
```

Each SAS procedure starts with the procedure specification (proc genmod) and ends with a run

Output 13.1 Results of a linear GEE analysis performed in SAS

The GENMOD Procedure

Model information		
Data set	chol_long	
Distribution	Normal	
Link function	Identity	
Dependent variable	Chol	cholesterol

Number of observations read	882
Number of observations used	882

GEE model information	
Correlation structure	Exchangeable
Subject effect	id (147 levels)
Number of clusters	147
Correlation matrix dimension	6
Maximum cluster size	6
Minimum cluster size	6

Exchangeable working correlation	
Correlation	0.515210383

Analysis of GEE parameter estimates						
Empirical standard error estimates						
Parameter	Estimate	Standard error	95% Confidence limits		Z	Pr > |Z|
Intercept	3.7993	0.0904	3.6221	3.9765	42.02	<.0001
skinf	0.1871	0.0201	0.1478	0.2265	9.31	<.0001

statement. The class statement in SAS is needed to indicate that the subject identifier is a categorical variable (class id). In the third line of the syntax the model to be analysed is specified (model chol = skinf), and in the fourth line the fact that the subjects are repeatedly measured (repeated subject=id), and that the correlation structure is exchangeable (type=exch).

13.2.3 R

R is a very popular software programme that can be downloaded for free from the Internet. R is developed from the commercial statistical software package S-plus and it uses the same programming environment (Venables and Ripley, 2000, 2002; Dalgaard, 2002; Fox, 2002; Maindonald and

Output 13.2 Results of a linear GEE analysis performed in R

```
Coefficients:

            Estimate  Std.err      Wald Pr(>|W|)
(Intercept) 3.79931   0.09043   1764.98 <2e-16 ***
skinf       0.18712   0.02010     86.69 <2e-16 ***
- - -
Signif. codes: 0 '***' 0.001 '**' 0.01 '*' 0.05 '.' 0.1 ' ' 1

Correlation structure = exchangeable
Estimated Scale Parameters:

            Estimate Std.err
(Intercept)   0.5693 0.0397
 Link = identity

Estimated Correlation Parameters:
      Estimate Std.err
alpha   0.5159 0.03779
Number of clusters:   147 Maximum cluster size: 6
```

Braun, 2003). Besides the fact that it is free, it is also recognised for its flexibility and excellent graphical features. Output 13.2 shows the output of a linear GEE analysis performed in R.

In the output of a linear GEE analysis performed in R, first the regression coefficients and the (robust) standard errors are given. Besides that, also the Wald statistics and the corresponding p-values are given. It should be noted that the Wald statistic is equal to the z-statistic squared and because the Chi-square distribution with one degree of freedom (which is used in the Wald-test) is equal to the standard normal distribution squared, the corresponding p-values are the same. Below the coefficients, the scale parameter is given (0.5693) and the magnitude of the correlation of the exchangeable working correlation matrix (0.5159). The syntax needed to perform a linear GEE analysis in R is as follows:

```
result <- geeglm(chol ~ skinf,
id=id, data=chol_long, family=
gaussian, corstr="exchangeable")
```

R is an object-oriented programme, which means that the result of the analysis must be linked to an object. The object for the analysis is named result and from the syntax it can be seen that this object is linked to the result of the GEE analysis. The other part of the syntax is straightforward and is comparable to the syntax used in STATA; i.e. after the GEE procedure specification, the outcome variable and the covariates are given. After the comma, additional information has to be specified, i.e. the subject identifier (id=id), the dataset used (data=chol_long), the distribution of the outcome variable (family= gaussian), and the correlation structure (corstr="exchangeable").

13.2.4 SPSS

Output 13.3 shows part of the output of a linear GEE analysis performed in SPSS.

The output of a linear GEE analysis performed in SPSS gives the same information as the outputs from the other software packages. First, some general model information is provided, i.e. the number of subjects, the minimum and maximum number of observations within the subject, the link function, the family (here the Probability Distribution) and the correlation structure that is used. The last part of the output contains the regression coefficients, the standard errors, the 95% confidence intervals and the results of the Wald-test for the regression coefficients. Although one of the best parts of SPSS is the fact that the programme is fully

Output 13.3   Results of a linear GEE analysis performed in SPSS

Model information	
Dependent variable	**Cholesterol**
Probability distribution	Normal
Link function	Identity
Subject effect	1	id number
Working correlation matrix structure	Exchangeable

Correlated data summary		
Number of levels	**Subject effect**	**id number**
Number of subjects		147
Number of measurements per subject	Minimum	6
	Maximum	6
Correlation matrix dimension		6

Parameter estimates							
Parameter	**B**	**Std. Error**	**95% Wald confidence interval**		**Hypothesis test**		
			Lower	**Upper**	**Wald Chi-Square**	**df**	**Sig.**
(Intercept)	3.799	.0904	3.622	3.976	1765.700	1	.000
Sum of skinfolds	.187	.0201	.148	.227	86.757	1	.000
(Scale)	.571						

Dependent variable: cholesterol
Model: (Intercept), sum of skinfolds

menu driven, it is also possible to use syntax to perform a GEE analysis. The following syntax was used to obtain the results presented in Output 13.3.

```
GENLIN chol WITH skinf
 /MODEL skinf INTERCEPT=YES
DISTRIBUTION=NORMAL LINK=IDENTITY
 /CRITERIA SCALE=MLE PCONVERGE=1E-
006(ABSOLUTE) SINGULAR=1E-012
ANALYSISTYPE=3(WALD) CILEVEL=95
LIKELIHOOD=FULL
 /REPEATED SUBJECT=id SORT=YES
CORRTYPE=EXCHANGEABLE
ADJUSTCORR=YES COVB=ROBUST
MAXITERATIONS=100 PCONVERGE=1e-006
(ABSOLUTE) UPDATECORR=1
 /MISSING CLASSMISSING=EXCLUDE
 /PRINT CPS DESCRIPTIVES MODELINFO
FIT SUMMARY SOLUTION.
```

13.2.5 Overview

Table 13.1 summarises the results of linear GEE analyses with an exchangeable correlation structure performed in different software packages.

From Table 13.1 it can be seen that the results of linear GEE analyses with an exchangeable correlation structure are exactly the same for all four software packages.

Table 13.1 Summary of the results for the relationship between cholesterol and sum of skinfolds derived from linear GEE analyses with an exchangeable correlation structure performed in different software packages

Package	Regression coefficient (se)
STATA	0.187 (0.020)
SPSS	0.187 (0.020)
SAS	0.187 (0.020)
R	0.187 (0.020)

13.3 GEE Analysis with a Dichotomous Outcome Variable

13.3.1 STATA

The syntax needed to perform a logistic GEE analysis in STATA is comparable to that needed to perform a linear GEE analysis, except for the part of the additional information where it is indicated that a logistic GEE analysis is performed (i.e. fam(bin) link(logit)):

```
xtgee hyperchol skinf, i(id) fam(bin)
link(logit) corr(exch) robust
```

Again, the standard errors are, by default, estimated by the model-based method. This can be changed by adding robust to the syntax (see Section 3.4.3).

13.3.2 SAS

Output 13.4 shows part of the output of a logistic GEE analysis with an exchangeable correlation structure performed in SAS. It is obvious that the output of a logistic GEE analysis is comparable to the output of a linear GEE analysis. The difference is the information in the first part of the output, where it is mentioned that a logit link is used with a binomial distribution, i.e. that a logistic GEE analysis is performed.

The syntax needed to perform a logistic GEE analysis in SAS is comparable to that discussed for the linear GEE analysis. The only difference is found in the third line, where it has to be specified that the outcome variable is dichotomous (link=logit and dist=binomial):

```
proc genmod data=chol_long;
class id;
model hyperchol = skinf /link=logit
dist=binomial;
repeated subject=id/type=exch;
run;
```

13.3.3 R

Output 13.5 shows the output of a logistic GEE analysis with an exchangeable correlation structure performed in R. As for STATA and SAS, the output of a logistic GEE analysis performed in R is comparable to that discussed for a linear GEE analysis.

The syntax needed to obtain a logistic GEE analysis is also fairly straightforward. The difference with the syntax needed to perform a linear GEE analysis is found in the family definition (family = binomial).

```
result <- gee(formula = hyperchol ~
skinf, id = id, data = chol_long,
family = binomial, corstr =
"exchangeable")
```

13.3.4 SPSS

Output 13.6 shows part of the output of a logistic GEE analysis performed in SPSS.

As for all the other software packages, the output of a logistic GEE analysis is comparable to the output of a linear GEE analysis. The syntax to obtain this result is also comparable to the syntax used to perform a linear GEE analysis. The difference is found in the third line where the distribution (BINOMIAL) and the link function (LOGIT) are defined.

```
GENLIN hyperchol (REFERENCE=FIRST)
WITH skinf
 /MODEL skinf INTERCEPT=YES
DISTRIBUTION=BINOMIAL LINK=LOGIT
 /CRITERIA METHOD=FISHER(1) SCALE=1
MAXITERATIONS=100 MAXSTEPHALVING=5
PCONVERGE=1E-006 (ABSOLUTE)
SINGULAR=1E-012 ANALYSISTYPE=3
(WALD) CILEVEL=95 LIKELIHOOD=FULL
    /REPEATED  SUBJECT=id  SORT=YES
CORRTYPE=EXCHANGEABLE
ADJUSTCORR=YES COVB=ROBUST
MAXITERATIONS=100 PCONVERGE=1e-006
(ABSOLUTE) UPDATECORR=1
 /MISSING CLASSMISSING=EXCLUDE
 /PRINT CPS DESCRIPTIVES MODELINFO
FIT SUMMARY SOLUTION.
```

13.3.5 Overview

Table 13.2 summarises the results of logistic GEE analyses with an exchangeable correlation structure performed in different software packages. As

Output 13.4 Results of a logistic GEE analysis performed in SAS

The GENMOD Procedure

Model information		
Data set	chol_long	
Distribution	Binomial	
Link function	Logit	
Dependent variable	hyperchol	Hypercholesterolemia

Number of observations read	882
Number of observations used	882
Number of events	587
Number of trials	882

GEE model information	
Correlation structure	Exchangeable
Subject effect	id (147 levels)
Number of clusters	147
Correlation matrix dimension	6
Maximum cluster size	6
Minimum cluster size	6

Exchangeable working correlation	
Correlation	0.4921003861

Analysis Of GEE parameter estimates						
Empirical standard error estimates						
Parameter	Estimate	Standard error	95% confidence limits		Z	Pr > |Z|
Intercept	1.7777	0.2680	1.2525	2.3029	6.63	<.0001
skinf	−0.2791	0.0539	−0.3848	−0.1734	−5.17	<.0001

Output 13.5 Results of a logistic GEE analysis performed in R

```
Coefficients:
             Estimate   Std.err   Wald   Pr(>|W|)
(Intercept)  -1.7773    0.2680    44.0   3.3e-11 ***
 skinf        0.2790    0.0539    26.8   2.3e-07 ***
- - -
Signif. codes: 0 '***' 0.001 '**' 0.01 '*' 0.05 '.' 0.1 ' ' 1

Correlation structure = exchangeable
Estimated Scale Parameters:

             Estimate   Std.err
(Intercept)  0.964      0.0563
 Link = identity

Estimated Correlation Parameters:
        Estimate   Std.err
 alpha   0.493     0.0503
Number of clusters:  147 Maximum cluster size: 6
```

---

was the case for the linear GEE analyses, the results obtained from the logistic GEE analyses in different software packages are exactly the same.

13.4 Mixed Model Analysis with a Continuous Outcome Variable

13.4.1 Introduction

In Section 3.3.5 it was argued that there is some debate about the use of maximum likelihood or restricted maximum likelihood for the estimation of the regression coefficients in a linear mixed model analysis. It was also argued that the default estimation method in STATA is maximum likelihood and therefore, the linear mixed model analyses used throughout the book were performed with maximum likelihood. However, in the other software packages used in this chapter, restricted maximum likelihood is the default estimation method. To obtain better comparisons between the results of the different software packages, the linear mixed model analyses will all be performed with maximum likelihood.

13.4.2 STATA

The syntax used for a linear mixed model analysis with only a random intercept is slightly different from the syntax used for the GEE analysis.

```
mixed chol skinf || id:
```

The first part of the syntax is the same for all STATA procedures. First the procedure is specified (i.e. mixed) and then the outcome variable and the covariates are given. Normally, after the variables a comma is given for some additional information. In the mixed procedure, however, first || id: is given in order to define the cluster variable. In a longitudinal study, the cluster variable is the variable indicating the subject. In the example dataset used throughout the book this identifier is the variable id. After the definition of the cluster variable, a comma can be given after which some additional information can be provided. In the syntax above there is no additional information needed. The following syntax can be used to perform a linear mixed model analysis with a random intercept and a random slope for the sum of skinfolds.

```
mixed chol skinf || id: skinf , cov
(unstruct)
```

The additional statement cov(unstruct) is necessary to obtain, besides the random intercept and the random slope for the sum of skinfolds, the covariance between the two (see Section 3.3.3).

Output 13.6 Results of a logistic GEE analysis performed in SPSS

Model information	
Dependent variable	Hypercholesterolemia[a]
Probability distribution	Binomial
Link function	Logit
Subject effect	1	id number
Working correlation matrix structure	Exchangeable

a. The procedure models 1 as the response, treating 0 as the reference category.

Correlated data summary			
Number of levels	Subject Effect	id number	147
Number of subjects			147
Number of measurements per subject	Minimum		6
	Maximum		6
Correlation matrix dimension			6

Parameter estimates							
Parameter	B	Std. Error	95% Wald confidence interval		Hypothesis test		
			Lower	Upper	Wald Chi-square	df	Sig.
(Intercept)	1.778	.2680	1.253	2.303	44.014	1	.000
Sum of skinfolds	.279	.0539	.385	.173	26.781	1	.000
(Scale)	1						

Dependent variable: hypercholesterolemia.
Model: (Intercept), sum of skinfolds.

Table 13.2 Summary of the results for the relationship between hypercholesterolemia derived from logistic GEE analyses with an exchangeable correlation structure performed in different software packages

Package	Regression coefficient (se)
STATA	0.279 (0.054)
SPSS	0.279 (0.054)
SAS	0.279 (0.054)
R	0.279 (0.054)

13.4.3 SAS

In SAS, the MIXED procedure can be used to perform a linear mixed model analysis. Output 13.7 shows part of the output of a linear mixed model analysis with only a random intercept performed in SAS.

In Output 13.7, it is first shown that the estimation method is maximum likelihood (ML). The next part of the output, which is of interest, is where the covariance parameter estimates are presented. The variance of the random intercept is equal to 0.2937, and the residual variance is equal to 0.2756.

In addition to the variance parameters, some model fit indicators are also provided. The −2 log likelihood, Akaike's Information Criterion (AIC), Hurvich and Tsai's Criterion (AICC) and Schwarz's Bayesian Information Criterion (BIC) are presented. AIC, AICC and BIC can be seen as adjusted values of the −2 log likelihood, i.e. adjusted for the number of parameters estimated by the particular model (Akaike, 1974; Schwarz, 1978; Hurvich and Tsai, 1989).

Output 13.7 Results of a linear mixed model analysis with only a random intercept performed in SAS

The Mixed Procedure

Model information	
Data set	chol_long
Dependent variable	chol
Covariance structure	Variance components
Subject effect	id
Estimation method	ML
Residual variance method	Profile
Fixed effects SE method	Model-based
Degrees of freedom method	Containment

Dimensions	
Covariance parameters	2
Columns in X	2
Columns in Z per subject	1
Subjects	147
Maximum observations per subject	6

Number of observations	
Number of observations read	882
Number of observations used	882

Covariance parameter estimates		
Covariance parameter	Subject	Estimate
Intercept	id	0.2937
Residual		0.2756

Fit statistics	
−2 log likelihood	1660.4
AIC (smaller is better)	1668.4
AICC (smaller is better)	1668.4
BIC (smaller is better)	1680.3

Solution for fixed effects					
Effect	Estimate	Standard error	DF	t Value	Pr > |t|
Intercept	3.7993	0.08387	146	45.30	<.0001
skinf	0.1871	0.01836	734	10.19	<.0001

The last part of the output shows the estimates of the regression coefficients, the standard errors, the degrees of freedom, the *t*-values and the corresponding *p*-values. It should be noted that in SAS the *t*-distribution is used instead of the standard normal distribution (*z*-distribution), which is used in STATA. Using the *t*-distribution instead of the *z*-distribution leads to slightly higher *p*-values, especially when the number of observations is low. However, when the number of observations is high, the *t*-distribution is almost equal to the *z*-distribution.

The following syntax can be used to perform a mixed model analysis with only a random intercept in SAS.

```
proc  mixed  data=chol_long  meth-
od=ml;
class id;
model chol = skinf/s;
random int/ subject=id;
run;
```

The syntax looks similar to that needed to perform a linear GEE analysis. The difference is firstly that the repeated statement is replaced by the random statement, which is necessary in order to identify the random part of the mixed model. Secondly, there is no specification of the correlation structure needed. Finally, it has to be mentioned that maximum likelihood has to be used (method=ML). This has to be done because the default estimation method in SAS is restricted maximum likelihood (see Section 13.4.1).

Output 13.8 shows part of the output of a linear mixed model analysis with both a random intercept and a random slope for the sum of skinfolds. The most important difference between Output 13.7 and Output 13.8 is the number of covariance parameters that are estimated. In the analysis with both a random intercept and a random slope, three covariance parameters are estimated: (1) UN(1,1) which is an estimate of the variance of the random intercept, (2) UN(2,2) which is an estimate of the variance of the random slope for the sum of skinfolds, and (3) UN(2,1) which is an estimate of the covariance between the random intercept and the random slope. The value of the -2 log likelihood can be used to evaluate the necessity of adding a random slope for the sum of skinfolds to the model by performing the likelihood ration test.

The following syntax can be used to perform a linear mixed model analysis with both a random intercept and a random slope for the sum of skinfolds in SAS.

```
proc  mixed  data=chol_long  meth-
od=ml;
class id;
model chol = skinf/s;
random  int  skinf/  subject=id
typ3=un;
run;
```

13.4.4 R

Output 13.9 shows the output of a linear mixed model analysis with only a random intercept performed in R.

The first line of Output 13.9 shows that the parameters of this linear mixed model analysis were estimated with maximum likelihood. In the same block of the output, the log likelihood of the model is shown, in addition to some other model fit indicators (i.e. AIC and BIC; see Section 13.4.3).

The next part of the output shows the random part of the model. In a model with only a random intercept, two variance parameters are estimated (given as standard deviations in the R output): the standard deviation of the random intercept (0.542) and the residual (or error) standard deviation (0.525). The following part of the output shows the estimates of the regression coefficients, the standard errors of the regression coefficients, the degrees of freedom, the *t*-values and the corresponding *p*-values. Note that in R, the *t*-distribution is used instead of the standard normal (*z*-)distribution.

The following syntax can be used to perform a linear mixed model analysis with only a random intercept in R.

```
result <- lme (chol~skinf, data=-
chol_long, random= ~1|id,
method="ML")
```

As for the GEE analysis, the results of the mixed model analysis are linked to the object result. In the last part of the syntax, the random part of the model is specified (random= ~1|id). Note that also in the R syntax it has to be mentioned that maximum likelihood must be used (method="ML"). Again, this is because in R, restricted maximum likelihood is the default estimation method.

Output 13.8 Results of a linear mixed model analysis with both a random intercept and a random slope for sum of skinfolds performed in SAS

The Mixed Procedure

Model information	
Data set	chol_long
Dependent variable	chol
Covariance structure	Unstructured
Subject effect	id
Estimation method	ML
Residual variance method	Profile
Fixed effects SE method	Model-based
Degrees of freedom method	Containment

Dimensions	
Covariance parameters	4
Columns in X	2
Columns in Z per subject	2
Subjects	147
Maximum observations per subject	6

Number of observations	
Number of observations read	882
Number of observations used	882
Number of observations not used	0

Covariance parameter estimates		
Covariance parameter	Subject	Estimate
UN(1,1)	id	0.4729
UN(2,1)	id	−0.04134
UN(2,2)	id	0.009403
Residual		0.2657

Fit statistics	
−2 log likelihood	1657.9
AIC (smaller is better)	1669.9
AICC (smaller is better)	1670.0
BIC (smaller is better)	1687.8

Solution for fixed effects					
Effect	Estimate	Standard error	DF	t Value	Pr > |t|
Intercept	3.7900	0.09271	146	40.88	<.0001
skinf	0.1920	0.02092	146	9.18	<.0001

Output 13.9 Results of a linear mixed model analysis with only a random intercept performed in R

```
Linear mixed-effects model fit by maximum likelihood
 Data: chol_long
  AIC BIC logLik
  1668 1688 -830

Random effects:
 Formula: ~1 | id
         (Intercept) Residual
StdDev:       0.542    0.525

Fixed effects: chol ~ skinf
             Value  Std.Error  DF  t-value  p-value
(Intercept)   3.80    0.0840  734    45.3        0
skinf         0.19    0.0184  734    10.2        0
 Correlation:
    (Intr)
skinf -0.819

Standardized Within-Group Residuals:
   Min       Q1       Med       Q3      Max
-2.7916  -0.6200  -0.0978   0.5229  4.2901

Number of Observations: 882
Number of Groups: 147
```

Output 13.10 shows the output of a linear mixed model analysis with both a random intercept and a random slope for the sum of skinfolds performed in R. It is obvious that the most important difference between Output 13.9 and Output 13.10 is the estimation of two more parameters in the random part of the model, i.e. the random slope for the sum of skinfolds and the correlation between the random intercept and random slope. Note the R provides the correlation between the random intercept and random slope instead of the covariance, which is provided by the other software programmes. Although the numbers are different, the general interpretation of the two is the same.

The following syntax can be used to perform a linear mixed model analysis with both a random intercept and a random slope for the sum of skinfolds in R.

```
result <- lme (chol~skinf, data=-
data, random= ~ skinf|id,
method="ML")
```

13.4.5 SPSS

Output 13.11 shows part of the output of a linear mixed model analysis with only a random intercept performed in SPSS.

Output 13.10 Results of a mixed model analysis with a both random intercept and a random slope for sum of skinfolds performed in R

```
Linear mixed-effects model fit by maximum likelihood
 Data: chol_long
  AIC BIC   logLik
  1670 1699   -829

Random effects:
 Formula: ~skinf | id
 Structure: General positive-definite, Log-Cholesky parametrization
           StdDev Corr
(Intercept) 0.688 (Intr)
skinf       0.097 -0.62
Residual    0.515

Fixed effects: chol ~ skinf
            Value  Std.Error  DF   t-value  p-value
(Intercept) 3.79   0.0928    734   40.8     0
skinf       0.19   0.0209    734    9.2     0
 Correlation:
      (Intr)
skinf -0.849

Standardized Within-Group Residuals:
   Min       Q1       Med       Q3        Max
 -2.4791  -0.6237  -0.0743   0.5176    4.2737

Number of observations: 882
Number of groups: 147
```

The first part of Output 13.11 shows some general information (Model Dimension) and the model fit indicators (Information Criteria). In the latter, first of all the –2 log likelihood is provided (1671.416). Besides the –2 log likelihood, AIC, AICC, and BIC were also provided. Again, they all can be seen as adjusted values of the –2 log likelihood. Bozdogan's criterion (CAIC) is slightly different but can be interpreted in more or less the same way (Bozdogan, 1987). The next part of the output shows the estimates of the fixed part of the model. In this part of the output, the regression coefficients, the standard errors, the degrees of freedom, the t-values, the corresponding p-values, and the 95% confidence intervals around the regression coefficients are provided. The last part of the output shows the estimates of the covariance parameters. Because only a random intercept was added to the model, only the variance of

the random intercept (0.293719) and the residual variance (0.275599) are provided.

The syntax to perform a linear mixed model analysis with only a random intercept in SPSS looks as follows:

```
MIXED chol WITH skinf
 /CRITERIA=DFMETHOD(SATTERTHWAITE)
CIN(95) MXITER(100) MXSTEP(10)
SCORING(1) SINGULAR
(0.000000000001) HCONVERGE(0,
ABSOLUTE) LCONVERGE(0, ABSOLUTE)
PCONVERGE(0.000001, ABSOLUTE)
 /FIXED=skinf | SSTYPE(3)
 /METHOD=ML
 /PRINT=SOLUTION
  /RANDOM=INTERCEPT  | SUBJECT(id)
COVTYPE(VC).
```

Output 13.11 Result of a linear mixed model analysis with only a random intercept performed in SPSS

Model dimension[a]		Number of levels	Covariance structure	Number of parameters	Subject variables
Fixed effects	Intercept	1		1	
	Skinf	1		1	
Random effects	Intercept	1	Variance components	1	id
Residual				1	
Total		3		4	

a. Dependent variable: cholesterol.

Information criteria[a]	
-2 log likelihood	1660.386
Akaike's Information Criterion (AIC)	1668.386
Hurvich and Tsai's Criterion (AICC)	1668.432
Bozdogan's Criterion (CAIC)	1691.515
Schwarz's Bayesian Information Criterion (BIC)	1687.515

The information criteria are displayed in smaller-is-better form.
a. Dependent variable: cholesterol.

Estimates of fixed effects[a]						95% confidence interval	
Parameter	Estimate	Std. Error	df	t	Sig.	Lower bound	Upper bound
Intercept	3.799312	.083867	505.237	45.301	.000	3.634540	3.964084
skinf	.187118	.018359	850.734	10.192	.000	.151084	.223152

a. Dependent variable: cholesterol.

Estimates of covariance parameters[a]		Estimate	Std. error
Residual		.275599	.014377
Intercept [subject = id]	variance	.293719	.039703

a. Dependent variable: cholesterol.

Output 13.12 shows part of the output of a linear mixed model analysis with both a random intercept and a random slope for the sum of skinfolds performed in SPSS. The output looks similar to the one discussed for the analysis with only a random intercept. The difference is found in the last part in which the estimates of covariance parameters are given. Besides the random intercept variance (UN(1,1)) and the remaining error variance, the random slope variance for the

Output 13.12 Result of a linear mixed model analysis with both a random intercept and a random slope for sum of skinfolds performed in SPSS

		Number of levels	Covariance structure	Number of parameters	Subject variables
Fixed effects	Intercept	1		1	
	Skinf	1		1	
Random effects	Intercept + skinf	2	Unstructured	3	id
Residual				1	
Total		4		6	

Model dimension[a]

a. Dependent variable: cholesterol.

Information criteria[a]

-2 log likelihood	1657.855
Akaike's Information Criterion (AIC)	1669.855
Hurvich and Tsai's Criterion (AICC)	1669.951
Bozdogan's Criterion (CAIC)	1704.548
Schwarz's Bayesian Information Criterion (BIC)	1698.548

The information criteria are displayed in smaller-is-better form.

a. Dependent variable: cholesterol.

Estimates of fixed effects[a]

Parameter	Estimate	Std. error	df	t	Sig.	95% confidence interval	
						Lower bound	Upper bound
Intercept	3.790026	.092707	99.069	40.882	.000	3.606076	3.973976
skinf	.191955	.020917	63.910	9.177	.000	.150169	.233742

a. Dependent variable: cholesterol.

Estimates of covariance parameters[a]

Parameter		Estimate	Std. error
Residual		.265658	.015143
Intercept + skinf [subject = id]	UN (1,1)	.472930	.154083
	UN (2,1)	-.041336	.030975
	UN (2,2)	.009403	.007130

a. Dependent variable: cholesterol.

sum of skinfolds (UN(2,2)) and the covariance between the random intercept and random slope (UN(2,1)) are also given.

The following syntax can be used to perform a linear mixed model analysis with a random intercept and a random slope for the sum of skinfolds in SPSS.

```
MIXED chol WITH skinf
 /CRITERIA=DFMETHOD
(SATTERTHWAITE) CIN(95) MXITER
(100) MXSTEP(10) SCORING(1)
SINGULAR(0.000000000001) HCONVERGE
(0, ABSOLUTE) LCONVERGE(0,
ABSOLUTE) PCONVERGE(0.000001,
ABSOLUTE)
 /FIXED=skinf | SSTYPE(3)
 /METHOD=ML
 /PRINT=SOLUTION
 /RANDOM=INTERCEPT skinf | SUBJECT
(id) COVTYPE(UN).
```

13.4.6 Overview

Table 13.3 summarises the results of the linear mixed model analyses with only a random intercept performed with different software packages, while Table 13.4 summarises the results of the linear mixed model analyses with both a random intercept and a random slope for the sum of skinfolds. From both tables it can be seen that using a different

Table 13.3 Summary of the results of linear mixed model analyses with only a random intercept performed in different software packages

Package	Regression coefficient (se)	Random intercept variance	−2 log likelihood
STATA	0.187 (0.018)	0.294	1660
SPSS	0.187 (0.018)	0.294	1660
SAS	0.187 (0.018)	0.294	1660
R	0.19 (0.018)	0.294	1660

software package does not lead to different results of the linear mixed model analyses.

13.5 Mixed Model Analysis with a Dichotomous Outcome Variable

13.5.1 Introduction

In Chapter 7 it has already been mentioned that a logistic mixed model analysis is quite difficult to perform (i.e. the mathematics behind a logistic mixed model analysis is complicated). Although there are different methods available to estimate the regression coefficients of a logistic mixed model analysis, the most straightforward method is the Gauss–Hermite method, which is based on Gaussian quadrature points (Rabe-Hesketh and Pickles, 1999; Rabe-Hesketh et al., 2000, 2001a, 2001b). In Chapter 7, it was shown that this method is the default method used in STATA. In a recent paper by Stroup and Claassen (2020), it was also shown that this method is the most appropriate for a logistic mixed model analysis. It should, however, be realised that different statistical software programmes can use a different default estimation method.

For more technical information about the different estimation methods, reference is made to the more technical literature (e.g. Goldstein, 1991; Schall, 1991; Breslow and Clayton, 1993; Longford, 1993; Liu and Pierce, 1994; Pinheiro and Bates, 1995; Goldstein and Rasbash, 1996; Agresti et al., 2000; Lesaffre and Spiessens, 2001).

13.5.2 STATA

In the examples discussed in Chapter 7, STATA was used to perform a logistic mixed model analysis. In STATA, the logistic mixed model analysis can be performed with the melogit procedure. The syntax to perform a logistic mixed model analysis with only a random intercept in STATA

Table 13.4 Summary of the results of linear mixed model analyses with both a random intercept and a random slope for the sum of skinfolds performed in different software packages

Package	Regression coefficient (se)	Random intercept variance	Random slope variance	−2 log likelihood
STATA	0.192 (0.021)	0.47	0.01	1658
SPSS	0.192 (0.021)	0.47	0.01	1658
SAS	0.192 (0.021)	0.47	0.01	1658
R	0.19 (0.021)	0.47	0.01	1658

is comparable to the syntax used to perform a linear mixed model analysis.

```
melogit hyperchol skinf || id:
```

In the examples presented in Chapter 7, the melogit procedure was used with the default number of integration points (i.e. 7). In the literature it is argued that the result of a logistic mixed model analysis can depend on the number of quadrature points used in the estimation (Lesaffre and Spiessens, 2001; Twisk, 2013). In the statistical literature, it is generally accepted that 10 quadrature points are sufficient for a valid logistic mixed model analysis, although others suggest that 20 quadrature points are needed (e.g. Hu et al., 1998; Rodriguez and Goldman, 2001). However, in the present example, as well as in examples presented by others (e.g. Lesaffre and Spiessens, 2001), neither of these suggestions is confirmed. In the example presented here, the default option of seven quadrature points seems to be very reasonable. See Table 13.5, which presents the results of logistic mixed model analyses with a different number of quadrature points.

The reason why the results from the melogit procedure with a different number of quadrature points are almost the same has to do with the use of adaptive quadrature, which leads to a much more accurate (numeric) integration and therefore to much more valid estimations of the parameters (Rice, 1975; Pinheiro and Bates, 1995; Gander and Gautschi, 2000).

For a mixed model analysis with a random intercept and a random slope for the sum of skinfolds, the following syntax can be used.

```
melogit hyperchol skinf || id:
skinf, cov(unstruct)
```

In Chapter 7, it has already been mentioned that this analysis did not converge, so it was not able to

Table 13.5 Summary of the results for the relationship between hypercholesterolemia and the sum of skinfolds derived from logistic mixed model analyses performed in STATA with a different number of integration points

Number of integration points	Regression coefficient (se)
7	0.561 (0.106)
10	0.563 (0.107)
15	0.561 (0.107)
20	0.561 (0.107)

add a random slope for the sum of skinfolds to the model.

13.5.3 SAS

In the nineties, a SAS macro called glimmix that can be used to perform logistic mixed model analysis became available (Breslow and Clayton, 1993). Although with the glimmix procedure in SAS it is possible to use the adaptive Gauss–Hermite quadrature method, the default option is the residual pseudo-likelihood method. When this method is used, the result of the logistic mixed model analysis is quite different from the one obtained from a logistic mixed model analysis using the Gauss–Hermite quadrature method. Output 13.13a shows part of the output of a logistic mixed model analysis with only a random intercept performed in SAS using the default estimation method, while Output 13.13b shows part of the output of a logistic mixed model analysis with only a random intercept performed in SAS using the Gauss–Hermite quadrature estimation method.

The output of the logistic mixed model analysis is comparable to the output obtained from a linear mixed model analysis performed in SAS.

The syntax needed to perform a logistic mixed model analysis is also comparable to the syntax used to perform a linear mixed model analysis.

```
proc glimmix data=chol_long;
class id;
model hyperchol = skinf/s dist=
binomial;
random int / subject=id;
run;
```

```
proc glimmix data=chol_long
method=quad (INITPL=7);
class id;
model hyperchol = skinf/s dist=
binomial;
random int / subject=id;
run;
```

Unfortunately, a logistic mixed model analysis with both a random intercept and a random slope for the sum of skinfolds could not be performed (the model did not converge). Nevertheless, the following syntax can be used to perform such an analysis (again performed with the Gauss–Hermite quadrature estimation method).

Output 13.13a Results of a logistic mixed model analysis with only a random intercept performed in SAS using the default estimation method

The GLIMMIX Procedure

Model information	
Data set	WORK.IMPORT
Response variable	hyperchol
Response distribution	Binomial
Link function	Logit
Variance function	Default
Variance matrix blocked by	id
Estimation technique	Residual PL
Degrees of freedom method	Containment

Dimensions	
G-side covariance parameters	1
Columns in X	2
Columns in Z per subject	1
Subjects (blocks in V)	147
Maximum observations per subject	6

Fit statistics	
−2 res log pseudo-likelihood	4263.38
Generalised Chi-square	533.72
Generalised Chi-square / DF	0.61

Covariance parameter estimates			
Covariance parameter	Subject	Estimate	Standard error
Intercept	id	3.2143	0.5662

Solutions for fixed effects					
Effect	Estimate	Standard error	DF	t Value	Pr > |t|
Intercept	−2.7221	0.3813	146	−7.14	<.0001
Skinf	0.4494	0.08629	734	5.21	<.0001

```
proc glimmix data=chol_long meth-      dist=binomial;
od=quad (INITPL=7);                     random int skinf/ subject=id
class id;                               typ3=un;
model hyperchol = skinf/s               run;
```

Output 13.13b Results of a logistic mixed model analysis with only a random intercept performed in SAS using the Gauss–Hermite quadrature estimation method

Model information	
Data set	WORK.IMPORT
Response variable	Hyperchol
Response distribution	Binomial
Link function	Logit
Variance function	Default
Variance matrix blocked by	id
Estimation technique	Maximum likelihood
Likelihood approximation	Gauss–Hermite quadrature
Degrees of freedom method	Containment

Dimensions	
G-side covariance parameters	1
Columns in X	2
Columns in Z per subject	1
Subjects (blocks in V)	147
Maximum observations per subject	6

Fit statistics	
−2 log likelihood	806.97
AIC (smaller is better)	812.97
AICC (smaller is better)	812.99
BIC (smaller is better)	821.94
CAIC (smaller is better)	824.94
HQIC (smaller is better)	816.61

Covariance parameter estimates			
Covariance parameter	Subject	Estimate	Standard error
Intercept	Id	6.7689	1.4910

Solutions for fixed effects					
Effect	Estimate	Standard error	DF	t Value	Pr > |t|
Intercept	−3.6087	0.5055	146	−7.14	<.0001
Skinf	0.5601	0.1063	734	5.27	<.0001

13.5.4 R

In R, the Gauss–Hermite quadrature estimation method is the default estimation method. However, the default method is the so-called Laplace method (Ju et al., 2020). Output 13.14a shows the output of a logistic mixed model analysis performed in R.

Output 13.14a is comparable to the output of a linear mixed model analysis performed in R (see Output 13.9).

With the following syntax a logistic mixed model analysis with only a random intercept can be performed in R.

```
result <- glmer(hyperchol ~ skinf +
(1|id), data=chol_long,
family=binomial)
```

It is also possible to perform the same logistic mixed model analysis in R as has been performed in STATA and in SAS, i.e. a logistic mixed model analysis with a Gauss–Hermite quadrature estimation method with seven integration points. Output 13.14b shows the results of that analysis.

The following syntax must be used to obtain the output shown in Output 13.14b.

```
result <- glmer(chol01 ~ skinf + (1|
id), data=chol_long, family=
binomial, nAGQ=7)
```

Comparable to the other software packages, a model with both a random intercept and a random slope for the sum of skinfolds did not converge. However, the following syntax can be used to perform such an analysis.

Output 13.14a Results of a logistic mixed model analysis with only a random intercept performed in R

```
Generalised linear mixed model fit by maximum likelihood (Laplace
Approximation) [
glmerMod]
  Family: binomial ( logit )
Formula: chol01 ~ skinf + (1 | id)
   Data: chol_long

  AIC    BIC  logLik deviance df.resid
  820    834   -407    814     879

Scaled residuals:
  Min      1Q Median     3Q    Max
-3.441 -0.306 -0.171 0.403 2.843

Random effects:
 Groups Name         Variance Std.Dev.
 id     (Intercept) 6.37      2.52
Number of obs: 882, groups:  id, 147

Fixed effects:
            Estimate Std. Error z value  Pr(>|z|)
(Intercept)  -3.693      0.511    -7.23 4.7e-13 ***
skinf         0.570      0.106     5.39 7.0e-08 ***
- - -
Signif. codes:  0 '***' 0.001 '**' 0.01 '*' 0.05 '.' 0.1 ' ' 1

Correlation of Fixed Effects:
      (Intr)
skinf -0.841
```

Output 13.14b Results of a logistic mixed model analysis with only a random intercept performed in R with a Gauss–Hermite quadrature estimation method with seven integration points

```
Generalised linear mixed model fit by maximum likelihood (Adaptive Gauss-
Hermite
 Quadrature, nAGQ = 7) [glmerMod]
 Family: binomial (logit)
Formula: chol01 ~ skinf + (1 | id)
   Data: chol_long

   AIC      BIC  logLik  deviance  df.resid
 813.0   827.3  -403.5     807.0       879

Scaled residuals:
   Min          1Q  Median        3Q      Max
-3.4462   -0.3059  -0.1711  0.3955  2.8128

Random effects:
 Groups Name          Variance  Std.Dev.
 id     (Intercept)   6.769     2.602
Number of obs: 882, groups:   id, 147

Fixed effects:
            Estimate Std. Error  z value  Pr(>|z|)
(Intercept) -3.6087      0.5055  -7.139  9.42e-13 ***
skinf        0.5601      0.1063   5.268  1.38e-07 ***
---
Signif. codes:  0 '***' 0.001 '**' 0.01 '*' 0.05 '.' 0.1 ' ' 1

Correlation of Fixed Effects:
      (Intr)
skinf -0.844
```

```
result <- glmer(chol01 ~ skinf +
(skinf|id), data=chol_long, family=
binomial, nAGQ=7)
```

13.5.5 SPSS

From version 19 onwards, SPPS provides the possibility to perform a logistic mixed model analysis. In SPSS, there is only one estimation method available and that is the residual pseudo-likelihood method (i.e. the same estimation method as the default estimation method used in SAS). Output 13.15 shows part of the output of a logistic mixed model analysis with only a random intercept performed in SPSS.

Like the SPSS output of a linear mixed model analysis, the first part of the output shows the

general information of the analysis performed, i.e. that a logit link function is used with a binomial probability distribution. In other words, it is mentioned that a logistic mixed model analysis is performed. Furthermore, two model fit indicators are given (AIC and BIC). The second part of the output shows the regression coefficients, the standard errors, t-values, corresponding p-values and the 95% confidence intervals around the regression coefficients, while the third part shows the random intercept variance.

The following syntax can be used to perform a logistic mixed model analysis with only a random intercept in SPSS.

```
GENLINMIXED
 /DATA_STRUCTURE SUBJECTS=id
 /FIELDS TARGET=hyperchol
```

Output 13.15 Results of a logistic mixed model analysis with only a random intercept performed in SPSS

Model summary	
Target	Hypercholesterolemia
Probability distribution	Binomial
Link function	Logit
Information criterion	Akaike Corrected	4265.384
	Bayesian	4270.159

Information criteria are based on the −2 log likelihood (4263,379) and are used to compare models. Models with smaller information criterion values fit better.

Fixed coefficients[a]

Model term	Coefficient	Std. error	T	Sig.	95% confidence interval	
					Lower	Upper
Intercept	-2.722	.3813	-7.139	.000	-3.471	-1.974
skinf	.449	.0863	5.208	.000	.280	.619

Model term	Coefficient	Exp(Coefficient)	95% confidence interval for Exp (Coefficient)	
			Lower	Upper
Intercept	-2.722	.066	.031	.139
skinf	.449	1.567	1.323	1.857

Probability distribution: binomial.
Link function: Logit.

Random effect

Random effect covariance	Estimate	Std. error	Z	Sig.	95% confidence interval	
					Lower	Upper
Var (Intercept)	3.214	.566	5.677	.000	2.276	4.540

Covariance structure: variance components.
Subject specification: id.

```
TRIALS=NONE OFFSET=NONE              COVARIANCE_TYPE=VARIANCE_COMPONE-
                /TARGET_OPTIONS      NTS SOLUTION=FALSE
DISTRIBUTION=BINOMIAL LINK=LOGIT                       /BUILD_OPTIONS
 /FIXED EFFECTS=skinf                TARGET_CATEGORY_ORDER=DESCENDING
USE_INTERCEPT=TRUE                   INPUTS_CATEGORY_ORDER=ASCENDING
 /RANDOM USE_INTERCEPT=TRUE                        MAX_ITERATIONS=100
SUBJECTS=id                          CONFIDENCE_LEVEL=95
```

Table 13.6 Summary of the results of logistic mixed model analyses with a random intercept to analyse the relationship between hypercholesterolemia and sum of skinfolds performed in different software packages

Package	Regression coefficient (se)	Random intercept variance	−2 log likelihood
STATA	0.561 (0.106) [1]	7.18	806
SPSS	0.449 (0.086) [2]	3.21	4263
SAS	0.449 (0.086) [2]	3.21	4263
	0.560 (0.106) [1]	6.77	806
R	0.570 (0.106) [3]	6.37	814
	0.560 (0.106) [1]	6.77	806

[1] Using the Gauss–Hermite quadrature method with seven quadrature points.
[2] Using the residual pseudo-likelihood method.
[3] Using the Gauss–Hermite quadrature Laplace method.

```
DF_METHOD=RESIDUAL COVB=MODEL
PCONVERGE=0.000001(ABSOLUTE)
                    SCORING=0
SINGULAR=0.000000000001
   /EMMEANS_OPTIONS SCALE=ORIGINAL
PADJUST=LSD.
```

Although it was possible to perform a logistic mixed model analysis with both a random intercept and a random slope for sum of skinfolds in SPSS, the programme gives a warning message indicating that the result cannot be trusted and therefore the output of the analysis will not be presented. However, the following syntax can be used to perform such an analysis.

```
GENLINMIXED
  /DATA_STRUCTURE SUBJECTS=id
  /FIELDS TARGET=hyperchol
TRIALS=NONE OFFSET=NONE
                  /TARGET_OPTIONS
DISTRIBUTION=BINOMIAL LINK=LOGIT
```

```
  /FIXED EFFECTS=skinf
USE_INTERCEPT=TRUE
  /RANDOM EFFECTS=skinf
USE_INTERCEPT=TRUE SUBJECTS=id
COVARIANCE_TYPE=UNSTRUCTURED
SOLUTION=FALSE
                /BUILD_OPTIONS
TARGET_CATEGORY_ORDER=DESCENDING
INPUTS_CATEGORY_ORDER=ASCENDING
            MAX_ITERATIONS=100
CONFIDENCE_LEVEL=95
DF_METHOD=RESIDUAL COVB=MODEL
PCONVERGE=0.000001(ABSOLUTE)
                    SCORING=0
SINGULAR=0.000000000001
   /EMMEANS_OPTIONS SCALE=ORIGINAL
PADJUST=LSD.
```

13.5.6 Overview

Table 13.6 summarises the results of the logistic mixed model analyses with only a random intercept performed with different software packages. From Table 13.6 it can be seen that there are (huge) differences between the results obtained with the different software packages, which are caused by the different estimation methods used. The results obtained from the residual pseudo-likelihood method is totally different from the results obtained from the Gauss–Hermite quadrature methods.

Although it has already been mentioned that the Gauss–Hermite quadrature methods are the most appropriate methods to estimate the parameters of a logistic mixed model analysis (Stroup and Claassen, 2020), the difference in results between the different estimation methods indicates that the results obtained from a logistic mixed model analysis must be interpreted with great caution.

References

Agresti, A., Booth, J.G., Hobart, J.P. and Caffo, B. (2000). Random-effects modelling of categorical response data. *Sociological Methodology*, **30**, 27–80.

Akaike, H. (1974). A new look at the statistical model identification. *IEEE Transactions on Automatic Control*, **19**, 716–723.

Albert, P.S. (1999). Longitudinal data analysis (repeated measures) in clinical trials. *Statistics in Medicine*, **18**, 1707–1732.

Altman, D.G. (1991). *Practical statistics for medical research*. London: Chapman and Hall.

Apeldoorn, A.T., Ostelo, R.W., Helvoirt, van H., Fritz, J.M., Knol, D.L., Tulder, van M.W. and Vet, de H.C.W. (2012) A randomized controlled trial on the effectiveness of a classification-based system for subacute and chronic low back pain. *Spine*, **37**, 1347–1356.

Austin, P.C., White, I.R., Lee, D.S. and Buuren van S.V. (2021). Missing data in clinical research: a tutorial on multiple imputation. *Canadian Journal of Cardiology*, **37**, 1322–1331.

Barbosa, M.F. and Goldstein, H. (2000). Discrete response multilevel models for repeated measures: an application to intentions data. *Quality and Quantity*, **34**, 323–330.

Barnard, J. and Meng, X-L. (1999). Applications of multiple imputation in medical studies: from AIDS to NHANES. *Statistical Methods in Medical Research*, **8**, 17–36.

Baybak, M.A. (2004). What you see may not be what you get: A brief, nontechnical introduction to overfitting in regression-type models. *Psychosomatic Medicine*, **66**, 411–421.

Basagaña, X. and Spiegelman, D. (2010). Power and sample size calculations for longitudinal studies comparing rates of change with a time-varying exposure *Statistics in Medicine*, **29**, 181–192.

Berkhof, J., Knol, D.J., Rijmen, F., Twisk, J.W.R., Uitdehaag, B.J.M. and Boers, M. (2009). Relapse – remission and remission – relapse switches in rheumatoid arthritis patients were modeled by random effects. *Journal of Clinical Epidemiology*, **62**, 1085–1094.

Bernaards, C.A., Belin, T.R. and Schafer, J.L. (2007). Robustness of a multivariate normal approximation for imputation of incomplete binary data. *Statistics in Medicine*, **26**, 1368–1382.

Blomquist, N. (1977). On the relation between change and initial value. *Journal of the American Statistical Association*, **72**, 746–749.

Boshuizen, H. (2005). Re: Twisk and Proper: Evaluation of the results of a randomized controlled trial: How to define changes between baseline and follow-up. *Journal of Clinical Epidemiology*, **58**, 209–210.

Box-Steffensmeier, J.M. and De Boef, S. (2006). Repeated events survival models: The conditional frailty model. *Statistics in Medicine*, **25**, 3518–3533.

Bozdogan, H. (1987). Model selection and Akaike's information criterion (AIC): The general theory and its analytical extensions. *Psychometrika*, **52**, 345–370.

Breslow, N.E. and Clayton, D.G. (1993). Approximate inference in generalised linear models. *Journal of the American Statistical Association*, **88**, 9–25.

Brown, C.A. and Lilford, R.J. (2006). The stepped wedge trial design: A systematic review. *BMC Medical Research Methodology*, **6**, 54.

Bruce, B. and Fries, J.F. (2003). The Stanford Health Assessment Questionnaire: Dimensions and practical applications. *Health Quality of Life Outcomes*, **1**, 20.

Burton, P., Gurrin, L. and Sly, P. (1998). Extending the simple linear regression model to account for correlated responses: An introduction to generalized estimating equations and multi-level mixed modelling. *Statistics in Medicine*, **17**, 1261–1291.

Burton, A., Altman, D.G., Royston, P. and Holder, R.L. (2006). The design of simulation studies in medical statistics. *Statistics in Medicine*, **25**, 4279–4292.

Buuren, van S.V. (2018). *Flexible imputation of missing data* (2nd edn.). London: Chapman and Hall/CRC.

Carey, V., Zeger, S.L. and Diggle, P.J. (1993). Modeling multivariate binary data with alternating logistic regression. *Biometrika*, **80**, 517–526.

Chen, P-L., Wong, E., Dominik, R. and Steiner, M.J. (2000). A transitional model of barrier methods compliance with unbalanced loss to follow-up. *Statistics in Medicine*, **19**, 71–82.

Cleves, M.A., Gould, W.W., Gutierrez, R.G. and Marchenko Y.V. (2010). *An introduction to survival analysis using Stata* (3rd edn.). College Station, TX: Stata Press.

Connell, A. and Frye, A. (2006a). Growth Mixture Modelling in developmental psychology: Overview and demonstration of heterogeneity in developmental trajectories of adolescent antisocial behaviour. *Infant and Child Development*, **15**, 609–621.

Connell, A. and Frye, A. (2006b). Response to commentaries on target paper, "Growth Mixture Modelling in Developmental Psychology". *Infant and Child Development*, **15**, 639–642.

Conway, M.R. (1990). A random effects model for binary data. *Biometrics*, **46**, 317–328.

Crowder, M.J. and Hand, D.J. (1990). *Analysis of repeated measures*. London: Chapman and Hall.

Crowther, M.J., Abrams, K.R. and Lambert, P.C. (2013). Joint modeling of longitudinal and survival data. *The Stata Journal*, **13**, 165–184.

Curren, P.J. and Bauer, D.J. (2001). The disaggregation of within-person and between-person effects in longitudinal models of change. *Annual Reviews in Psychology*, **62**, 583–619.

Dalgaard, P. (2002). *Introductory statistics with* R. New York: Springer.

Deeg, D.J.H. and Westendorp-de Serière, M. (eds.) (1994). *Autonomy and well-being in the aging population I: Report from the Longitudinal Aging Study Amsterdam 1992–1993*. Amsterdam: VU University Press.

Demirtas, H., Freels, S.A. and Yucel, R.M. (2008). Plausibility of multivariate normality assumption when multiple imputing non-Gaussian continuous outcomes: A simulation assessment. *Journal of Statistical Computation and Simulation*, **78**, 69–84.

Demirtas, H. and Schafer, J.L. (2003). On the performance of random-coefficient pattern-mixture models for non-ignorable drop-out. *Statistics in Medicine*, **22**, 2553–2575.

Diggle, P.J. (1989). Testing for random dropouts in repeated measurement data. *Biometrics*, **45**, 1255–1258.

Dik, M.G., Jonker, C., Comijs, H.C., Bouter, L.M., Twisk, J.W.R., van Kamp, G.J. and Deeg, D.J.H. (2001). Memory complaints and Apo E ε4 accelerate cognitive decline in cognitively normal elderly. *Neurology*, **57**, 2217–2222.

Duncan, T., Duncan, S., Stryker, L., Li, F. and Alpert, A. (1999). *An introduction to latent variable modelling. Concepts, issues and applications*. Mahwah, NJ: Lawrence Erlbaum Associated Publishers.

Enders, C.K. (2010). *Applied missing data analysis*. New York: The Guilford Press.

Fairclough, D.L., Thijs, H., Huang, I-C., Finnern, H.W. and, Wu, A.W. (2008). Handling missing quality of life data in HIV clinical trials: What is practical? *Quality of Life Research*, **17**, 61–73.

Feldman, B., Masyn, K. and Conger, R. (2009). New approaches to studying problem behaviors: A comparison of methods for modeling longitudinal, categorical adolescent drinking data. *Developmental Psychology*, **45**, 652–676.

Fitzmaurice, G.M., Laird, N.M. and Lipsitz, S.R. (1994). Analysing incomplete longitudinal binary responses: A likelihood-based approach. *Biometrics*, **50**, 601–612.

Fitzmaurice, G.M., Laird, N.M. and Ware, J.H. (2004) *Applied longitudinal data analysis*. Hoboken, NJ: Wiley.

Fleiss, J.L. (1981). *Statistical methods for rates and proportions*. New York: Wiley.

Forbes, A.B., Carlin, J.B. (2005). "Residual change" analysis is not equivalent to analysis of covariance. *Journal of Clinical Epidemiology*, **58**, 540–541.

Fox, J. (2002). *An R and S-Plus comparison to applied regression*. New York: Sage Publications.

Gandar, W. and Gautschi, W. (2000). Adaptive quadrature – revisited. *BIT Numerical Mathematics*, **40**, 84–101

Gebski, V., Leung, O., McNeil, D. and Lunn, D. (eds.) (1992). *SPIDA user manual*, version 6. Sydney, NSW: Macquarie University.

Gibbons, R.D. and Hedeker, D. (1997). Random effects probit and logistic regression models for three level data. *Biometrics*, **53**, 1527–1537.

Glynn, R.J., Stukel, T.A., Sharp, S.M, Bubolz, T.A., Freeman, J.L. and Fisher, E.S. (1993). Estimating the variance of standardized rates of recurrent events, with application to hospitalizations among the elderly in New England. *American Journal of Epidemiology*, **137**, 776–786.

Goldstein, H. (1986). Multilevel mixed linear model analysis using iterative generalised least squares. *Biometrika*, **73**, 43–56.

Goldstein, H. (1989). Restricted unbiased iterative generalised least squares estimation. *Biometrika*, **76**, 622–623.

Goldstein, H. (1991). Nonlinear multilevel models with an application to discrete response data. *Biometrika*, **78**, 45–51.

Goldstein, H. (1995). *Multilevel statistical models*. London: Edward Arnold.

Goldstein, H. and Rasbash, J. (1996). Improved approximation for multilevel models with binary responses. *Journal of the Royal Statistical Society*, **159**, 505–513.

Goldstein, H., Rasbash, J., Plewis, I., Draper, D., Browne, W., Yang, M., Woodhouse, G. and Healy, M. (1998). *A user's guide to MLwiN*. London: Institute of Education.

Graham, J.W. (2009). Missing data analysis: Making it work in the real world. *Annual Review of Psychology*, **60**, 549–576.

Green, J.A. (2021). Too many zeros and/or highly skewed? A tutorial on modelling health behavior as count data with Poisson and negative binomial regression. *Health Psychology and Behavioral Medicine*, **9**, 436–455.

Greenland, S. and Finkle, D. (1995). A critical look at methods for handling missing covariates in epidemiologic regression analysis. *American Journal of Epidemiology*, **142**, 1255–1264.

Guo, Y., Logan, H.L., Glueck, D.H. and Muller, K.E. (2013). Selecting a sample size for studies with repeated measures. *BMC Medical Research Methodology*, **13**, 100

Guo, Y. and Pandis, N. (2015). Sample-size calculation for repeated-measures and longitudinal studies. *The American Journal of Orthodontics and Dentofacial Orthopedics*, **147**, 146–149.

Haan, M.N., Shemanski, L., Jagust, W.J., Manolio, T.A. and Kuller, L. (1999). The role of APOE ε4 in modulating effects of other risk factors for cognitive decline in elderly persons. *Journal of the American Medical Association*, **282**, 40–46.

Hajos T.R.S., Pouwer F., de Grooth R., Holleman F., Twisk J.W.R., Diamant M. and Snoek F. (2011). Initiation of insulin glargine in patients with type 2 diabetes in suboptimal glycaemic control positively impacts health-related quality of life: A prospective cohort study in primary care. *Diabetic Medicine*, **28**, 1096–1102.

Hand, D.J. and Crowder, M.J. (1996). *Practical longitudinal data analysis*. London: Chapman and Hall.

Harville, D.A. (1977). Maximum likelihood approaches to variance component estimation and to related problems. *Journal of the American Statistical Association*, **72**, 320–340.

Hedeker, D., Gibbons, R.D. and Waternaux, C. (1999). Sample size estimation for longitudinal designs with attrition: Comparing time-related contrasts between groups. *Journal of Education and Behavioral Statistics*, **24**, 70–93.

Hoeksma, J. and Kelderman, H. (2006). On growth curves and mixture models. *Infant and Child Development*, **15**, 627–634.

Hogan, J.W., Roy, J. and Korkontzelou, C. (2004). Handling drop-out in longitudinal studies. *Statistics in Medicine*, **23**, 1455–1497.

Hogan, J.W. and Laird, N.M. (1997). Mixture models for the joint distribution of repeated measures and event times. *Statistics in Medicine*, **16**, 239–257.

Holford, T.R. (1992). Analysing the temporal effects of age, period and cohort. *Statistical Methods in Medical Research*, **1**, 317–337.

Holford, T.R., Armitage, P. and Colton, T. (2005). *Age-period-cohort analysis encyclopedia of biostatistics* (2nd vol., pp. 82–99). New York: John Wiley & Sons, Ltd.

Hosmer, D.W. and Lemeshow, S. (1989). *Applied logistic regression*. New York: Wiley.

Hu, F.B., Goldberg, J., Hedeker, D., Flay, B.R. and Pentz, M.A. (1998). Comparison of population-averaged and subject specific approaches for analyzing repeated measures binary outcomes. *American Journal of Epidemiology*, **147**, 694–703.

Hurvich, C.M. and Tsai, C-L. (1989). Regression and time series model selection in small samples. *Biometrika*, **76**, 297–307.

Imlach Gunasekara, F., Richardson, K., Carter, K. and Blakely, T. (2014). Fixed effects analysis of repeated measures data. *International Journal of Epidemiology*, **43**, 264–269.

Jennrich, R.I. and Schluchter, M.D. (1986). Unbalanced repeated measures models with structured covariance matrices. *Biometrics*, **42**, 805–820.

Jones, B., Nagin, D. and Roeder, K. (2001). A SAS procedure based on mixed models for estimating developmental trajectories. *Social Methods Research*, **229**, 374–393.

Ju, K., Lin, L., Chu, H., Cheng, L-L. and Xu, C. (2020). Laplace approximation, penalized quasilikelihood, and adaptive Gauss–Hermite quadrature for generalized linear mixed models: towards meta-analysis of binary outcome with sparse data. *BMC Medical Research Methodology*, **20**, 152.

Judd, C.M., Smith, E.R. and Kidder, L.H. (1991). *Research methods in social relations*. Fort Worth, TX: Harcourt Brace Jovanovich College Publishers.

Jung, T. and Wickrama, K.A.S. (2008). Introduction to latent class growth analysis and growth mixture modelling. *Social and Personality Psychology Compass*, **2**, 302–317.

Kelly, P.J. and Lim, L-Y. (2003). Survival analysis for recurrent event data: An application to childhood infectious diseases. *Statistics in Medicine*, **19**, 13–33.

Kemper, H.C.G. (ed.) (1995). *The Amsterdam growth study: a longitudinal analysis of health, fitness and lifestyle*. HK Sport Science Monograph Series, vol. 6. Champaign, IL: Human Kinetics Publishers.

Kenward, M.G. (1998). Selection models for repeated measurements with non-random dropout: An illustration of sensitivity. *Statistics in Medicine*, **17**, 2723–2732.

Kenward, M.G. and Carpenter, J. (2007). Multiple imputation: Current perspectives. *Statistical Methods in Medical Research*, **16**, 199–218.

Kenward, M.G. and Molenberghs, G. (1999). Parametric models for incomplete continuous and categorical longitudinal data. *Statistical Methods in Medical Research*, **8**, 51–84.

Kleinbaum, D.G. (1994). *Logistic regression: A self-learning text*. New York: Springer-Verlag.

Kotz, D., Spigt, M., Arts, I.C.W., Crutzen, R. and Viechtbauer, W. (2012). Use of the stepped wedge design cannot be recommended: A critical appraisal and comparison with the classic cluster randomised controlled trial design. *Journal of Clinical Epidemiology*, **65**, 1249–1252.

Krieger, N. and Davey Smith, G.D. (2016). The tale wagged by the DAG: Broadening the scope of causal inference and explanation for epidemiology. *International Journal of Epidemiology*, **45**, 1787–1808.

Kristman, V.L., Manno, M, and Côté, P. (2005). Methods to account for attrition in longitudinal data: do they work? A simulation study. *European Journal of Epidemiology*, **20**, 657–662.

Kupper, L.L., Janis, J.M., Karmous, A. and Greenberg, B.G. (1985). Statistical age–period–cohort analysis: A review and critique. *Journal of Chronic Diseases*, **38**, 811–830.

Kwakkel, G., Wagenaar, R.C., Twisk, J.W.R., Lankhorst, G.J. and Koetsier, J.C. (1999). Intensity of leg and arm training after primary middle-cerebral artery stroke: A randomised trial. *Lancet*, **354**, 191–196.

Laird, N.M. and Ware, J.H. (1982). Random effects models for longitudinal data. *Biometrics*, **38**, 963–974.

Lambert, P.C. and Royston, P. (2009). Further development of flexible parametric models for survival analysis. *Stata Journal*, **9**, 265–290.

Lebowitz, M.D. (1996). Age, period, and cohort effects: Influences on differences between cross-sectional and longitudinal pulmonary function results. *American Journal of Respiratory and Critical Care Medicine*, **154**, S273–277.

Lee, E.W. and Durbin, N. (1994). Estimation and sample size considerations for clustered binary responses. *Statistics in Medicine*, **13**, 1241–1252.

Lee, I.-M., Paffenbarger Jr., R.S. and Hsieh, C-C. (1992). Time trends in physical activity among college alumni, 1962–1988. *American Journal of Epidemiology*, **135**, 915–925.

Lee, K.J., Tilling, K.M., Cornish, R.P., Little, R.J.A., Bell, M.L., Goetghebeur, E., Hogan, J.W. and Carpenter, J.R. (2021). STRATOS initiative. Framework for the treatment and reporting of missing data in observational studies: The Treatment and Reporting of Missing Data in Observational Studies framework. *Journal of Clinical Epidemiology*, **134**, 79–88.

Lesaffre, E. and Spiessens, B (2001). On the effect of the number of quadrature points in a logistic random-effects model: An example. *Applied Statistics*, **50**, 325–335.

Liang, K-Y. and Zeger, S.L. (1986). Longitudinal data analysis using generalised linear models. *Biometrica*, **73**, 45–51.

Liang, K-Y. and Zeger, S.L. (1993). Regression analysis for correlated data. *Annual Review of Public Health*, **14**, 43–68.

Liang, K-Y., Zeger, S.L. and Qaqish, B. (1992). Multivariate regression analysis for categorical data. *Journal of the Royal Statistical Society*, **54**, 3–40.

Lingsma, H. (2010). Covariate adjustment increases statistical power in randomised controlled trials. *Journal of Clinical Epidemiology*, **63**, 1391.

Lipsitz, S.R. and Fitzmaurice, G.M. (1994). Sample size for repeated measures studies with binary responses. *Statistics in Medicine*, **13**, 1233–1239.

Lipsitz, S.R. and Fitzmaurice, G.M. (1996). Estimating equations for measures of association between repeated binary responses. *Biometrics*, **52**, 903–912.

Lipsitz, S.R., Fitzmaurice, G.M., Orav, E.J. and Laird, N.M. (1994a). Performance of generalised estimating equations in practical situations. *Biometrics*, **50**, 270–278.

Lipsitz, S.R., Kim, K. and Zhao, L. (1994b). Analysis of repeated categorical data using generalised estimating equations. *Statistics in Medicine*, **13**, 1149–63.

Lipsitz, S.R., Laird, N.M. and Harrington, D.P. (1991). Generalized estimating equations for correlated binary data: using the odds ratio as a measure of association. *Biometrika*, **78**, 153–160.

Littel, R.C., Freund, R.J. and Spector, P.C. (1991). *SAS system for linear models* (3rd edn.). Cary, NC: SAS Institute Inc.

Littel, R.C., Milliken, G.A., Stroup, W.W. and Wolfinger, R.D. (1996). *SAS system for mixed models*. Cary, NC: SAS Institute Inc.

Littel, R.C., Pendergast, J. and Natarajan, R. (2000). Modelling covariance structures in the analysis of repeated measures data. *Statistics in Medicine*, **19**, 1793–1819.

Little, R.J.A. (1993). Pattern-mixture models for multivariate incomplete data. *Journal of the American Statistical Association*, **88**, 125–134.

Little, R.J.A. (1994). A class of pattern-mixture models for normal incomplete data. *Biometrika*, **81**, 471–483.

Little, R.J.A. (1995). Modelling the drop-out mechanism repeated measures studies. *Journal of the American Statistical Association*, **90**, 1112–1121.

Liu, Q. and Pierce, D.A. (1994). A note on Gauss–Hermite quadrature. *Biometrika*, **81**, 624–629.

Liu, G. and Liang, K-Y. (1997). Sample size calculations for studies with correlated observations. *Biometrics*, **53**, 937–947.

Loeys, T., Moerkerke, B. and Vansteelandt, S. (2015). A cautionary note on the power of the test for the indirect effect in mediation analysis. *Frontiers in Psychology*, **5**, 1549.

Longford, N.T. (1993). *Random coefficient models*. Oxford: Oxford University Press.

Lui, K-J. and Cumberland, W.G. (1992). Sample size requirement for repeated measurements in continuous data. *Statistics in Medicine*, **11**, 633–641.

Maindonald, J. and Braun, J. (2003). *Data analysis and graphics using R: An example-based approach*. Cambridge: Cambridge University Press.

Mansournia, M.A., Etminan, M., Danaei, G., Kaufman, J.S. and Collins, G. (2017). Handling time varying confounding in observational research. *British Medical Journal*, **359**, j4587.

MathSoft (2000). *S-PLUS 2000 guide to statistics*, Vol. 1. Data analysis product division. Seattle, WA: MathSoft Inc.

Mayer, K.U. and Huinink, J. (1990). Age, period, and cohort in the study of the life course: a comparison of classical A-P-C-analysis with event history analysis, or Farewell to Lexis? In *Data quality in longitudinal research*, ed. D. Magnusson and L.R. Bergman, pp. 211–232. Cambridge: Cambridge University Press.

Mazumdar, S., Tang, G., Houck, P.R., Dew, M.A., Begley, A.E., Scott, J., Mulsant, B.H. and Reynolds III, C.F. (2007). Statistical analysis of longitudinal psychiatric data with dropouts. *Journal of Psychological Research*, **41**, 1032–1041.

McCullagh, P. (1983). Quasi-likelihood functions. *Annals of Statistics*, **11**, 59–67.

Mchunu, N.N., Mwambi, H.G., Reddy, T., Yende-Zuma, N. and Naidoo K. (2020). Joint modelling of longitudinal and time-to-event data: an illustration using CD4 count and mortality in a cohort of patients initiated on antiretroviral therapy. *BMC Infectious Diseases*, **20**, 256.

McNally, R.J., Alexander, F.E., Strains, A. and Cartaright, R.A. (1997). A comparison of three methods of analysis age–period–cohort models with application to incidence data on non-Hodgkin's lymphoma. *International Journal of Epidemiology*, **26**, 32–46.

Mdege, N.D., Man, M-S., Taylor, C.A. and Torgerson, D.J. (2011). Systematic review of stepped wedge cluster randomized trials shows that design is particularly used to evaluate interventions during routine implementation. *Journal of Clinical Epidemiology*, **64**, 936–948.

Miller, M.E., Davis, C.S. and Landis, J.R. (1993). The analysis of longitudinal polytomous data: Generalized estimating equations and connections with weighted least squares. *Biometrics*, **49**, 1033–1044.

Molenberghs, G., Michiels, B., Kenward, M.G. and Diggle, P.J. (1998). Monotone missing data and pattern-mixture models. *Statistica Neerlandica*, **52**, 153–161.

Muthén B. (2004). Latent variable analysis: Growth mixture modeling and related techniques for longitudinal data. In *Handbook of quantitative methodology for the social sciences*, ed. D. Kaplan. Newbury Park, CA: Sage Publications.

Muthén, B. (2006). The potential of growth mixture modelling. *Infant and Child Development*, **15**, 623–625.

Muthén, B. and Asparouhov, B. (2008). Growth mixture modeling: Analysis with non-Gaussian random effects. In *Longitudinal data analysis*, eds. G. Fitmaurice, M. Davidian, G. Vebeke and G. Molenberghs. pp. 143–165. Boca Raton: Chapman & Hall/CRC Press.

Muthén, B. and Muthén, L. (2000). Integrating person-centered and variable-centered analyses: Growth mixture modeling with latent trajectory classes. *Alcoholism. Clinical and Experimental Research*, **24**, 882–891.

Muthén, B. and Shedden, K. (1999). Finite mixture modeling with mixture outcomes using the EM algorithm. *Biometrics*, **55**, 463–469.

Nagin, D. (1999). Analyzing developmental trajectories. A semi-parametric group-based approach. *Psychological Methods*, **6**, 18–34.

Nagin, D. and Tremblay, R. (2001). Analyzing developmental trajectories of distinct but related behaviors: A group-based method. *Psychological Methods*, **6**, 18–34.

Naimi, A.I., Cole, S.R. and Kennedy, E.H. (2017). An introduction to g methods. *International Journal of Epidemiology*, **46**, 756–762.

Nelder, J.A. and Lee, Y. (1992). Likelihood, quasi-likelihood and psuedo-likelihood: Some comparisons. *Journal of the Royal Statistical Society Series B*, **54**, 273–284.

Nelder, J.A. and Pregibon, D. (1987). An extended quasi-likelihood function. *Biometrika*, **74**, 221–232.

Neuhaus, J.M., Kalbfleisch, J.D. and Hauck, W.W. (1991). A comparison of cluster-specific and population-averaged approaches for analyzing correlated binary data. *International Statistical Reviews*, **59**, 25–36.

Omar, R.Z., Wright, E.M., Turner, R.M. and Thompson, S.G. (1999). Analysing repeated measurements data: A practical comparison of methods. *Statistics in Medicine*, **18**, 1587–1603.

Pinheiro, J.C. and Bates, D.M. (1995). Approximations to the log-likelihood function in the non-linear mixed-effects model. *Journal of Computational and Graphical Statistics*, **4**, 12–35.

Pinheiro, J.C. and Bates, D.M. (2000). *Mixed-effects models in S and S-PLUS*. New York: Springer-Verlag.

Porkka, K.V.K., Viikari, J.S.A. and Åkerblom, H.K. (1991). Tracking of serum HDL-cholesterol and other lipids in children and adolescents: The cardiovascular risk in young Finns study. *Preventive Medicine*, **20**, 713–724.

Potthoff, R.F., Tudor, G.E., Pieper, K.S. and Hasselblad, V. (2006) Can one assess whether missing data are missing at random in medical studies? *Statistical Methods in Medical Research*, **15**, 213–234.

Prentice, R.L. (1988). Correlated binary regression with covariates specific to each binary observation. *Biometrics*, **44**, 1033–1048.

Proper, K.I., Hildebrandt, V.H., Beek van de, A.J., Twisk, J.W.R. and Mechelen van, W. (2003). Individual counseling and physical activity, fitness and health: a randomised controlled trial in a worksite setting. *American Journal of Preventive Medicine*, **24**, 218–226.

Rabe-Hesketh, S. and Pickles, A. (1999). Generalised linear latent and mixed models. In *Proceedings of the 14th International workshop on statistical modelling*, ed. H. Friedl, A. Berghold and G. Kauermann, pp. 332–339. Graz, Austria.

Rabe-Hesketh, S., Pickles, A. and Skrondal, A. (2001a). *GLAMM manual technical report 2001/01*. Department of Biostatistics and Computing, Institute of Psychiatry, King's College, University of London.

Rabe-Hesketh, S., Pickles, A. and Skrondal, A. (2001b). GLLAMM: a class of models and a Stata program. *Multilevel Modelling Newsletter*, **13** (1), 17–23.

Rabe-Hesketh, S., Pickles, A. and Taylor, C. (2000). sg129: generalized linear latent and mixed models. *Stata Technical Bulletin*, **53**, 47–57.

Rabe-Hesketh, S. and Skrondal, A. (2001). Parameterisation of multivariate random effects models for categorical data. *Biometrics*, **57**, 1256–1264.

Rabe-Hesketh, S., Skrondal, A. and Pickles, A. (2002). Reliable estimation of generalized linear mixed models using adaptive quadrature. *The Stata Journal*, **2**, 1–21.

Rabe-Hesketh, S., Skrondal A. and Pickles A. (2005). Maximum likelihood estimation of limited and discrete dependent variable models with nested random effects. *Journal of Econometrics*, **128**, 301–323.

Rasbash, J., Browne, W., Goldstein, H., Yang, M., Plewis, I., Healy, M., Woodhouse, G. and Draper, D. (1999). *A user's guide to MLwiN* (2nd edn.). London: Institute of Education.

Rhian, D.M., De Stavola, B.L. and Cousens, S.N. (2011). gformula: Estimating causal effects in the presence of time-varying confounding or mediation using the g-computational formula. *The Stata Journal*, **11**, 479–517.

Rice, J.C. (1975). A metalgorithm for adaptive quadrature. *Journal of the Association for Computing Machinery*, **22**, 61–82.

Ridout, M.S. (1991). Testing for random dropouts in repeated measurement data. Reader reaction. *Biometrics*, **47**, 1617–1621.

Rijnhart, J.J.M., Lamp, S.J., Valente, M.J., MacKinnon, D.P., Twisk, J.W.R. and Heymans, M.W. (2021). Mediation analysis methods used in observational research: A scoping review and recommendations. *BMC Medical Research Methodology*, **21**, 226.

Rizopoulos, D. (2011). Dynamic predictions and prospective accuracy in joint models for longitudinal and time-to-event data. *Biometrics*, **67**, 819–829.

Robertson, C. and Boyle, P. (1998). Age–period–cohort analysis of chronic disease rates; I modelling approach. *Statistics in Medicine*, **17**, 1302–1323.

Robertson, C., Gandini, S. and Boyle, P. (1999). Age–period–cohort models: A comparative study of available methodologies, *Journal of Clinical Epidemiology*, **52**, 569–583.

Robins, J.M., Hernan, M.A. and Brumback, B. (2000). Marginal structural models and causal inference in epidemiology. *Epidemiology*, **11**, 550–560.

Robins, J. and Wang, N. (2000). Inference for imputation estimators. *Biometrika*, **87**, 113–124.

Rodriguez, G. and Goldman, N. (1995). An assessment of estimation procedures for multilevel models with binary responses. *Journal of the Royal Statistical Association*, **158**, 73–89.

Rodriguez, G. and Goldman, N. (2001). Improved estimation procedures for multilevel models with binary responses: A case study. *Journal of the Royal Statistical Association*, **164**, 339–355.

Rogossa, D. (1995). Myths and methods: "Myths about longitudinal research" plus supplemental questions. In *The analysis of change*, ed. J.M. Gottman, pp. 3–66. Mahwah, NJ: Lawrence Erlbaum.

Rosenberg, P.S. and Anderson, W.F. (2010). Proportional hazards models and age-period-cohort analysis of cancer rates. *Statistics in Medicine*, **20**, 1228–1238.

Rosner, B. and Munoz, A. (1988). Autoregressive modelling for the analysis of longitudinal data with unequally spaced examinations. *Statistics in Medicine*, **7**, 59–71.

Rosner, B., Munoz, A., Tager, I., Speizer, F. and Weiss, S. (1985). The use of an autoregressive model for the analysis of longitudinal data in epidemiologic studies. *Statistics in Medicine*, **4**, 457–467.

Royston, P. 2001. Flexible parametric alternatives to the Cox model, and more. *Stata Journal*, **1**, 1–28.

Royston, P. (2004). Multiple imputation of missing values. *Stata Journal*, **4**, 227–241.

Royston, P., Carlin, J.B., and White, I.R. (2009). Multiple imputation of missing values: New features for mim. *Stata Journal*, **2**, 252-264.

Royston, P., and Lambert P.C. (2011). *Flexible parametric survival analysis using stata: Beyond the cox model*. College Station, TX: Stata Press.

Rubin, D. B. (1976). Inference and missing data. *Biometrika*, **63**, 581–592.

Rubin, D.B. (1987). *Multiple imputation for nonresponse in surveys*. New York: Wiley.

Rubin, D.B. (1996). Multiple imputation after 18+ years. *Journal of the American Statistical Association*, **91**, 473–489.

Schafer, J.L. (1999). Multiple imputation: a primer. *Statistical Methods in Medical Research*, **8**, 3–15.

Schall, R. (1991). Estimation in generalized linear models with random effects. *Biometrika*, **40**, 719–727.

Schwarz, G. (1978). Estimating the dimensions of a model. *Annals of Statistics*, **6**, 461–464.

Shih, W.J. and Quan, H. (1997). Testing for treatment differences with dropouts present in clinical trials: A composite approach. *Statistics in Medicine*, **16**, 1225–1239.

Skrondal, A. and Rabe-Hesketh, S. (2004). *Generalized latent variable modeling: multilevel, longitudinal and structural equation models*. Boca Raton, FL: Chapman & Hall/ CRC Press.

Snijders, T.A.B. and Bosker, R.J. (1993). Standard errors and sample sizes for two-level research. *Journal of Educational Statistics*, **18**, 237–259.

Spriensma, A.S., Hajos, T.R.S., Boer de M.R., Heymans, M.W. and Twisk J.W.R. (2013) A new approach to analyse longitudinal epidemiological data with an excess of zeros. *BMC Medical Research Methodology*, **13**, 27.

Stanek III, E.J., Shetterley, S.S., Allen, L.H., Pelto, G.H. and Chavez, A. (1989). A cautionary note on the use of autoregressive models in analysis of longitudinal data. *Statistics in Medicine*, **8**, 1523–1528.

STATA (2009). *Multiple-imputation reference manual. Release 11*. College Station, TX: StataCorp LP.

Stevens, J. (1996). *Applied multivariate statistics for the social sciences* (3rd edn.). Mahway, NJ: Lawrence Erlbaum.

Steyerberg, E.W. (2000) Clinical trials in acute myocardial infarction: Should we adjust for baseline characteristics? *American Heart Journal*, **139**, 745–751.

Stroup, W. and Claassen, E. (2020). Pseudo-likelihood or quadrature? What we thought we knew, what we think we know, and what we are still trying to figure out. *Journal of Agricultural, Biological, and Environmental Statistics*, **25**, 639–656.

Sun, J. and Song, P.X-K. (2001). Statistical analysis of repeated measurements with informative censoring times. *Statistics in Medicine*, **20**, 63–73.

Tobin, J. (1958). Estimation of relationships for limited dependent variables. *Econometrics*, **26**, 24–36.

Twisk, J.W.R. (1997). Different statistical models to analyze epidemiological observational longitudinal data: an example from the Amsterdam Growth and Health Study. *International Journal of Sports Medicine*, **18** (Suppl. 3), S216–224.

Twisk, J.W. (2004). Longitudinal data analysis. A comparison between generalized estimating equations and random coefficient analysis. *European Journal of Epidemiology*, **19**, 769–776.

Twisk, J.W.R. (2006). *Applied multilevel analysis. A practical guide*. Cambridge: Cambridge University Press.

Twisk, J.W.R. (2013). *Applied longitudinal data analysis for epidemiology: A practical guide*. Cambridge: Cambridge University Press.

Twisk, J.W.R. (2014). Is it necessary to classify developmental trajectories over time? A critical note. *Annals of Nutrition and Metabolism*, **65**, 236–240.

Twisk, J.W.R. (2019). *Applied mixed model analysis. A practical guide*. Cambridge: Cambridge University Press.

Twisk, J.W.R. (2022). *Analysis of data from randomized controlled trials: A practical guide*. Cham, Switzerland: Springer Nature.

Twisk, J., Bosman, L., Hoekstra, T., Rijnhart, J., Welten, M., Heymans, M. (2018). Different ways to estimate treatment effects in randomised controlled trials.

Contemporary Clinical Trials Communications, **10**, 80–85.

Twisk, J.W.R. and de Vente, W. (2002). Attrition in longitudinal studies: How to deal with missing data. *Journal of Clinical Epidemiology*, **55**, 329–337.

Twisk, J.W.R., de Vente, W. Apeldoorn, A.T. and de Boer, MR. (2017). Should we use logistic mixed model analysis for the effect estimation in a longitudinal RCT with a dichotomous outcome variable? *Epidemiology Biostatistics and Public Health*, **3**, e12613–12621.

Twisk, J.W.R. and Hoekstra, T. (2012). Classifying developmental trajectories over time should be done with great caution; a comparison between methods. *Journal of Clinical Epidemiology*, **65**, 1078–1087.

Twisk, J.W.R., Hoogendijk, E.O., Zwijsen, S.A., Boer, M.R. de. (2016). Different methods to analyze stepped wedge trial designs revealed different aspects of intervention effects. *Journal of Clinical Epidemiology*, **72**, 75–83.

Twisk, J.W.R., Kemper, H.C.G., van Mechelen, W. and Post, G.B. (2001). Clustering of risk factors for coronary heart disease: The longitudinal relationship with lifestyle. *Annals of Epidemiology*, **11**, 157–165.

Twisk, J. and Proper, K. (2005). Evaluation of the results of a randomized controlled trial: How to define changes between baseline and follow-up. *Journal of Clinical Epidemiology*, **57**, 223–228.

Twisk, J. and Rijmen, F. (2009). Longitudinal tobit regression: A new approach to analyze outcome variables with floor or ceiling effects. *Journal of Clinical Epidemiology*, **62**, 953–958.

Twisk, J.W.R., Staal, B.J., Brinkman, M.N., Kemper, H.C.G. and van Mechelen, W. (1998). Tracking of lung function parameters and the longitudinal relationship with lifestyle. *European Respiratory Journal*, **12**, 627–634.

VanderWeele, T.J. (2015). *Explanation in causal inference: Methods for mediation and interaction.* Oxford: Oxford University Press.

Venables, W.N. and Ripley, B.D. (1997). *Modern applied statistics with S-PLUS* (2nd edn.). New York: Springer-Verlag.

Venables, W.N. and Ripley, B.D. (2000). *S programming.* New York: Springer.

Venables, W.N. and Ripley, B.D. (2002). *Modern applied statistics with S* (4th edn.). New York: Springer.

Verbeke, G. and Molenberghs, G. (2000). *Linear mixed models for longitudinal data.* New York: Springer-Verlag.

Vermeulen, E.G.J., Stehouwer, C.D.A., Twisk, J.W.R., van den Berg, M., de Jong, S., Mackaay, A.J.C., van Campen, C.M.C., Visser, F.J., Jakobs, C.A.J.M., Bulterijs, E.J. and Rauwerda, J.A. (2000). Effect of homocysteine-lowering treatment with folic acid plus vitamin B6 on progression of subclinical atherosclerosis: A randomised, placebo-controlled trial. *Lancet*, **355**, 517–522.

Vickers, A.J. and Altman, D.G. (2001). Analysing controlled trials with baseline and follow up measurements. *British Medical Journal*, **323**, 1123–1124.

Wiliamson, J.M., Kim, K. and Lipsitz, S.R. (1995). Analyzing bivariate ordinal data using a global odds ratio. *Journal of the American Statistical Association*, **90**, 1432–1437.

Wing, D., Simon, K. and Bello-Gomez, R.A. (2018). Designing difference in difference studies: Best practices for public health policy research. *Annual Review of Public Health*, **39**, 453–469.

Wolfinger, R.D. (1998). Towards practical application of generalized linear mixed models. In *Proceedings of the 13th International workshop on statistical modelling*, ed. B. Marx and H. Friedl, pp. 388–395. New Orleans, LA.

Yang, M. and Goldstein, H. (2000). Multilevel models for repeated binary outcomes: Attitudes and voting over the electoral cycle. *Journal of the Royal Statistical Society*, **163**, 49–62.

Yang, X., Li, J. and Shoptaw, S. (2008). Imputation-based strategies for clinical trial longitudinal data with nonignorable missing values. *Statistics in Medicine*, **27**, 2826–2849.

Yucel, R.M., He, Y. and Zaslavsky, A.M. (2008). Using calibration to improve rounding in imputation. *American Statistician*, **62**, 1–5.

Zeger, S.L. and Liang, K-Y. (1986). Longitudinal data analysis for discrete and continuous outcomes. *Biometrics*, **42**, 121–130.

Zeger, S.L. and Liang, K-Y. (1992). An overview of methods for the analysis of longitudinal data. *Statistics in Medicine*, **11**, 1825–1839.

Zeger, S.L., Liang, K-Y. and Albert, P.S. (1988). Models for longitudinal data: a generalised estimating equation approach. *Biometrics*, **44**, 1049–1060.

Zeger, S.L. and Qaqish, B. (1988). Markov regression models for time series: A quasi-likelihood approach. *Biometrics*, **44**, 1019–1031.

Index

Printed in the United States
by Baker & Taylor Publisher Services